Molecular and Translational Medicine

Series Editors
William B. Coleman
Gregory J. Tsongalis

For further volumes:
http://www.springer.com/series/8176

Daniel Gioeli

Editor

Targeted Therapies

Mechanisms of Resistance

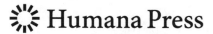 Humana Press

Editor
Daniel Gioeli, Ph.D.
Department of Microbiology and Cancer Center
University of Virginia
Charlottesville, VA
USA
dgg3f@virginia.edu

1006613298

ISBN 978-1-60761-477-7   e-ISBN 978-1-60761-478-4
DOI 10.1007/978-1-60761-478-4
Springer New York Dordrecht Heidelberg London

Library of Congress Control Number: 2011928683

Printed on acid-free paper

Humana Press is part of Springer Science+Business Media (www.springer.com)

Foreword

The spectacular success of the first tyrosine kinase inhibitor imatinib, approved just 10 years ago, has transformed oncology drug development. Nearly all drug discovery efforts today have shifted away from conventional cytotoxic therapies toward the development of molecularly-targeted agents. Much of the emphasis is on finding drugs that inhibit "driver" oncogenes in tumors, with the expectation that these new compounds will have single agent activity in appropriately selected patients whose tumors contain "driver" mutations in the gene or pathway targeted by the new agent. The list of successes using this approach continues to grow, including two examples in the past year – BRAF-mutant melanoma and ALK-mutant lung cancer – that are likely to result in two new drug approvals.

Yet all these successes are accompanied by the problem of drug resistance, which has plagued cancer drug development beginning with the very first success using antimetabolites to treat childhood acute lymphocytic leukemia. The drug resistance problem in acute lymphocytic leukemia, as well as other chemotherapy-sensitive tumors such as Hodgkin's lymphoma and testicular cancer, was overcome through the use of combination of chemotherapy agents with nonoverlapping toxicities. But this success required decades of clinical trials – mixing and matching various agents through a largely empiric approach.

Unlike the early days of chemotherapy, molecular understanding of resistance to targeted therapies is progressing at a remarkably rapid rate – and offers the promise of more rapid evolution of successful combinations of molecularly-targeted agents. In the case of chronic myeloid leukemia, second generation agents that circumvent many of the resistance mechanisms that tumors exploit to escape first generation compounds, have already proven effective. *Mechanisms of Resistance to Molecular-Targeted Therapies* is the first book that deals with these and other issues in a focused way – and it does so at just the right time. As readers, we owe a great debt to Dr. Daniel Gioeli for tackling this important new topic and to the authors of the many excellent chapters that provide important guidance for the future development of this exciting field of oncology that offers great hope for cancer patients around the world.

28 December, 2010   Charles L. Sawyers

Preface

The scientific community has made tremendous strides in understanding the molecular basis of cancer since the pioneering work that culminated in the identification of the first human cellular oncogene in 1978 and tumor suppressor gene in 1987. It is this knowledge of the molecular underpinnings of cancer that has led to the advent of small molecule and antibody therapies targeting proteins that drive carcinogenesis. The preeminent example of these molecular-targeted therapies is imatinib, a selective inhibitor of ABL, KIT, and PDGFR, which is effective for the treatment of chronic myelogenous leukemia and gastrointestinal stromal tumors. However, the overall therapeutic response to the molecular-targeted therapies evaluated has been much less than initially hoped. The clinical response of patients to imatinib seems the exception, not the rule. Of the molecular-targeted therapies approved by the Food and Drug Administration, most work on only a subset of patients and ultimately resistance emerges for all molecular-targeted agents. The extensive cross talk between signaling pathways, the multiple mutations, and the genetic plasticity of cancer all contribute to the inherent and acquired resistance to molecular-targeted therapies that leads to the inevitable relapse for patients.

The fundamental hurdle to developing more effective, durable treatments for cancer is overcoming the robustness of cancer. Robustness is the quality of being able to withstand perturbations, coping well with unpredictable variations with minimal loss of functionality. In the case of cancer, this is continued survival and growth. It is important to note that the robustness of the cancer system applies to cancer as a disease and not individual tumor cells. The machinery that maintains cellular and tissue robustness in a healthy individual is hijacked to maintain the dysfunction of cancer, even in response to molecular-targeted therapies that disrupt signaling events that drive carcinogenesis. Thus, responses to molecular-targeted therapies, which are often very dramatic, do not endure.

This book presents examples of the major mechanisms of resistance to targeted agents, new tools for studying the cell signaling network, and emerging fields addressing the mechanism of resistance. The goal is to provide the reader with both an overview as well as a detailed perspective on the mechanisms of resistance to targeted therapeutics. Chapters 1 and 2 of this book address two fundamental mechanisms of resistance to molecular-targeted agents. Chapter 1, "Resistance to

Targeted Therapies As a Result of Mutation(s) in the Target", describes acquired resistance through the acquisition of new mutations within the protein target. This discovery has critical implications for the development of new, molecular-targeted agents that will be effective as second-line treatments for patients with resistance mutations. Alternative mechanisms for resistance include compensatory and redundant signaling events such as the upregulation or preexistence of bypass signaling. In Chapter 2, "The Dynamics of the Cell Signaling Network; Implications for Targeted Therapies", specific examples of compensatory and redundant signaling leading to therapeutic resistance are discussed along with the general implications of the cell signaling network on the design of effective drug treatments.

Not discussed in this book is how multidrug resistance efflux pumps contribute to the resistance of molecular-targeted agents. In general, the same knowledge of how these pumps can facilitate resistance to conventional chemotherapy can be applied to kinase inhibitors. The reader is directed to the book "Multi-Drug Resistance in Cancer" edited by Jun Zhou and published by Springer for in-depth information on this subject. Also not discussed in this book is the potential role of cancer progenitor cells in resistance to molecular-targeted agents. The topic is not without controversy, although the controversy may be largely due to: (1) semantics, (2) the question of how fluid intratumoral cell populations are, and (3) how applicable this concept is to cancers originating from different tissues. The attributes of cancer progenitor cells that facilitate resistance include their rarity, ability to undergo asynchronous DNA synthesis, as well as increased expression in enzymes for DNA repair and antiapoptotic proteins. The reader is directed to the book "Stem Cells and Cancer", edited by Rebecca Bagley and Beverly Teicher, and published by Springer for information on this subject.

The next three chapters (Chapters 3–5) describe cutting edge technologies for evaluating the cell signaling network. Chapter 3, "Cancer Signaling Network Analysis by Quantitative Mass Spectrometry", details advances in both mass spectrometry instrumentation and methodology for identifying and quantifying protein phosphorylation in the cell signaling network. Chapter 4, "Development and Implementation of Array Technologies for Proteomics: Clinical Implications and Applications", describes how tissue and protein microarrays are enabling researchers to assess signaling network activation and broad-scale pathway mapping in a relatively large number of samples, including patient tissue samples where sample material is limited. This section ends with Chapter 5, "Using Phosphoflow to Study Signaling Events of Subpopulations Resistant to Current Therapies", which details how phosphoflow cytometry can be used to study signaling events in cell subpopulations resistant to molecular-targeted therapies. This chapter illustrates how it is now possible to study signal transduction in single cell populations, enabling the study of signaling events in subpopulations of cells that are resistant to targeted therapeutics. These three chapters represent the significant progress in phosphoproteomic research that has occurred in the last decade. Implementing and integrating the approaches described in these chapters will enhance our understanding of cell signaling networks involved in cancer and how cell signaling networks respond to perturbations such as molecular-targeted therapeutics.

These early chapters illustrate the enormous complexity of the problem facing therapeutic resistance. Not only is it difficult to effectively measure changes in the cell signaling network, the network complexity obscures interpretation of such data. One tactic to address this issue is to integrate quantitative experiments with computational modeling. Mathematical modeling of cell signaling and mutation rates provides important insights into how resistance to targeted therapies arises. Such models are uncovering new areas of exploration such as the need for better quantitative tools for measuring patient samples. Importantly, mathematical models also predict the numbers of drug combinations (or targets) required for effective treatment. The application of mathematical modeling found in systems biology is presented in Chapter 6, "Mathematical and Computational Models in Cancer". This highly approachable presentation of this complex subject introduces the reader to how the application of mathematical models can facilitate tracking and interpreting more variables than an individual investigator's cognitive ability can achieve. It also introduces the critical issue that the cancer response to molecular-targeted agents is a multiscale problem not only of many signaling pathways (microscale) but also of different cell and tissue types (macroscale).

Increasingly complex in vitro cancer models and in vivo models of cancer are important tools for studying the mechanism of resistance to targeted therapies. The "gold standard" for the integrated study of micro- and macroscale is the animal model. However, animal models are not without their limitations, since the experimental system chosen may elicit unpredicted escape mechanisms. Chapter 7, "Interrogating Resistance to Targeted Therapy Using Genetically Engineered Mouse Models of Cancer", describes how the engineering of mouse cancer models can be utilized to model molecular-targeted therapies and how in vivo cancers respond to modifications in specific molecular pathways.

Fully addressing the challenge of therapeutic resistance will require incorporating broad-based concepts such as somatic evolution. After all, it is the evolutionary response of the cancer to the molecular-targeted agents that form the basis of resistance. Chapter 8, "Somatic Evolution of Acquired Drug Resistance in Cancer", addresses the role of somatic selection in resistance to targeted therapies and suggests therapeutic modalities that do not impose strong somatic selection pressure.

In our final two chapters, we explore possible ways to inhibit multiple therapeutic targets simultaneously, either with novel therapeutics or combinations of molecular-targeted agents. Chapter 9, "MicroRNA: A Potential Therapy Able to Target Multiple Cancer Pathways", explores the role of miRNAs in cancer and discusses the potential for miRNA-based therapeutic strategies. The discovery of noncoding microRNAs as regulators of development and disease has ushered in a new area of research. MicroRNAs target multiple genes, and therefore are potential therapies for the simultaneous inhibition of multiple oncogenes. Such multi-target therapies will be an important tool for addressing resistance to targeted therapies. It is becoming increasingly clear that, for many cancers, the most effective use of molecular-targeted therapies for cancer will require a combination of several such agents. Our final chapter, Chapter 10, "Rational Combination of Targeted Agents to Overcome Cancer Cell Resistance", describes some of the ongoing work using combinations of molecular-targeted agents. The argument is that the rational combination of targeted agents, and in particular those that block complementary cell survival or cell cycle regulatory pathways, will be an effective therapeutic strategy.

There are many people to thank and whose help was critical for completing this book. First and foremost are the contributing authors, who always responded politely to the continuous inquires on progress. Most importantly, they have written outstanding pieces describing the latest information in their fields of inquiry. I would like to thank Drs Gregory Tsongalis and William Coleman for presenting the opportunity to edit a book in their series *Molecular and Translational Medicine* and Richard Hruska of Humana Press/Springer SBM for helping make it happen. I am especially appreciative of the efforts of Barbara Lopez-Lucio who kept my feet to the fire and made certain that all the pieces were in place for the final book manuscript. Barbara was always polite and professional, even in the face of delays and authorship withdrawals. I would also like to thank my mentor and collaborator, Dr Michael Weber for countless helpful discussions on signal transduction and science in general. Finally, I would like to thank my family for putting up with the additional level of stress that accompanies such an endeavor; their love and support make anything possible.

I hope that the insights and perspective shared in this book will not only aid in your understanding of the subject matter, but also inspire your science well into the future. Enjoy.

Charlottesville, VA   Daniel Gioeli

Contents

Contributors

Sudhir Chowbina, MS
Department of Biomedical Engineering, University of Virginia,
Charlottesville, VA, USA

Alexis B. Cortot, MD
Lowe Center for Thoracic Oncology, Dana Farber Cancer Institute,
Boston, MA, USA

Yun Dai, MD, PhD
Department of Internal Medicine, Hematology/Oncology,
Virginia Commonwealth University, Richmond, VA, USA

Daniel Gioeli, PhD
Department of Microbiology and Cancer Center, University of Virginia,
Charlottesville, VA, USA

Steven Grant, MD
Department of Internal Medicine, Hematology/Oncology,
Virginia Commonwealth University, Richmond, VA, USA

Edward Gunther, MD
Department of Medicine, Pennsylvania State College of Medicine;
Jake Gittlen Cancer Research Foundation, Pennsylvania State College
of Medicine, Hershey, PA, USA

Kevin A. Janes, PhD
Department of Biomedical Engineering, University of Virginia,
Charlottesville, VA, USA

Pasi A. Jänne, MD, PhD
Harvard Medical School, Lowe Center for Thoracic Oncology,
Dana Faber Cancer Institute, Boston, MA, USA

Benjamin Kefas, B Pharm, Msc, PhD
Department of Neurology, University of Virginia, Charlottesville, VA, USA

Menawar Khalil, MD
Department of Neurosciences, Inova Fairfax Hospital, Falls Church, VA, USA

Lance A. Liotta, MD, PhD
Center for Applied Proteomics and Molecular Medicine,
George Mason University, Manassas, VA, USA

Jason R. Neil, PhD
Department of Biological Engineering, Massachusetts Institute
of Technology, Cambridge, MA, USA

Jason A. Papin, PhD
Department of Biomedical Engineering, University of Virginia,
Charlottesville, VA, USA

Shayn M. Peirce, PhD
Department of Biomedical Engineering, University of Virginia,
Charlottesville, VA, USA

John W. Pepper, PhD
Division of Cancer Prevention, National Cancer Institute, Bethesda, MD, USA

Omar D. Perez, PhD
Preclinical Development, Tocagen, Inc., San Diego, CA, USA

Emanuel F. Petricoin III, PhD
Center for Applied Proteomics and Molecular Medicine,
George Mason University, Manassas, VA, USA

Benjamin W. Purow, MD
Department of Neurology, University of Virginia, Charlottesville, VA, USA

Joseph C. Watson, MD
Inova Regional Neurosurgery Service, Department of Neurosciences,
Inova Fairfax Hospital, Falls Church, VA, USA

Forest M. White, PhD
Department of Biological Engineering, Massachusetts Institute of Technology,
Cambridge, MA, USA

Julia D. Wulfkuhle, PhD
Center for Applied Proteomics and Molecular Medicine,
George Mason University, Manassas, VA, USA

Chapter 1
Resistance to Targeted Therapies As a Result of Mutation(s) in the Target

Alexis B. Cortot and Pasi A. Jänne

Keywords Tyrosine kinase inhibitor • Resistance • Mutation • Gatekeeper residue • T790M • T315I

Introduction

Targeted therapies launched a new era in the treatment of cancer. Spectacular successes have been obtained with these agents, for example in chronic myelogenous leukemia (CML) or in gastrointestinal stromal tumors (GIST) with imatinib (Gleevec™; Novartis) [1, 2]. The efficacy of these therapies is usually associated with the presence of a genetic alteration which renders the cancer cell "addicted" to an oncoprotein which is targeted by the treatment. Efficacy of imatinib relies on the presence of the BCR-ABL translocation in CML, and KIT or platelet-derived growth factor receptor alpha (PDGFRA) mutations in GIST. In non-small cell lung cancer (NSCLC), the epidermal growth factor receptor (EGFR) kinase inhibitors gefitinib (Iressa™; AstraZeneca) and erlotinib (Tarceva™; OSI pharmaceuticals/ Genentech/Roche) are clinically most effective in NSCLC patients that harbor an *EGFR* tyrosine kinase domain mutation. However, some patients never achieve any clinical response with these treatments, a situation usually referred to as "de novo" resistance and those who respond will ultimately develop a tumor relapse which is the consequence of an "acquired" resistance. Known mechanisms of acquired resistance include point mutations of the targeted kinase and activation of alternative pathways that bypass the targeted kinase. Drug efflux and epigenetic mechanisms have also been implicated. In this chapter, we will focus on acquired resistance through acquisition of a new mutation within the protein target. This kind

P.A. Jänne (✉)
Harvard Medical School, Lowe Center for Thoracic Oncology,
Dana Faber Cancer Institute, Boston, MA, USA
e-mail: pasi_janne@dfci.harvard.edu

D. Gioeli (ed.), *Targeted Therapies: Mechanisms of Resistance*,
Molecular and Translational Medicine, DOI 10.1007/978-1-60761-478-4_1,
© Springer Science+Business Media, LLC 2011

1

of resistance mechanism has been mostly observed and studied in CML and GIST following imatinib treatment, and in NSCLC following gefitinib or erlotinib treatment. It is important to note that most, if not all, of the data about acquired resistance mutations come from studies with kinase inhibitors. Acquired resistance mutations have not been described with other targeted therapies so far, especially with monoclonal antibodies, even when they are designed to inhibit the same target (for example EGFR, cetuximab). Thus, in this chapter, we will address the question of how acquired mutations in the kinase provide resistance to kinase inhibitors.

Kinases in Cancer

Kinase Structure and Function

The human kinome encompasses more than 500 human protein kinases that are encoded by 2% of all human genes. Kinases transiently phosphorylate specific amino acids on 30% of all human proteins, including molecules that are in charge of key cellular processes such as growth, differentiation, proliferation, survival, and migration, which makes the kinome an increasingly attractive therapeutic target, especially for anticancer drug development.

The role of kinases is to transfer a phosphate from adenosine triphosphate (ATP) to a target protein that usually contains a serine, threonine, or tyrosine residue. This phosphorylation usually affects enzyme activity or association with other proteins [3].

The catalytic structures of kinases are highly conserved. The adenosine ring of ATP usually forms hydrogen bonds with the kinases that are typically composed of 12 subdomains that fold into a bilobed catalytic core structure with ATP binding in a deep cleft located between the lobes. Some key regions of the ATP-binding site include the hydrophobic purine-binding cavity; the hinge segment, which connects the N- and C-terminal kinase domains. The P-loop corresponds to the "ceiling" of the ATP-binding site, whereas the activation loop (A-loop) modulates kinase activity by switching between a phosphorylated, catalytically-competent "active" form (often referred as "DFG-in" conformation, in reference to the orientation of a highly-conserved amino acid motif), and an inactive form ("DFG-out" conformation) which prevents substrate binding [4].

Oncogenic Kinases in Cancer

Kinases are involved in cancer through several different mechanisms [5]. The therapeutically most successful kinases have acquired an increased activity, independent of normal regulatory mechanisms, through acquisition of genetic alterations.

They are usually essential for survival and/or proliferation of the cancer cell; this phenomenon has been called "oncogene addiction" [6, 7]. This addiction renders the cells particularly sensitive to the specific inhibition of the oncogenic kinase. Given these critical functions, inhibition of oncogenic kinases, using small molecule kinase inhibitors, has been therapeutically successful in cancer patients [5]. Examples of such kinases include the BCR-ABL chimeric oncoprotein in CML, the KIT and PDGFRA mutants in GIST, and the EGFR mutants in NSCLC.

BCR-ABL Translocation in CML

CML is usually regarded as an exemplary model for understanding the molecular pathogenesis of malignancy, since 95% of affected individuals express the chimeric BCR-ABL oncoprotein, which results from the balanced translocation of *c-ABL* (which encodes the tyrosine kinase ABL) from chromosome 9 and *BCR* on chromosome 22 [8, 9]. The resulting shortened chromosome 22 is referred as the Philadelphia (Ph) chromosome. Deregulated BCR-ABL displays constitutive tyrosine kinase activity that results in enhanced cellular proliferation, resistance to apoptosis, and altered adhesion, key characteristics of CML cells [10, 11].

EGFR Mutations in NSCLC

EGFR (HER1) is a transmembrane tyrosine kinase receptor that belongs to the ErbB (HER) family which includes four members. Ligand binding induces EGFR homo- or heterodimerization with other HER receptors, which, in turn, induces phosphorylation of tyrosine residues within the cytoplasmic domain and activation of downstream pathways. These include the phosphatidylinositol-3-kinase (PI3K)-Akt pathway or the STAT pathway, which are mainly associated with cell survival, and the RAS-RAF-MAP kinase pathway, which is mainly associated with cell cycle progression [12, 13]. Mutations in the tyrosine kinase domain of *EGFR* were first described in 2004, mostly in patients with lung adenocarcinoma who were female, never-smokers, and of Asian ethnicity [14–20]. The most common oncogenic mutations are small, in-frame deletions in exon 19, and a point mutation that substitutes leucine at codon 858 with arginine (L858R). These mutations both account for 90% of all *EGFR* mutations [21]. They confer constitutive activation of the receptor in the absence of ligand binding, by destabilizing the auto-inhibited conformation, which is normally maintained in the absence of ligand stimulation. *EGFR* mutated cancer cells are highly dependent on the EGFR pathway for survival and proliferation, which makes them exquisitely vulnerable to EGFR inhibition. It is reported that the PI3K-Akt signaling pathway is mainly activated in EGFR mutant cells where ERBB3 acts as a dimer partner of EGFR, and the downregulation of this pathway is required for gefitinib-induced apoptosis in these cells [22].

KIT and PDGFRA Mutations in GIST

KIT is a transmembrane receptor tyrosine kinase. Binding of its ligand, the stem cell factor induces homodimerization of the receptor and activation of the kinase activity and downstream intracellular signal transduction pathways, especially the MAPKinase and PI3K-AKT-mTOR pathways [23–25]. Approximately, 85% of GISTs have oncogenic mutations in *KIT*, which result in constitutive kinase activation. The most commonly mutated region of *KIT* is exon 11 (found mutated in approximately 70% of tumors) which encodes the juxtamembrane domain known to stabilize the autoinhibited conformation of KIT [26–28]. Autoinhibited KIT is stabilized by this domain, which inserts into the kinase-active site and disrupts formation of the activated structure [29]. In-frame deletions, insertions, or point mutations of this region disrupt this autoinhibitory motif and allow ligand-independent receptor activation. Most of the other *KIT* mutations occur in exon 9. In 5–7% of GIST, mutations are found in *PDGFRA*, a gene that encodes a receptor tyrosine kinase (PDGFRα(alpha)) that is highly homologous to KIT. These mutations occur in the juxtamembrane domain (exon 12) or activation loop (exon 18). *PDGFRA* mutations are mutually exclusive with KIT mutations, but activate the same signal transduction pathways [30].

Kinase Inhibitors

Kinases are highly amenable to inhibition by small molecule drugs, and several of these have already demonstrated clinical success. The most dramatic clinical responses to kinase inhibitors are observed for the tumors that are the most addicted to the targeted oncogenic kinase [31]. In such cases, acute inhibition induces an apoptotic response or growth arrest, which translates into tumor shrinkage or disease stabilization in treated patients [32]. In fact in the three above mentioned diseases harboring kinase mutations, GIST, CML and EGFR mutant NSCLC, kinase inhibitors now represent the standard first-line systemic therapy.

Clinical Activity of Kinase Inhibitors

Imatinib in CML

The "oncogene addiction" concept has been clinically validated with the success of imatinib as an inhibitor of the BCR-ABL kinase in CML [1]. Imatinib is a phenylaminopyrimidine which principally targets the tyrosine kinase activity of BCR-ABL. It binds to the inactive conformation of BCR-ABL and occupies the ATP-binding pocket of the ABL kinase domain, thus preventing a change in conformation of the protein to the active form of the molecule [33]. The recent update of the phase III randomized IRIS study (International Randomized Study of Interferon-α(alpha) plus Ara-C vs. STI571) prospectively comparing imatinib with interferon-α and cytarabine in previously untreated patients in first chronic phase showed the best observed rate for a complete cytogenetic response or an undetectable number of Ph+ chromosomes by conventional metaphase analysis on imatinib of 82% at 6 years [34].

EGFR Tyrosine Kinase Inhibitors in NSCLC

Erlotinib and gefitinib are reversible ATP-competitive inhibitors of EGFR that suppress receptor phosphorylation and activation of downstream pathways. The first results of clinical trials with these agents were either disappointing (as first-line, in combination with chemotherapy) or modest (as second- or third-line, in mono-therapy). However, identification of clinical (female gender, never-smoking status, adenocarcinoma histology and Asian ethnicity) and molecular (*EGFR* mutation and high copy number) predictive factors highlighted the potential benefit of these compounds in selected populations [15–17]. Erlotinib was approved for the second- or third-line treatment of patients with advanced NSCLC, following the results of the randomized phase III trial BR.21 showing a significant improvement in overall survival among patients who were given erlotinib alone compared with placebo [35]. Recently, gefitinib has received approval from the European Medicines Agency (EMEA) for first-line treatment in patients harboring an *EGFR* mutation, following the results of the IPASS trial [36]. This trial compared gefitinib to chemotherapy for first-line treatment in East Asian patients who were never or light smokers with advanced NSCLC and showed superiority of gefitinib with respect to progression-free survival. Response rate in *EGFR* mutation-positive patients was 71% with gefitinib, and progression-free survival was significantly longer among patients receiving gefitinib than among those receiving chemotherapy in the mutation-positive group, whereas the contrary was observed in the mutation-negative group [36]. These results were further confirmed in another phase III study in which 177 patients harboring *EGFR* mutations were randomly assigned to receive either gefitinib or chemotherapy (cisplatin and docetaxel). The gefitinib group had significantly longer progression-free survival compared with the cisplatin plus docetaxel group (9.2 months vs. 6.3 months; Hazard Ratio=0.489, $p<0.0001$) [37].

Imatinib in GIST

Beside its ability to inhibit ABL kinase, imatinib also targets the KIT and PDGFRA kinases, which makes it an effective agent for treatment of GIST. As observed with BCR-ABL, imatinib only binds to the inactive conformation of KIT [29]. Phase I and II trials of imatinib in GIST reported partial response rates of 54 and 68%, respectively, with most remaining patients achieving stable disease. In two large phase III studies comparing imatinib dose levels (400 mg per day vs. 800 mg per day), the median progression-free survival for either arm was approximately 20 months, and median overall survival was approximately 50 months [2, 38].

Different Types of Kinase Inhibitors

Kinase inhibitors can be classified depending upon the activity state of the kinase they recognize, and their reversibility.

Classical kinase inhibitors, also referred as "type 1 inhibitors," are ATP-competitive and bind in the ATP-binding site of the enzyme in the active form, which is characterized by an open conformation of the activation loop (DFG "in") [39]. They usually form at least one hydrogen bond with the amino acids located in the hinge region of the target kinase, thereby mimicking the hydrogen bonds that are normally formed by the adenine ring of ATP. The type 1 inhibitors constitute the majority of ATP-competitive inhibitors, including gefitinib, erlotinib, dasatinib, and sunitinib. These inhibitors are expected to have low selectivity since the DFG "in" conformation that they recognize is similar among many kinases.

Some kinase inhibitors bind to an extended ATP-binding site of the inactive form of the kinase characterized by a closed conformation of the activation loop (DFG "out") which prevents binding of both nucleotide and protein substrates. These "type 2 inhibitors" not only bind to the same area occupied by the type 1 compounds but also extend to an additional hydrophobic site available only in the inactive form. The mechanism of action of type 2 inhibitors was discovered fortuitously while studying imatinib binding [40], but some new compounds are now deliberately designed to bind to the DFG "out" conformation of their target.

Allosteric inhibitors, sometimes known as "type 3 inhibitors," bind at an allosteric site, outside the ATP-binding site (even though in some cases they may bind in proximity to it), which modifies kinase activity. These inhibitors have high selectivity since the site they bind to is usually specific of a certain kinase. Among the best known allosteric inhibitors are MEK inhibitors such as CI-1040, which inhibits MEK1 and MEK2 by occupying a pocket adjacent to the ATP-binding site [41]. GNF-2 is another allosteric inhibitor, which binds to the myristate binding site of BCR–ABL [42].

Covalent inhibitors represent a fourth class of kinase inhibitors that bind covalently to a cysteine residue within the catalytic pocket of the kinase. This irreversible, covalent bond confers infinite affinity for the ATP-binding site [43, 44]. As a result, the inhibitor irreversibly blocks binding of ATP to the kinase, thereby rendering the kinase inactive.

Resistance Mutations

Tyrosine kinase inhibitors have yielded exciting results both in hematological and solid malignancies. However, even among the most responsive patients, one of the major factors limiting the long-term efficacy of selective kinase inhibitors is drug resistance. Kinase inhibition induces a strong selective pressure for the emergence of resistance, especially through acquired mutations. These mutations can confer resistance through various mechanisms, including abrogation of drug binding and increased affinity of the kinase for ATP. Additional cell autonomous mechanisms of resistance to TKIs have been described, such as target amplification in the case of *BCR-ABL* in CML patients [45] and upregulation of alternative kinase pathways such as the MET pathway in the acquisition of resistance to EGFR TKI in NSCLC [46].

Clinical Findings

Resistance to Imatinib in CML

The emergence of mutations within the kinase domain of *BCR-ABL* is regularly associated with resistance to TKI therapy. Gorre et al. were the first to document the development of *BCR-ABL* mutations in 11 patients with advanced-phase CML or Ph+ Acute Lymphoblastic Leukemia (ALL) who relapsed on imatinib [47]. In 6 of 9 assessable patients, resistance was associated with the presence of a T315I mutation (substitution of a threonine residue by an isoleucine residue at codon 315, due to a C to T single nucleotide change) occurring at the gatekeeper residue of ABL. The T315I mutation was further shown to be one of the most frequent mutations arising in patients on imatinib therapy, occurring between 4 and 19% of resistant cases [48–50] and to confer resistance to all ABL kinase inhibitors. This mutation is associated with a poor outcome (median survival 12.6 months) [51, 52]. The detailed mechanisms by which T315I confers resistance to imatinib are discussed further. Frequency of *BCR-ABL* mutations in patients resistant to imatinib ranges from 40 to 90%, depending on the definition of resistance, the methodology of detection, and CML phase [47, 53–58]. Despite the wide variety of point mutations found in *BCR-ABL*, most mutants are rare. Actually, amino acid substitutions at only seven residues – M244V, G250E, Y253F/H, E255K/V (P-loop), T315I (imatinib binding site), M351T, and F359V (catalytic domain) – account for 85% of all resistance-associated mutations [59]. Certain mutations seem to occur more often in different disease phases. For example, substitutions at M244, L248, F317, H396, and S417 are more likely to occur in patients with chronic phase disease, whereas those at Q252, Y253, E255, T315, E459, and F486 are associated with advanced-phase disease [60].

Resistance to EGFR TKI in NSCLC

Patients whose tumors harbor sensitizing mutations in the *EGFR* kinase domain typically initially respond to gefitinib and erlotinib but invariably develop progressive disease, which is termed "acquired resistance," after a progression-free period of approximately 10 months. In analogy with the T315I gatekeeper mutation of *BCR-ABL*, researchers investigated whether the same C to T single nucleotide change, resulting in a T790M substitution at the gatekeeper residue of EGFR, could confer resistance to gefitinib and showed that this was the case [61]. Two groups of investigators further confirmed that the T790M mutation is detected in patients who develop acquired resistance to EGFR TKI treatment [62, 63]. The EGFR T790M mutation occurs in *cis* with the primary activating mutation, and is found in approximately 50% of patients with acquired resistance to EGFR TKI treatment [64, 65]. Introduction of T790M in a gefitinib-sensitive cell line confers resistance to gefitinib [30], which is mediated by maintenance of phosphoinositide 3-kinase (PI3K) activation in the presence of gefitinib [30]. The T790M mutation accounts for >90% of secondary EGFR mutations. So far, three other resistance mutations have been described – D761Y, L747S and T854A – with a very low prevalence [65–67]. Other mechanisms of resistance to EGFR TKIs have also been identified, especially with the development of EGFR-independent activation of key growth and survival pathways such as the MET pathway [46].

Resistance to Imatinib in GIST

In GIST, approximately 40–50% of patients develop imatinib resistance within 2 years, after enjoying a partial response or at least disease stabilization during initial follow-up. These patients are classified as having "delayed" resistance [68]. Analysis from a phase II trial evaluating imatinib revealed that 67% of patients with delayed resistance had acquired one or more secondary mutations, including mutation at the gatekeeper residue T670I. No secondary mutations were identified in wild-type GIST (GIST that lack *KIT* or *PDGFRA* primary mutation) [69]. Interestingly, secondary *KIT* mutations develop more frequently in association with primary *KIT* exon 11 mutations, which confer the most sustained clinical response to imatinib. Secondary mutations were found in 73–86% of imatinib-resistant patients harboring exon 11 primary mutations and only 19–33% of patients with exon 9 primary mutation developed secondary mutations [70–72]. This may be due to the longer exposure to the drug in patients with exon 11 primary mutation [73]. The secondary *KIT* mutations involved either the ATP-binding pocket of the kinase domain (exons 13 and 14) or the kinase activation loop (exons 17 and 18) [69].

Tools to Study Resistance Mutations

The study of mechanisms of resistance is usually based on two strategies [4, 74]. The first one is to compare the molecular characteristics, especially the appearance of new mutations, between samples obtained before and after the patient has relapsed after TKI treatment. This strategy is limited by the difficulty to obtain postrelapse samples, which sometimes requires invasive investigations, and if so, by the quality and amount of cancer cells. The second strategy is to use TKI-sensitive cell lines and to make them resistant by progressively increasing the concentration of the drug [4]. This approach offers a useful tool that has allowed, for example, to model various mechanisms of resistance to gefitinib or erlotinib in EGFR TKI-sensitive cell lines, such as the T790M mutation or the MET amplification [46, 75, 76].

The study of mechanisms of resistance to kinase inhibitors also requires the most sensitive and accurate methods for detection of mutations. Indeed, detection of resistance mutations can be challenging when only a small subset of cells is implicated [77]. These technical limitations may explain the variations observed in the incidence of resistance mutations among various studies. Direct sequencing is an easy and widespread tool that offers a low sensitivity (about 10–20%) for mutation detection [78]. This results in high rates of false negatives [54, 79]. The development of highly-sensitive PCR-based screening assays has greatly facilitated the detection and identification of point mutations in TKI-resistant patients [54, 79–81]. Moreover, several studies have shown that denaturing high-performance liquid chromatography, with a sensitivity of 1–10%, or pyrosequencing, with a sensitivity of 5%, and the possibility of quantifying the mutant clone, may be successfully used for clinical purposes [82–85]. More recently, highly-sensitive detection methods such as SARMS (Scorpion Amplification Refractory Mutation System) allowed the detection of the T790M resistance mutation on DNA recovered from circulating tumor cells [86].

Mutations of the Gatekeeper Residue

The gatekeeper residue plays a key role in resistance to TKIs because it is located at the back of the ATP-binding site, the properties of which (size, charge and hydrophobicity) regulate the binding of inhibitors [87]. Mutations at the gatekeeper residue usually have little effect on the kinase activity since most of the time this residue is not in direct contact with ATP but they have the potential to confer inhibitor resistance [39]. However, the precise mechanism implicated in resistance to TKI differs among these mutant kinases (Table 1.1). For example, the T315I gatekeeper mutation in *BCR-ABL* impairs drug binding through loss of a crucial hydrogen bond with the inhibitor and introduction of a steric clash, whereas the T790M mutation in *EGFR* is responsible for a change in the biochemical property of the kinase, resulting in an increased affinity for ATP, and thus a decreased efficacy of EGFR TKIs (Figs. 1.1 and 1.2). These two examples are detailed below.

An Example of Steric Hindrance: The T315I Mutation

As aforementioned, imatinib binds to a catalytically inactive conformation of ABL kinase, often referred to as the "DFG-out" conformation, in which the DFG motif is swung out of its position in the active kinase conformation. The threonine 315 residue

Table 1.1 Analogous gatekeeper mutations and their mechanisms

Mechanism of resistance	Mutation	Target kinase	Disease	Clinical resistance to
Steric hindrance	T315I	BCR-ABL	CML	Imatinib, dasatinib, nilotinib
	T670I	KIT	GIST	Imatinib
	T674I	FIP1L1-PDGFRA	HES	Imatinib
Change in ATP affinity	T790M	EGFR	NSCLC	Gefitinib, erlotinib

T threonine; *I* isoleucine; *M* methionine; *BCR-ABL* breakpoint cluster region-Abelson kinase; *KIT* mast-stem cell growth factor receptor kinase; *PDGFRA* platelet-derived growth factor receptor; *EGFR* epidermal growth factor receptor; *CML* chronic myelogenous leukemia; *GIST* gastrointestinal stromal tumor; *HES* hypereosinophilic syndrome; *NSCLC* non-small cell lung cancer

WILD-TYPE   T315I MUTANT

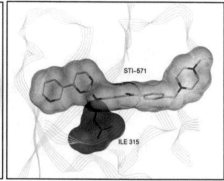
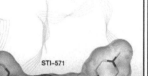
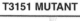

Fig. 1.1 Model of wild-type Abl in complex with STI-571 (imatinib mesylate, *left*) and predicted structure of T315I mutant Abl creating steric hindrance interfering with STI-571 (*right*). From Gorre et al. [47]. Used with permission

is located at the gatekeeper position at the periphery of the nucleotide-binding site of the protein, and participates, through the hydroxymethylene side-chain, in a crucial hydrogen bonding interaction between imatinib and ABL, as well as BCR-ABL [40, 88, 89]. Mutation to isoleucine abrogates the possibility of this hydrogen bonding interaction, which, combined with the additional bulk of the isoleucine side-chain, sterically hinders imatinib binding and leads to imatinib insensitivity and consequently resistance (Fig. 1.1). Substitution of the threonine residue by an isoleucine residue is the most potent potential resistance mutation at the gatekeeper residue, as shown by Negri et al. who explored all possible point mutations in the DNA triplet codon of the gatekeeper residue T670 of *KIT* (equivalent to the T315 of *BCR-ABL*) that could result in amino acid substitutions (T670R, T670I, T670K, T670A, T670S, T670P) and showed that only the T670I mutant was fully active (autophosphorylated) and resistant to imatinib [90]. Of note, second-generation TKIs dasatinib and nilotinib are also ineffective on the T315I mutant BCR-ABL kinase [87].

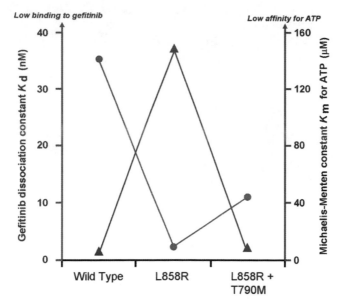

Fig. 1.2 Gefitinib dissociation constants K_d (*red*) and Michaelis–Menten constants K_m (*blue*) for the WT and mutant EGFR kinases. Based on data from Yun et al. [91]

An Example of Change of ATP Affinity: The T790M Mutation

The substitution of a bulky methionine residue for threonine at the gatekeeper residue in position 790 in the kinase domain of EGFR was initially thought to cause resistance by steric interference with binding of TKIs, in analogy with the T315I mutation in BCR-ABL [44, 62, 63]. However, contrary to the T315I mutant, the T790M mutant kinase remains sensitive to irreversible inhibitors, which is in contradiction with the hypothesis of steric hindrance as the mechanism of resistance, since it should affect binding of both reversible and irreversible anilinoquinazoline inhibitors [91].

Indeed, Yun et al. used a direct binding assay to show that the T790M mutation only modestly affects binding of gefitinib in the context of the L858R mutant, which cannot explain the clinically observed drug resistance [91]. The resistant L858R/T790M mutant was shown to bind gefitinib with Kd (dissociation constant) = 10.9 nM, which is only fourfold weaker than the exquisitely sensitive L858R mutant (Kd = 2.4 nM, Fig. 1.2). Moreover, the crystal structures clearly demonstrated that the gatekeeper mutation does not sterically block binding of reversible inhibitors (Fig. 1.3). Taken together, these data confirmed that the mechanism underlying resistance to gefitinib in T790M mutant was not due to a steric hindrance. Interestingly, the authors performed kinetic characterization of the wild-type and mutant EGFR kinases which revealed a marked decrease in the Michaelis–Menten constant (*K*m) for ATP (inversely proportional to ATP affinity)

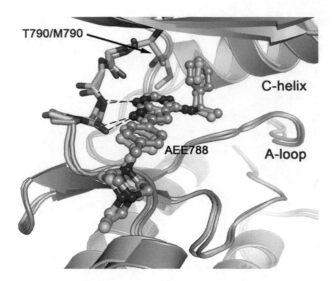

Fig. 1.3 Superposition of crystal structures of EGFR T790M/AEE788 (ATP-competitive inhibitor) complex (*yellow*) and WT/AEE788 complex (*light blue*) showing good accommodation of the inhibitor in the presence of the gatekeeper mutation. From Yun et al. [91]. Used with permission

in the drug-resistant L858R/T790M mutant as compared with the drug-sensitive L858R mutant. As already known, the L858R mutant activates EGFR, but also reduces the apparent affinity for ATP. Strikingly, the T790M mutation restores the ATP affinity to near wild-type levels in the L858R/T790M double mutant (Km[ATP]=8.4 μ(mu)M, as compared with Km[ATP]=148 μM for the L858R mutant, Fig. 1.2). Of note, the T790M mutation alone, in absence of L858R mutation, did not increase affinity for ATP. In accordance with the finding that T315I mutation in the ABL kinase confers resistance to imatinib through a different mechanism, i.e., steric hindrance, the authors did not observe a major difference in Km[ATP] between the T315I mutant and the wild-type ABL kinase [91]. Thus, as highlighted by the authors, the L858R mutation opens a therapeutic window by decreasing affinity of the kinase for ATP, and the addition of the T790M mutation merely closes this therapeutic window by restoring ATP affinity to its baseline level [91].

Mutations Outside the Gatekeeper Residue

Mutations at the gatekeeper residue have been the subject of numerous studies and are now better understood, as shown previously. The resistance mutations that occur outside the gatekeeper residue have been less extensively studied. Some of the mechanisms by which these mutations confer resistance to kinase inhibitors are discussed below.

Destabilization of the Inactive Conformation of the Kinase

Some mutations impede kinase inhibitors binding through an indirect mechanism that exploits the particular binding mode of the drug to its target protein. Type 2 inhibitors such as imatinib bind to a catalytically inactive conformation of the kinase domain in which the DFG motif is flipped out of its usual position in active kinase conformations. In addition, the inactive conformation of the P-loop stabilizes binding of imatinib. Point mutations in the *ABL* kinase domain that destabilize the inactive conformations of the P-loop and the DFG motif with respect to the catalytically active conformation reduce the imatinib binding affinity. This leads to a shift in the equilibrium between the inactive and active states and a restoration of BCR-ABL kinase activity. Mutations in the P-loop (residues 244–255 of *ABL*) account for up to 48% of all mutations in imatinib-resistant cases and have been associated with an increased transforming potential. For example, the mutation of tyrosine 253 to phenylalanine or histidine results in the loss of an hydrogen bonding interaction between this residue and asparagine 322 which is thought to be important in stabilizing the inactive P-loop conformation [92, 93].

The same kinds of mutations, which result in a shift in equilibrium toward the active kinase conformation, have also been described in KIT mutants resistant to imatinib or sunitinib [94].

Mutations in the Allosteric Site

It is anticipated that allosteric inhibitors, which have a different mechanism of action from ATP-competitive inhibitors, will induce specific mechanisms of resistance. Although data concerning these kinase inhibitors are still sparse, a few studies tend to confirm this assumption. Thus, mechanisms of resistance to the allosteric MEK1 inhibitor AZD6244 in melanoma have been recently studied using massively parallel sequencing of resistant clones generated from a MEK1 random mutagenesis screen in vitro as well as tumors obtained from relapsed patients [95]. Resistance mutations could be divided into two classes identified by the authors as "primary" mutations, occurring within or directly perturbating the allosteric binding site, and "secondary" mutations that resided outside of the drug binding region.

Arylamine MEK inhibitors function by locking the kinase into a "closed" inactive conformation, in which the activation loop causes α(alpha)-helix C to become externally rotated and displaced [41]. "Primary" *MEK1* resistance mutations were situated directly within the arylamine binding pocket or in a distinct set located in the second protein shell, along and adjacent to the α(alpha)-C helix. Notably, the MEK1 hydrophobic pocket includes residues from both α(alpha)-helix C and the activation loop. Binding of arylamine inhibitors within this pocket prevents the structural reorganization of α(alpha)-helix C and other motifs, which generates a catalytically active MEK1 conformation. Thus, primary *MEK1* mutations may introduce resistance through direct interference of drug binding or by forcing α(alpha)-C helix toward a closed conformation that disrupts the binding pocket. Specific ATP-competitive inhibitors may overcome resistance conferred by these resistance mutations [95].

The "secondary" mutations resided outside of the drug binding pocket, localizing to regions such as the C-terminal kinase domain or the interface between the N-terminal negative regulatory domain known as helix A and the core kinase domain. The proline residue at codon 124 (P124) is uniquely positioned such that it may exert an indirect influence on α(alpha)-C helix conformation while also interfacing directly with helix A which acts as a negative regulatory motif. Interestingly, a P124L substitution was identified in one out of 5 patients with melanoma who relapsed following MEK inhibitor treatment [95]. This mutation occurred in the postrelapse samples but was absent in the pretreatment sample. Mutation of this proline may disrupt a key regulatory interaction between helix A and the rest of the kinase, while simultaneously altering helix C indirectly through loss of a turn motif proximal to this segment. Of note, this mutation was shown to provide cross-resistance to BRAF inhibitors. These results illuminate clinical mechanisms of resistance to both MEK and B-RAF inhibition and confirm the specificity of mechanisms of resistance to allosteric inhibitors [95].

Oncogenic Potential of the Resistance Mutations

As mentioned above, resistance mutations usually impair drug binding or induce conformational change, but typically don't interact with ATP binding. Consequently, these mutations have the potential to confer inhibitor resistance through a variety of biochemical mechanisms, and maintain kinase activity. However, there are variations of the oncogenic potential among the different resistance mutations.

Griswold et al. studied the transformation potential, kinase activity, and substrate specificity of five of the most frequent mutations arising in BCR-ABL following imatinib treatment for CML: Y253F, E255K, T315I, M351T, and H396P [96]. The P-loop mutations Y253F and E255K exhibited increased transformation potency, whereas M351T and H396P were less potent, with a rank order being Y253F, E255K>native BCR-ABL>T315I>H396P>M351T. Interestingly, the development of E255K is associated with poorer prognosis among patients with CML receiving imatinib. Notably, the kinase activity of E255K, H396P, and T315I did not correlate with transforming potency. Indeed, the proliferative advantage of a given mutant seems multifactorial and determined by intrinsic kinase activity, substrate specificity, and extrinsic factors including growth factors and cytokines [78]. Analysis of the phosphotyrosine proteome by mass spectroscopy confirmed the presence of differences in the tyrosine phosphorylation patterns of the various mutants, confirming that different mutations determine substrate specificity leading to activation of different downstream pathways [96].

As far as *EGFR* is concerned, several cases of patients who carry both the T790M and L858R mutations before any treatment with EGFR TKI have been reported [97, 98]. Moreover, germline transmission of the T790M mutation has been described in a family with multiple cases of lung cancer with four of the six tumors analyzed showing a secondary somatic activating EGFR mutation (either L858R, del L747-T751, or G719A) occurring in *cis* with the germline T790M mutation [99]. These results suggest the proliferative advantage associated with the T790M mutation, beside its role in the resistance to EGFR TKI. Although it was initially reported that the kinase activity of the EGFR T790M mutant was indistinguishable from wild-type EGFR [61–63], Vikis et al. further showed that the T790M mutation alone is responsible for increased phosphorylation levels of EGFR and growth advantage with respect to wild-type EGFR [100]. Recent work showed a substantial increase in autophosphorylation at several sites in the L858R/T790M mutant cells compared with the L858R mutant cells, suggesting that T790M confers enhanced catalytic phosphorylating activity and cooperates to produce a more potent kinase [101]. In mice models with inducible expression in type II pneumocytes of EGFR T790M alone or together with a L858R mutation, both transgenic lines develop lung adenocarcinomas that require mutant EGFR for tumor maintenance [102]. Notably, mice expressing EGFR T790M develop tumors with longer latency than those with EGFR L858R+T790M [102]. These results indicate that the T790M mutation is not only a cause of resistance to gefitinib/erlotinib but is also an oncogenic mutation that confers growth advantage to cancer cells. Its oncogenic potential is maximized when the mutation arises in combination with other common EGFR-activating mutations [103].

Mutational Heterogeneity

Heterogeneity of resistance mutations within and between tumor sites is an important feature of certain types of cancer, especially GIST. Liegl et al. have highlighted this phenomenon. They showed substantial interlesional heterogeneity of drug resistance mutations in patients treated with imatinib alone or imatinib followed by sunitinib. In this study, 9 patients out of 11 (83%) had secondary drug-resistant *KIT* mutations, and in 6 patients (67%), there were two to five different secondary mutations among separate metastases. More strikingly, 3 patients (34%) showed two different secondary *KIT* mutations within the same metastasis [104]. Thus, at least in GIST, a biopsy of one progressing lesion may not be representative of others.

In NSCLC, analysis of various progressive lesions in an autopsy case from an individual with acquired resistance to EGFR TKI revealed that the seven different sites all harbored the exon 19 deletion, whereas the T790M mutation was found in six out of seven sites, but was not detected in the brain metastasis, despite the use of highly-sensitive methods [65]. These results suggest that the selection pressure for resistant tumor cells that grow in the presence of EGFR TKI may be different among the different tumor sites.

Origins of Resistance Mutations

Resistance mutations may arise through two different mechanisms: either the mutation is acquired through selective pressure during treatment, or it exists before treatment and grows in prevalence owing to the selective pressure of treatment.

First studies conducted in imatinib-resistant CML or ALL compared mutational status between pre- and posttreatment samples. In these studies, the resistance mutations were only found in the posttreatment samples, suggesting that the mutation had been acquired during treatment [105, 106]. The method used to detect mutations in these studies was usually the same for pre- and posttreatment samples, and had a low sensitivity for detection of mutations. Therefore, it was only possible to detect highly prevalent mutations but not mutations present in a small subset of cells. However, with improvement of detection thresholds thanks to techniques with increasing sensitivity, it became clear that in some cases, the resistance mutation was detectable before and after treatment with imatinib. For example, using PCR-single strand conformation polymorphism (PCR-SSCP) technique, Hoffman et al. were able to detect the E255K resistance mutation of *BCR-ABL* in the pretreatment samples of 2 out of 4 patients with imatinib-resistant ALL [107], whereas the same team, in a previous study using direct sequencing, had not been able to detect any resistance mutation in the pretreatment samples of six imatinib-resistant patients with ALL for whom the E255K had been found in posttreatment samples [106]. These results highlight the crucial importance of the sensitivity of the detection techniques when studying emergence of resistance mutations. In some cases, no resistance mutations are found in the pretreatment samples despite the use of highly-sensitive techniques. Whether the mutation is present at undetectable level or has been acquired during treatment remains unknown.

In NSCLC, it remains unclear how tumor cells harboring the T790M mutation arise in patients receiving gefitinib or erlotinib. Here again, the sensitivity of the techniques used to detect the resistance mutation seems to be critical. This is even truer since a phenomenon named "allelic dilution" has been observed in TKI-resistant models, which is responsible for some biologically significant resistance mutations being undetectable using traditional means [108]. Allelic dilution has been observed in gefitinib-sensitive lung cancer cells with *EGFR* mutations and amplifications that acquire resistance through acquisition of a T790M mutation which is present only in a small subset of the amplified alleles and can be detected only with highly-sensitive techniques such as denaturing high-performance liquid chromatography. This phenomenon intensifies the need to improve sequencing techniques to assure accuracy.

Using the SARMS technology (DxS), Maheswaran et al. were able to detect low levels of T790M in pretreatment samples from 10 of 26 patients (38%), in addition to the known activating *EGFR* mutation [86]. The high number of amplification cycles needed to detect T790M suggests that the mutation was present in a small subset of cells. Interestingly, although the presence of the T790M mutation didn't affect the response rate, the progression-free survival was significantly shorter in these patients compared to those without T790M mutation (7.7 vs. 16.5 months, hazard ratio for progression for the T790M allele, 11.5; 95% confidence interval, 2.94–45.1; $p < 0.001$) [86]. Thus, T790M may initially arise by virtue of its oncogenicity and may rapidly emerge as a dominant allele after treatment. These results suggest that T790M may be a useful pretreatment biomarker for identifying patients who are unlikely to achieve durable responses with reversible EGFR TKIs.

Therapeutic Approaches to Overcome Resistant Mutants

The important role of acquired drug resistance in limiting the clinical efficacy of kinase inhibitors has prompted considerable effort to develop next generation treatments to surmount resistance. The better understanding of how these mutations confer resistance to kinase inhibitors enables the development of new compounds specifically designed to overcome resistant mutants. Several therapeutic approaches to overcome resistant mutants are being developed (Table 1.2) [109–133]. The first one is to target the mutant kinase with more potent inhibitors, such as irreversible or mutant-selective inhibitors. The second approach is to target signaling pathways downstream of the mutant kinase. It is also important to consider the possibility that multiple distinct resistance mechanisms might develop simultaneously in individual patients, thereby challenging our ability to overcome acquired resistance with single agent therapy.

Targeting of the Mutant Kinase

ATP-Competitive Inhibitors

Second-Generation ATP-Competitive Inhibitors

One strategy for overcoming resistance mutations is to design new ATP-competitive inhibitors that derive potency and selectivity from alternative binding modes. In CML, two second-generation inhibitors, nilotinib (Tasigna™; Novartis) and dasatinib (Sprycel™; Bristol–Myers Squibb), which are capable of inhibiting most *BCR-ABL* mutations, with the exception of the T315I gatekeeper, have been approved for clinical use [74]. Nilotinib is a phenylaminopyrimidine with a selectivity profile similar to imatinib (BCR-ABL, PDGFR and KIT) that binds to the inactive conformation of the kinase and has approximately 20-fold higher cellular activity than imatinib. Dasatinib is a thiazole-derived compound with a pan-tyrosine kinase inhibitor profile that binds to the active conformation of the kinase. The development of these inhibitors demonstrates that by increasing affinity to the ATP-binding site through more extensive and complementary hydrogen bonding and hydrophobic interactions, it is possible to overcome most of the resistant mutations in *BCR-ABL*. Two new inhibitors that are capable of inhibiting T315I BCR-ABL have recently been reported, they are: PPY-A101 and PHA-739358 [134].

Table 1.2 Therapeutic strategies against gatekeeper mutations

Mechanism of action / Compound	Mutant kinase	Effective in cellular assays	Effective in murine models	Tested in clinical trials including resistant patients	References
Targeting of the mutant kinase					
ATP-competitive inhibitors					
Irreversible inhibitors					
HKI272, PF00299804, BIBW2992	EGFR T790M	Y	Y	Y	[110]
Mutant-selective inhibitors					
WZ4002	EGFR T790M	Y	Y	N	[111]
Other inhibitors					
SGX393	BCR-ABL T315I	Y	Y	Y	[125]
AP24534	BCR-ABL T315I	Y	Y	Y	[112]
Non-ATP-competitive inhibitors					
Allosteric inhibitors					
GNF-2 + ATP-competitive ABL inhibitor	BCR-ABL T315I	Y	Y	N	[113]
Switch pocket inhibitors					
DCC2036, DCC2157	BCR-ABL T315I	Y	Y	Y	[114]
Other inhibitors					
ON012380	BCR-ABL T315I	Y	Y	N	[109]
Multikinase inhibitors					
VEGFR/EGFR inhibitors					
Vandetanib	EGFR T790M	Y	Y	N	[116, 117]
EXEL-7647	EGFR T790M	Y	Y	N	[118]
Aurora/ABL kinase inhibitors					
MK-0457, XL228, PHA-739358, KW-2449	BCR-ABL T315I	Y	Y	Y	[115]

Monoclonal antibodies					
Cetuximab + BIBW2992	EGFR T790M	Y	Y	N	[126]
Panitumumab	EGFR T790M	Y	Y	N	[127]
Targeting of downstream or alternative signaling pathways					
Alternative kinase inhibitors					
MET inhibitors					
MET inhibitor + ATP-competitive EGFR inhibitor	EGFR T790M	Y	Y	N	[128]
RAF inhibitors					
BMS-214662, tipifarnib + imatinib	BCR-ABL T315I	Y	N	N	[119]
MEK inhibitors					
MEK 1/2 inhibitor + ATP-competitive EGFR inhibitor	EGFR T790M	Y	N	N	[120]
MEK 1/2 inhibitor + PI3K inhibitor	EGFR T790M	Y	Y	N	[121]
mTOR inhibitors					
Rapamycin + HKI-272	EGFR T790M	Y	Y	N	[122]
RAC inhibitors					
NSC2376664	BCR-ABL T315I	Y	Y	N	[129]
PP2A activators					
FTY720	BCR-ABL T315I	Y	Y	Y	[130]
Apoptosis inducers					
Homoharringtonine Omacetaxine mepesuccinate	BCR-ABL T315I	Y	Y	Y	[123]
BH3 mimetic					
ABT-737	BCR-ABL T315I	Y	N	N	[124]

(continued)

Table 1.2 (continued)

Mechanism of action	Compound	Mutant kinase	Effective in cellular assays	Effective in murine models	Tested in clinical trials including resistant patients	References
Targeting of both the mutant kinase and downstream signaling						
	HSP90 inhibitors					
	Geldanamycins					
	17-DMAG	EGFR T790M	Y	Y	N	[131]
	17-AAG, 17-DMAG + MEK inhibitor	BCR-ABL T315I	Y	N	N	[132]
	HDAC inhibitors					
	LBH583, vorinostat + MK-0457	BCR-ABL T315I	Y	N	N	[133]

Both inhibitors recognize the active conformation of the kinase (type 1, DFG in). The selectivity profile of PPY-A has not been reported but PHA-739358 is reported to have a broad selectivity profile, which may impair its safety profile [5, 135]. Another approach for overcoming resistance to ATP-competitive inhibitors in CML has been to target the kinase with inhibitors that bind at alternative binding sites. For example, the substrate binding site has been targeted by On012380, a vinyl sulfone-containing inhibitor [109, 136], and the myristate binding site has been targeted by the GNF-2 class of inhibitors, which will be discussed later [42].

Irreversible ATP-Competitive Inhibitors

Irreversible EGFR inhibitors such as HKI-272 (Wyeth), BIBW2992 (Tovok™; Boehringer Ingelheim), and PF00299804 (Pfizer) are currently being evaluated in clinical trials [110]. These agents covalently bind a cysteine residue in EGFR at amino acid position 797; once covalently bound, they are no longer in a competitive, reversible equilibrium with ATP, which allows them to overcome EGFR T790M in preclinical models [44, 137]. The irreversible inhibitors inhibit EGFR driven signaling and lung cancer cell survival in vitro and in vivo [138]. However, the efficacy of these agents may be impaired due to various reasons. First, all current irreversible inhibitors are less potent in cell line models harboring *EGFR* T790M than those with an *EGFR*-activating mutation alone and, at clinically achievable concentrations, these agents do not inhibit EGFR T790M in vitro [137–141]. T790M has even been found to mediate resistance to low (clinically achievable) concentrations of irreversible inhibitors [140]. Moreover, because the ATP affinity of EGFR T790M is similar to wild-type EGFR, the concentration of quinazoline-based EGFR inhibitors required to inhibit EGFR T790M will also effectively inhibit wild-type EGFR. In patients, this concurrent inhibition of wild-type EGFR will result in skin rash and diarrhea, and limit the ability to achieve plasma concentrations sufficient to inhibit EGFR T790M. Indeed, the clinical efficacy of the irreversible EGFR inhibitors has been limited, especially in patients with gefitinib or erlotinib resistant NSCLC, and the dose-limiting toxicity has been diarrhea and skin rash [142, 143]. Finally, covalent inhibitors may yield high toxicity caused by off-target effects, since at least 10 kinases in addition to EGFR have a reactive cysteine residue in the position equivalent to cysteine 797 in EGFR [5].

Mutant-Selective ATP-Competitive Inhibitors

An alternative approach has been recently proposed for the development of EGFR TKIs effective against the T790M mutant EGFR, based on a functional pharmacological screen against mutant kinases [111]. In this study, it was hypothesized that the anilinoquinazoline scaffold of gefitinib and erlotinib may not be the most potent or specific for inhibiting EGFR T790M because it relies on the small size and hydrogen bonding interactions with the gatekeeper threonine of wild-type EGFR. By screening an irreversible kinase inhibitor library specifically against EGFR T790M, a novel structural class of EGFR kinase inhibitors that are effective against EGFR T790M was identified [111]. The anilinopyrimidine scaffold is an intrinsically better fit for the mutant gatekeeper methionine. The compound binds within the ATP-binding cleft of the enzyme, forming the expected covalent bond with cysteine at position 797. The anilinopyrimidine core forms a hydrogen bonding interaction with the "hinge" residue methionine 793. The chlorine substituent on the pyrimidine ring contacts the mutant gatekeeper residue, methionine 790. The hydrophobicity conferred by this mutation likely contributes to the potency of these compounds against the T790M mutant. These agents are 30–100-fold more potent against EGFR T790M, and up to 100-fold less potent against wild-type EGFR, than quinazoline-based EGFR inhibitors in vitro. They are also effective in murine models of lung cancer driven by EGFR T790M [111]. These mutant-selective irreversible EGFR kinase inhibitors may be clinically more effective and better tolerated than quinazoline-bases compounds. These results demonstrate that cellular screens expressing the mutant kinase of interest represent a powerful strategy to identify new classes of mutant-selective kinase inhibitors.

Structure-Based Drug Design of Next Generation Inhibitors

O'Hare et al. have recently reported encouraging results from the new BCR-ABL inhibitor AP24534, which was obtained among several compounds designed by introducing a vinyl and ethyl linkages into a purine-based inhibitor scaffold [112]. This compound binds the DFG-out conformation of the kinase and accommodates the T315I side-chain by virtue of a carbon–carbon triple bond (ethynyl) linkage. A total of five hydrogen bonds are made between the inhibitor and the protein, which confers high potency and balance and distribute the overall binding affinity. As a result, AP24534 retains potency against all tested resistance mutations, including the T315I gatekeeper mutation. The compound has been shown to be effective on CML primary cells and in mouse xenografts models driven either by native BCR-ABL or by BCR-ABL with the T315I mutation. Moreover, in an accelerated muta-genesis assay used to characterize the resistance profile to AP24534, the compound was found to induce a concentration-dependent reduction in both the frequency and in the range of mutations observed [112]. Finally, given its structure, AP24534 has a relatively broad kinase specificity profile which includes VEGFR, FGFR, PDGFR, and SRC family kinases, but not Aurora kinases, which makes it an inter-esting therapeutic approach for the treatment of other malignancies.

Non-ATP-Competitive Inhibitors

Allosteric Inhibitors

A potential alternative approach to ATP-competitive inhibition is to use molecules that inhibit the kinase activity either by a non-ATP-competitive allosteric mecha-nism or by preventing the binding of substrates to the kinase. This strategy has the advantage that the mutants resistant to ATP-competitive inhibitors are unlikely to be resistant to allosteric inhibitors, owing to the different binding sites. High-throughput screening for inhibitors of BCR-ABL-dependent cell proliferation has already resulted in the identification of a lead compound that was subsequently modified to give GNF-2 as a prototype inhibitor, which bound to the myristate binding site of BCR-ABL, located near the C terminus of the kinase domain, resulting in the allosteric inhibition of ABL tyrosine kinase activity. A recent study showed that combination of an allosteric inhibitor such as GNF-2 or related compounds with an ATP-competitive inhibitor of BCR-ABL suppressed the emergence of resistance mutations in vitro, displayed additive inhibitory activity in biochemical and cellular assays against T315I mutant, and displayed in vivo efficacy against the same mutant in a murine bone-marrow transplantation model [113]. The authors propose that binding of GNF-2 compound and its analogs to the myristate binding site causes structural reorganization, possibly communicated by means of a conformational rearrangement of other parts of ABL, which disrupts the catalytic machinery located in the ATP-binding site. Although these compounds lack significant biochemical and cellular potency against the T315I gatekeeper mutation, they can act cooperatively with an ATP-competitive inhibitor to inhibit both wild-type and T315I BCR-ABL [113].

Switch Pocket Inhibitors

The conformational change between the active and inactive form of the kinase is controlled by the phosphorylation of key regions called "switch pockets." Targeting of these pockets blocks conformational activation of the kinase and thus appears as an interesting therapeutic approach. Moreover, since the switch pockets are quite unique for each kinase, these compounds are expected to have a good selectivity profile. DCC-2036 is a switch pocket inhibitor of BCR-ABL that impaired proliferation and induced apoptosis of Ba/F3 cells expressing a wide variety of BCR-ABL imatinib-resistant mutants, including the T315I mutant [114]. It also prolonged survival in mice injected with Ba/F3 cells harboring the T315I mutant. This compound is now being evaluated in early-phase clinical studies.

Multikinase Inhibitors

Multikinase inhibitors are TKIs that can target several various kinases. They can be exploited for the treatment of resistant tumors through two different ways. The first way is to use inhibitors that have been initially designed to target a certain kinase and also display inhibitory effect against another kinase, even in the presence of a resistance mutation. For example, Aurora kinases inhibitors such as MK-0457, XL228, PHA-739358, and KW-2449 also fit into the ATP-binding pocket of BCR-ABL, even in the presence of the T315I mutation. They have shown potency against both wild-type and mutant isoforms BCR-ABL in in vitro and murine models [115].

Another way to exploit the multiple spectrum of some inhibitors is to target several relevant kinases with synergistic effects. For example, vandetanib and EXEL-7647 are inhibitors of both EGFR and VEGFR, and showed increased efficacy against T790M EGFR mutants in vitro and in vivo compared to gefitinib or erlotinib alone [116–118].

Targeting of Downstream Signaling

Downstream signaling of deregulated kinases such as EGFR or BCR-ABL is transmitted through several pathways, such as the MAPKinase pathway, that plays a key role in the growth and proliferation of cancer cells, and the PI3Kinase/AKT/mTOR pathway that plays a key role in cell survival. RAF and MEK inhibitors (targeting the MAPKinase pathway) and mTOR inhibitors (targeting the PI3K/AKT/mTOR pathway) have shown potency against models harboring the mutant isoforms of EGFR and BCR-ABL, mostly in combination with ATP-competitive inhibitors [119–122].

Apoptosis induction is also an emerging therapeutic approach that showed encouraging results in TKI-resistant models. Omacetaxine mepesuccinate is a semisynthetic formulation of homoharringtonine, which interrupts chain elongation during translation by targeting the 60S ribosome subunit. It induces apoptosis in CML cells (with or without a T315I mutation) by inhibition of protein synthesis, particularly Mcl-1, which leads to mitochondrial disruption and release of cytochrome c, leading to caspase-9 and caspase-3 activation [123]. An ongoing phase 2/3 clinical study of omacetaxine in BCR-ABL T315I-positive CML showed promising preliminary results, with a reduction of the BCR-ABL T315I clone below the level of detection in 64% of evaluable patients with chronic phase CML [123].

Apoptosis can also be targeted trough BH3 mimetics, which act by binding to and inhibiting members of the prosurvival Bcl-2 family. ABT-737 is the leading compound of this new therapeutic class, and has been shown to be effective in several various cancer cell lines, most of the times in combination with a second antineoplastic agent. In CML cell lines, ABT-737 enhanced apoptosis induced by an ATP-competitive ABL inhibitor, even in the presence of point mutations conferring resistance to imatinib, with the exception of the T315I gatekeeper mutation [124].

Conclusion

Kinase inhibitors are effective clinical therapies for several human malignancies. However, their clinical efficacy is ultimately limited by the development of drug resistance. Recent studies have identified resistance mechanisms to kinase inhibitors and used these findings to develop more effective therapeutic approaches. By inhibiting a specific kinase that plays a crucial role in the cancer cell, kinase inhibitors induce a strong selective pressure on their target for emergence of resistance mechanisms.

Among these mechanisms, resistance mutations have a predominant place. Not surprisingly, the type of resistance mutations depends on the type of inhibitors used to target the kinase. The ATP-competitive inhibitors are likely to induce mutations within or close to the ATP-binding site, especially at the gatekeeper residue, whereas allosteric inhibitors are likely to induce mutations close to the allosteric site. Recent studies offered new insights into the precise mechanisms implicated in resistance, such as the finding that the T790M mutation in *EGFR* confers resistance through a change in ATP affinity rather than because of steric hindrance. Such findings allow development of adequate new generation inhibitors. However, it is expected that resistance will also occur with these inhibitors. For example, some mechanisms of resistance to irreversible EGFR TKIs have already been identified in vitro and implicate the amplification of a T790M allele [144]. In CML, sequential treatment with imatinib and dasatinib induced the development of multiple resistance mutations [79, 145]. As new kinase inhibitors enter the clinical area, it will be necessary to prospectively study drug resistance to these agents. The continued interaction of drug development, basic biology, and translational studies will make new therapeutic approaches emerge, that will further improve clinical outcomes for these patients [125–133].

References

1. Druker BJ et al. Efficacy and safety of a specific inhibitor of the BCR-ABL tyrosine kinase in chronic myeloid leukemia. N Engl J Med. 2001;344(14):1031–7.
2. Verweij J et al. Progression-free survival in gastrointestinal stromal tumours with high-dose imatinib: randomised trial. Lancet. 2004;364(9440):1127–34.
3. Lahiry P et al. Kinase mutations in human disease: interpreting genotype-phenotype relationships. Nat Rev Genet. 2010;11(1):60–74.
4. Janne PA, Gray N, Settleman J. Factors underlying sensitivity of cancers to small-molecule kinase inhibitors. Nat Rev Drug Discov. 2009;8(9):709–23.
5. Zhang J, Yang PL, Gray NS. Targeting cancer with small molecule kinase inhibitors. Nat Rev Cancer. 2009;9(1):28–39.
6. Weinstein IB et al. Disorders in cell circuitry associated with multistage carcinogenesis: exploitable targets for cancer prevention and therapy. Clin Cancer Res. 1997;3(12 Pt 2):2696–702.
7. Weinstein IB, Joe AK. Mechanisms of disease: Oncogene addiction–a rationale for molecular targeting in cancer therapy. Nat Clin Pract Oncol. 2006;3(8):448–57.
8. Hantschel O, Superti-Furga G. Regulation of the c-Abl and Bcr-Abl tyrosine kinases. Nat Rev Mol Cell Biol. 2004;5(1):33–44.
9. Milojkovic D, Apperley J. State-of-the-art in the treatment of chronic myeloid leukaemia. Curr Opin Oncol. 2008;20(1):112–21.
10. Melo J. Inviting leukemic cells to waltz with the devil. Nat Med. 2001;7(2):156–7.
11. Quintas-Cardama A, Cortes J. Molecular biology of bcr-abl1-positive chronic myeloid leukemia. Blood. 2009;113(8):1619–30.
12. Hynes NE, Lane HA. ERBB receptors and cancer: the complexity of targeted inhibitors. Nat Rev Cancer. 2005;5(5):341–54.
13. Yarden Y, Sliwkowski MX. Untangling the ErbB signalling network. Nat Rev Mol Cell Biol. 2001;2(2):127–37.
14. Gazdar AF et al. Mutations and addiction to EGFR: the Achilles 'heal' of lung cancers? Trends Mol Med. 2004;10(10):481–6.

15. Lynch TJ et al. Activating mutations in the epidermal growth factor receptor underlying responsiveness of non-small-cell lung cancer to gefitinib. N Engl J Med. 2004;350(21): 2129–39.
16. Paez JG et al. EGFR mutations in lung cancer: correlation with clinical response to gefitinib therapy. Science. 2004;304(5676):1497–500.
17. Pao W et al. EGF receptor gene mutations are common in lung cancers from "never smokers" and are associated with sensitivity of tumors to gefitinib and erlotinib. Proc Natl Acad Sci USA. 2004;101(36):13306–11.
18. Johnson BE, Janne PA. Epidermal growth factor receptor mutations in patients with non-small cell lung cancer. Cancer Res. 2005;65(17):7525–9.
19. Shigematsu H, Gazdar AF. Somatic mutations of epidermal growth factor receptor signaling pathway in lung cancers. Int J Cancer. 2006;118(2):257–62.
20. Chan SK, Gullick WJ, Hill ME. Mutations of the epidermal growth factor receptor in non-small cell lung cancer–search and destroy. Eur J Cancer. 2006;42(1):17–23.
21. Mitsudomi T, Yatabe Y. Mutations of the epidermal growth factor receptor gene and related genes as determinants of epidermal growth factor receptor tyrosine kinase inhibitors sensitivity in lung cancer. Cancer Sci. 2007;98(12):1817–24.
22. Engelman JA et al. ErbB-3 mediates phosphoinositide 3-kinase activity in gefitinib-sensitive non-small cell lung cancer cell lines. Proc Natl Acad Sci USA. 2005;102(10):3788–93.
23. Heinrich MC et al. Inhibition of c-kit receptor tyrosine kinase activity by STI 571, a selective tyrosine kinase inhibitor. Blood. 2000;96(3):925–32.
24. Heinrich MC et al. Biology and genetic aspects of gastrointestinal stromal tumors: KIT activation and cytogenetic alterations. Hum Pathol. 2002;33(5):484–95.
25. Tsujimura T et al. Activating mutation in the catalytic domain of c-kit elicits hematopoietic transformation by receptor self-association not at the ligand-induced dimerization site. Blood. 1999;93(4):1319–29.
26. Corless CL, Fletcher JA, Heinrich MC. Biology of gastrointestinal stromal tumors. J Clin Oncol. 2004;22(18):3813–25.
27. Heinrich MC et al. Kinase mutations and imatinib response in patients with metastatic gastrointestinal stromal tumor. J Clin Oncol. 2003;21(23):4342–9.
28. Debiec-Rychter M et al. KIT mutations and dose selection for imatinib in patients with advanced gastrointestinal stromal tumours. Eur J Cancer. 2006;42(8):1093–103.
29. Mol CD et al. Structural basis for the autoinhibition and STI-571 inhibition of c-Kit tyrosine kinase. J Biol Chem. 2004;279(30):31655–63.
30. Heinrich MC et al. PDGFRA activating mutations in gastrointestinal stromal tumors. Science. 2003;299(5607):708–10.
31. Sharma SV, Settleman J. Oncogene addiction: setting the stage for molecularly targeted cancer therapy. Genes Dev. 2007;21(24):3214–31.
32. Shah NP et al. Transient potent BCR-ABL inhibition is sufficient to commit chronic myeloid leukemia cells irreversibly to apoptosis. Cancer Cell. 2008;14(6):485–93.
33. Deininger M, Buchdunger E, Druker BJ. The development of imatinib as a therapeutic agent for chronic myeloid leukemia. Blood. 2005;105(7):2640–53.
34. Hochhaus A et al. Six-year follow-up of patients receiving imatinib for the first-line treatment of chronic myeloid leukemia. Leukemia. 2009;23(6):1054–61.
35. Shepherd FA et al. Erlotinib in previously treated non-small-cell lung cancer. N Engl J Med. 2005;353(2):123–32.
36. Mok TS et al. Gefitinib or carboplatin-paclitaxel in pulmonary adenocarcinoma. N Engl J Med. 2009;361(10):947–57.
37. Mitsudomi T et al. Gefitinib versus cisplatin plus docetaxel in patients with non-small-cell lung cancer harbouring mutations of the epidermal growth factor receptor (WJTOG3405): an open label, randomised phase 3 trial. Lancet Oncol. 2010;11(2):121–8.
38. Blanke CD et al. Phase III randomized, intergroup trial assessing imatinib mesylate at two dose levels in patients with unresectable or metastatic gastrointestinal stromal tumors expressing the kit receptor tyrosine kinase: S0033. J Clin Oncol. 2008;26(4):626–32.

39. Liu Y, Gray NS. Rational design of inhibitors that bind to inactive kinase conformations. Nat Chem Biol. 2006;2(7):358–64.
40. Schindler T et al. Structural mechanism for STI-571 inhibition of abelson tyrosine kinase. Science. 2000;289(5486):1938–42.
41. Ohren JF et al. Structures of human MAP kinase kinase 1 (MEK1) and MEK2 describe novel noncompetitive kinase inhibition. Nat Struct Mol Biol. 2004;11(12):1192–7.
42. Adrian FJ et al. Allosteric inhibitors of Bcr-abl-dependent cell proliferation. Nat Chem Biol. 2006;2(2):95–102.
43. Cohen MS et al. Structural bioinformatics-based design of selective, irreversible kinase inhibitors. Science. 2005;308(5726):1318–21.
44. Kwak EL et al. Irreversible inhibitors of the EGF receptor may circumvent acquired resistance to gefitinib. Proc Natl Acad Sci USA. 2005;102(21):7665–70.
45. le Coutre P et al. Induction of resistance to the Abelson inhibitor STI571 in human leukemic cells through gene amplification. Blood. 2000;95(5):1758–66.
46. Engelman JA et al. MET amplification leads to gefitinib resistance in lung cancer by activating ERBB3 signaling. Science. 2007;316(5827):1039–43.
47. Gorre ME et al. Clinical resistance to STI-571 cancer therapy caused by BCR-ABL gene mutation or amplification. Science. 2001;293(5531):876–80.
48. Jabbour E et al. Frequency and clinical significance of BCR-ABL mutations in patients with chronic myeloid leukemia treated with imatinib mesylate. Leukemia. 2006;20(10):1767–73.
49. Nicolini FE et al. Mutation status and clinical outcome of 89 imatinib mesylate-resistant chronic myelogenous leukemia patients: a retrospective analysis from the French intergroup of CML (Fi(phi)-LMC GROUP). Leukemia. 2006;20(6):1061–6.
50. Jabbour E et al. Characteristics and outcomes of patients with chronic myeloid leukemia and T315I mutation following failure of imatinib mesylate therapy. Blood. 2008;112(1):53–5.
51. Nicolini FE et al. Clinical outcome of 27 imatinib mesylate-resistant chronic myelogenous leukemia patients harboring a T315I BCR-ABL mutation. Haematologica. 2007;92(9):1238–41.
52. Soverini S et al. Contribution of ABL kinase domain mutations to imatinib resistance in different subsets of Philadelphia-positive patients: by the GIMEMA Working Party on Chronic Myeloid Leukemia. Clin Cancer Res. 2006;12(24):7374–9.
53. Hochhaus A, La Rosee P. Imatinib therapy in chronic myelogenous leukemia: strategies to avoid and overcome resistance. Leukemia. 2004;18(8):1321–31.
54. Shah NP et al. Multiple BCR-ABL kinase domain mutations confer polyclonal resistance to the tyrosine kinase inhibitor imatinib (STI571) in chronic phase and blast crisis chronic myeloid leukemia. Cancer Cell. 2002;2(2):117–25.
55. Lowenberg B. Minimal residual disease in chronic myeloid leukemia. N Engl J Med. 2003;349(15):1399–401.
56. Corbin AS et al. Several Bcr-Abl kinase domain mutants associated with imatinib mesylate resistance remain sensitive to imatinib. Blood. 2003;101(11):4611–4.
57. Gambacorti-Passerini CB et al. Molecular mechanisms of resistance to imatinib in Philadelphia-chromosome-positive leukaemias. Lancet Oncol. 2003;4(2):75–85.
58. Hughes T, Branford S. Molecular monitoring of BCR-ABL as a guide to clinical management in chronic myeloid leukaemia. Blood Rev. 2006;20(1):29–41.
59. Soverini S et al. ABL mutations in late chronic phase chronic myeloid leukemia patients with up-front cytogenetic resistance to imatinib are associated with a greater likelihood of progression to blast crisis and shorter survival: a study by the GIMEMA Working Party on Chronic Myeloid Leukemia. J Clin Oncol. 2005;23(18):4100–9.
60. Apperley JF. Part I: mechanisms of resistance to imatinib in chronic myeloid leukaemia. Lancet Oncol. 2007;8(11):1018–29.
61. Blencke S, Ullrich A, Daub H. Mutation of threonine 766 in the epidermal growth factor receptor reveals a hotspot for resistance formation against selective tyrosine kinase inhibitors. J Biol Chem. 2003;278(17):15435–40.
62. Kobayashi S et al. EGFR mutation and resistance of non-small-cell lung cancer to gefitinib. N Engl J Med. 2005;352(8):786–92.

63. Pao W et al. Acquired resistance of lung adenocarcinomas to gefitinib or erlotinib is associated with a second mutation in the EGFR kinase domain. PLoS Med. 2005;2(3):e73.

64. Kosaka T et al. Analysis of epidermal growth factor receptor gene mutation in patients with non-small cell lung cancer and acquired resistance to gefitinib. Clin Cancer Res. 2006;12(19):5764–9.

65. Balak MN et al. Novel D761Y and common secondary T790M mutations in epidermal growth factor receptor-mutant lung adenocarcinomas with acquired resistance to kinase inhibitors. Clin Cancer Res. 2006;12(21):6494–501.

66. Costa DB et al. BIM mediates EGFR tyrosine kinase inhibitor-induced apoptosis in lung cancers with oncogenic EGFR mutations. PLoS Med. 2007;4(10):1669–79. discussion 1680.

67. Bean J et al. Acquired resistance to epidermal growth factor receptor kinase inhibitors associated with a novel T854A mutation in a patient with EGFR-mutant lung adenocarcinoma. Clin Cancer Res. 2008;14(22):7519–25.

68. Gramza AW, Corless CL, Heinrich MC. Resistance to Tyrosine Kinase Inhibitors in Gastrointestinal Stromal Tumors. Clin Cancer Res. 2009;15(24):7510–8.

69. Heinrich MC et al. Molecular correlates of imatinib resistance in gastrointestinal stromal tumors. J Clin Oncol. 2006;24(29):4764–74.

70. Antonescu CR et al. Acquired resistance to imatinib in gastrointestinal stromal tumor occurs through secondary gene mutation. Clin Cancer Res. 2005;11(11):4182–90.

71. Heinrich MC et al. Primary and secondary kinase genotypes correlate with the biological and clinical activity of sunitinib in imatinib-resistant gastrointestinal stromal tumor. J Clin Oncol. 2008;26(33):5352–9.

72. Nishida T et al. Secondary mutations in the kinase domain of the KIT gene are predominant in imatinib-resistant gastrointestinal stromal tumor. Cancer Sci. 2008;99(4):799–804.

73. Guo T et al. Mechanisms of sunitinib resistance in gastrointestinal stromal tumors harboring KITAY502–3ins mutation: an in vitro mutagenesis screen for drug resistance. Clin Cancer Res. 2009;15(22):6862–70.

74. Engelman JA, Settleman J. Acquired resistance to tyrosine kinase inhibitors during cancer therapy. Curr Opin Genet Dev. 2008;18(1):73–9.

75. Koizumi F et al. Establishment of a human non-small cell lung cancer cell line resistant to gefitinib. Int J Cancer. 2005;116(1):36–44.

76. Ogino A et al. Emergence of epidermal growth factor receptor T790M mutation during chronic exposure to gefitinib in a non small cell lung cancer cell line. Cancer Res. 2007;67(16):7807–14.

77. Janne PA. Challenges of detecting EGFR T790M in gefitinib/erlotinib-resistant tumours. Lung Cancer. 2008;60 Suppl 2:S3–9.

78. Quintas-Cardama A, Kantarjian HM, Cortes JE. Mechanisms of primary and secondary resistance to imatinib in chronic myeloid leukemia. Cancer Control. 2009;16(2):122–31.

79. Quintas-Cardama A, et al. Mutational analysis of chronic myeloid leukemia (cml) clones reveals heightened BCR-ABL1 genetic instability and wild-type BCR-ABL1 exhaustion in patients failing sequential imatinib and dasatinib therapy. ASH Annual Meeting Abstracts. 2007;110(11):1938.

80. Nardi V et al. Quantitative monitoring by polymerase colony assay of known mutations resistant to ABL kinase inhibitors. Oncogene. 2008;27(6):775–82.

81. Willis SG et al. High-sensitivity detection of BCR-ABL kinase domain mutations in imatinib-naive patients: correlation with clonal cytogenetic evolution but not response to therapy. Blood. 2005;106(6):2128–37.

82. Khorashad JS et al. The presence of a BCR-ABL mutant allele in CML does not always explain clinical resistance to imatinib. Leukemia. 2006;20(4):658–63.

83. Deininger MW et al. Detection of ABL kinase domain mutations with denaturing high-performance liquid chromatography. Leukemia. 2004;18(4):864–71.

84. Soverini S et al. Denaturing-HPLC-based assay for detection of ABL mutations in chronic myeloid leukemia patients resistant to Imatinib. Clin Chem. 2004;50(7):1205–13.

85. Ernst T et al. Dynamics of BCR-ABL mutated clones prior to hematologic or cytogenetic resistance to imatinib. Haematologica. 2008;93(2):186–92.
86. Maheswaran S et al. Detection of mutations in EGFR in circulating lung-cancer cells. N Engl J Med. 2008;359(4):366–77.
87. Weisberg E et al. Second generation inhibitors of BCR-ABL for the treatment of imatinib-resistant chronic myeloid leukaemia. Nat Rev Cancer. 2007;7(5):345–56.
88. Manley PW et al. Imatinib: a selective tyrosine kinase inhibitor. Eur J Cancer. 2002;38 Suppl 5:S19–27.
89. Nagar B et al. Crystal structures of the kinase domain of c-Abl in complex with the small molecule inhibitors PD173955 and imatinib (STI-571). Cancer Res. 2002;62(15):4236–43.
90. Negri T et al. T670X KIT mutations in gastrointestinal stromal tumors: making sense of missense. J Natl Cancer Inst. 2009;101(3):194–204.
91. Yun CH et al. The T790M mutation in EGFR kinase causes drug resistance by increasing the affinity for ATP. Proc Natl Acad Sci USA. 2008;105(6):2070–5.
92. Roumiantsev S et al. Clinical resistance to the kinase inhibitor STI-571 in chronic myeloid leukemia by mutation of Tyr-253 in the Abl kinase domain P-loop. Proc Natl Acad Sci USA. 2002;99(16):10700–5.
93. Cowan-Jacob SW et al. Structural biology contributions to the discovery of drugs to treat chronic myelogenous leukaemia. Acta Crystallogr D Biol Crystallogr. 2007;63(Pt 1):80–93.
94. Gajiwala KS et al. KIT kinase mutants show unique mechanisms of drug resistance to imatinib and sunitinib in gastrointestinal stromal tumor patients. Proc Natl Acad Sci USA. 2009;106(5):1542–7.
95. Emery CM et al. MEK1 mutations confer resistance to MEK and B-RAF inhibition. Proc Natl Acad Sci USA. 2009;106(48):20411–6.
96. Griswold IJ et al. Kinase domain mutants of Bcr-Abl exhibit altered transformation potency, kinase activity, and substrate utilization, irrespective of sensitivity to imatinib. Mol Cell Biol. 2006;26(16):6082–93.
97. Toyooka S, Kiura K, Mitsudomi T. EGFR mutation and response of lung cancer to gefitinib. N Engl J Med. 2005;352(20):2136. author reply 2136.
98. Inukai M et al. Presence of epidermal growth factor receptor gene T790M mutation as a minor clone in non-small cell lung cancer. Cancer Res. 2006;66(16):7854–8.
99. Bell DW et al. Inherited susceptibility to lung cancer may be associated with the T790M drug resistance mutation in EGFR. Nat Genet. 2005;37(12):1315–6.
100. Vikis H et al. EGFR-T790M is a rare lung cancer susceptibility allele with enhanced kinase activity. Cancer Res. 2007;67(10):4665–70.
101. Mulloy R et al. Epidermal growth factor receptor mutants from human lung cancers exhibit enhanced catalytic activity and increased sensitivity to gefitinib. Cancer Res. 2007;67(5):2325–30.
102. Regales L et al. Development of new mouse lung tumor models expressing EGFR T790M mutants associated with clinical resistance to kinase inhibitors. PLoS One. 2007;2(8):e810.
103. Suda K et al. EGFR T790M mutation: a double role in lung cancer cell survival? J Thorac Oncol. 2009;4(1):1–4.
104. Liegl B et al. Heterogeneity of kinase inhibitor resistance mechanisms in GIST. J Pathol. 2008;216(1):64–74.
105. Branford S et al. High frequency of point mutations clustered within the adenosine triphosphate-binding region of BCR/ABL in patients with chronic myeloid leukemia or Ph-positive acute lymphoblastic leukemia who develop imatinib (STI571) resistance. Blood. 2002;99(9):3472–5.
106. Hofmann WK et al. Ph(+) acute lymphoblastic leukemia resistant to the tyrosine kinase inhibitor STI571 has a unique BCR-ABL gene mutation. Blood. 2002;99(5):1860–2.
107. Hofmann WK et al. Presence of the BCR-ABL mutation Glu255Lys prior to STI571 (imatinib) treatment in patients with Ph+ acute lymphoblastic leukemia. Blood. 2003;102(2):659–61.

108. Engelman JA et al. Allelic dilution obscures detection of a biologically significant resistance mutation in EGFR-amplified lung cancer. J Clin Invest. 2006;116(10):2695–706.
109. Gumireddy K et al. ON01910, a non-ATP-competitive small molecule inhibitor of Plk1, is a potent anticancer agent. Cancer Cell. 2005;7(3):275–86.
110. Riely GJ. Second-generation epidermal growth factor receptor tyrosine kinase inhibitors in non-small cell lung cancer. J Thorac Oncol. 2008;3(6 Suppl 2):S146–9.
111. Zhou W et al. Novel mutant-selective EGFR kinase inhibitors against EGFR T790M. Nature. 2009;462(7276):1070–4.
112. O'Hare T et al. AP24534, a pan-BCR-ABL inhibitor for chronic myeloid leukemia, potently inhibits the T315I mutant and overcomes mutation-based resistance. Cancer Cell. 2009;16(5):401–12.
113. Zhang J et al. Targeting Bcr-Abl by combining allosteric with ATP-binding-site inhibitors. Nature. 2010;463(7280):501–6.
114. Van Etten RA, et al. Switch pocket inhibitors of the ABL tyrosine kinase: distinct kinome inhibition profiles and in vivo efficacy in mouse models of CML and B-lymphoblastic leukemia induced by BCR-ABL T315I. ASH Annual Meeting Abstracts. 2008;112(11):576.
115. Noronha G et al. Inhibitors of ABL and the ABL-T315I mutation. Curr Top Med Chem. 2008;8(10):905–21.
116. Naumov GN et al. Combined vascular endothelial growth factor receptor and epidermal growth factor receptor (EGFR) blockade inhibits tumor growth in xenograft models of EGFR inhibitor resistance. Clin Cancer Res. 2009;15(10):3484–94.
117. Ichihara E et al. Effects of vandetanib on lung adenocarcinoma cells harboring epidermal growth factor receptor T790M mutation in vivo. Cancer Res. 2009;69(12):5091–8.
118. Gendreau SB et al. Inhibition of the T790M gatekeeper mutant of the epidermal growth factor receptor by EXEL-7647. Clin Cancer Res. 2007;13(12):3713–23.
119. Copland M et al. BMS-214662 potently induces apoptosis of chronic myeloid leukemia stem and progenitor cells and synergizes with tyrosine kinase inhibitors. Blood. 2008;111(5):2843–53.
120. Balko JM, et al. Combined MEK and EGFR inhibition demonstrates synergistic activity in EGFR-dependent NSCLC. Cancer Biol Ther. 2009;8(6):522–530.
121. Faber AC et al. Differential induction of apoptosis in HER2 and EGFR addicted cancers following PI3K inhibition. Proc Natl Acad Sci USA. 2009;106(46):19503–8.
122. Li D et al. Bronchial and peripheral murine lung carcinomas induced by T790M-L858R mutant EGFR respond to HKI-272 and rapamycin combination therapy. Cancer Cell. 2007;12(1):81–93.
123. Quintas-Cardama A, Kantarjian H, Cortes J. Homoharringtonine, omacetaxine mepesuccinate, and chronic myeloid leukemia circa 2009. Cancer. 2009;115(23):5382–93.
124. Kuroda J et al. Apoptosis-based dual molecular targeting by INNO-406, a second-generation Bcr-Abl inhibitor, and ABT-737, an inhibitor of antiapoptotic Bcl-2 proteins, against Bcr-Abl-positive leukemia. Cell Death Differ. 2007;14(9):1667–77.
125. Freeman DJ et al. Activity of panitumumab alone or with chemotherapy in non-small cell lung carcinoma cell lines expressing mutant epidermal growth factor receptor. Mol Cancer Ther. 2009;8(6):1536–46.
126. O'Hare T et al. SGX393 inhibits the CML mutant Bcr-AblT315I and preempts in vitro resistance when combined with nilotinib or dasatinib. Proc Natl Acad Sci USA. 2008;105(14):5507–12.
127. Regales L et al. Dual targeting of EGFR can overcome a major drug resistance mutation in mouse models of EGFR mutant lung cancer. J Clin Invest. 2009;119(10):3000–10.
128. Tang Z et al. Dual MET-EGFR combinatorial inhibition against T790M-EGFR-mediated erlotinib-resistant lung cancer. Br J Cancer. 2008;99(6):911–22.
129. Thomas EK et al. Rac guanosine triphosphatases represent integrating molecular therapeutic targets for BCR-ABL-induced myeloproliferative disease. Cancer Cell. 2007;12(5):467–78.
130. Neviani P et al. FTY720, a new alternative for treating blast crisis chronic myelogenous leukemia and Philadelphia chromosome-positive acute lymphocytic leukemia. J Clin Invest. 2007;117(9):2408–21.

131. Shimamura T et al. Epidermal growth factor receptors harboring kinase domain mutations associate with the heat shock protein 90 chaperone and are destabilized following exposure to geldanamycins. Cancer Res. 2005;65(14):6401–8.

132. Nguyen TK et al. Synergistic interactions between DMAG and mitogen-activated protein kinase kinase 1/2 inhibitors in Bcr/abl+ leukemia cells sensitive and resistant to imatinib mesylate. Clin Cancer Res. 2006;12(7 Pt 1):2239–47.

133. Dai Y et al. Vorinostat synergistically potentiates MK-0457 lethality in chronic myelogenous leukemia cells sensitive and resistant to imatinib mesylate. Blood. 2008;112(3):793–804.

134. Modugno M et al. Crystal structure of the T315I Abl mutant in complex with the aurora kinases inhibitor PHA-739358. Cancer Res. 2007;67(17):7987–90.

135. Carpinelli P et al. PHA-739358, a potent inhibitor of Aurora kinases with a selective target inhibition profile relevant to cancer. Mol Cancer Ther. 2007;6(12 Pt 1):3158–68.

136. Gumireddy K et al. A non-ATP-competitive inhibitor of BCR-ABL overrides imatinib resistance. Proc Natl Acad Sci USA. 2005;102(6):1992–7.

137. Engelman JA et al. PF00299804, an irreversible pan-ERBB inhibitor, is effective in lung cancer models with EGFR and ERBB2 mutations that are resistant to gefitinib. Cancer Res. 2007;67(24):11924–32.

138. Li D et al. BIBW2992, an irreversible EGFR/HER2 inhibitor highly effective in preclinical lung cancer models. Oncogene. 2008;27(34):4702–11.

139. Yuza Y et al. Allele-dependent variation in the relative cellular potency of distinct EGFR inhibitors. Cancer Biol Ther. 2007;6(5):661–7.

140. Godin-Heymann N et al. The T790M "gatekeeper" mutation in EGFR mediates resistance to low concentrations of an irreversible EGFR inhibitor. Mol Cancer Ther. 2008;7(4):874–9.

141. Sos ML et al. Chemogenomic profiling provides insights into the limited activity of irreversible EGFR inhibitors in tumor cells expressing the T790M EGFR resistance mutation. Cancer Res. 2010;70(3):868–74.

142. Janne PA, et al. Preliminary activity and safety results from a phase I clinical trial of PF-00299804, an irreversible pan-HER inhibitor, in patients (pts) with NSCLC. ASCO Meeting Abstracts. 2008;26(15_suppl):8027.

143. Janne PA et al. Multicenter, randomized, phase II trial of CI-1033, an irreversible pan-ERBB inhibitor, for previously treated advanced non small-cell lung cancer. J Clin Oncol. 2007;25(25):3936–44.

144. Ercan D et al. Amplification of EGFR T790M causes resistance to an irreversible EGFR inhibitor. Oncogene. 2010;29:2346–56.

145. Shah NP et al. Sequential ABL kinase inhibitor therapy selects for compound drug-resistant BCR-ABL mutations with altered oncogenic potency. J Clin Invest. 2007;117(9):2562–9.

Chapter 2
The Dynamics of the Cell Signaling Network; Implications for Targeted Therapies

Daniel Gioeli

Keywords Signal transduction • Signaling network • Feedback • Resistance • Molecular targeted therapeutics • Systems theory • PI3K • AKT • mTOR • RAS • RAF • MEK • ERK • S6K

Introduction

There are four major mechanisms of resistance to molecular targeted therapies that have been identified thus far (Fig. 2.1). Mutations in the ATP binding pocket result in resistance to small molecule ATP mimetics [1] and this mechanism is discussed in Chap. 1 of this book [2]. The other identified mechanisms are consequences of changes in the cell signaling network. Intrinsic resistance to molecular targeted therapies may exist due to the activity of redundant signaling pathways within the network at the time of initial treatment. Similarly, there can be preexisting activating mutations in effector proteins downstream of the targeted kinase. Compensatory signaling events within the cell signaling network can also result in acquired resistance. These include upregulation of alternate signaling pathways controlling growth and survival as well as the loss of feedback control, which triggers activation of secondary growth and survival signaling pathways. The mechanisms that are dependent on changes within the cell signaling network are discussed in this chapter. The references cited are in no way comprehensive of the field, rather they illustrate the major points presented; apologies for any omissions.

D. Gioeli (✉)
Department of Microbiology and Cancer Center,
University of Virginia, Charlottesville, VA 22908, USA
e-mail: dgg3f@virginia.edu

D. Gioeli (ed.), *Targeted Therapies: Mechanisms of Resistance*,
Molecular and Translational Medicine, DOI 10.1007/978-1-60761-478-4_2,
© Springer Science+Business Media, LLC 2011

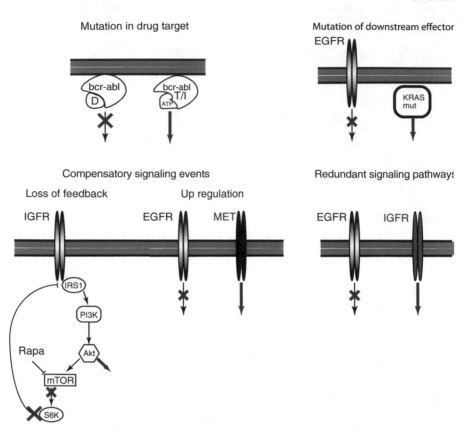

Fig. 2.1 The major mechanisms of resistance to molecular targeted therapies. These include (1) mutation in the drug target preventing binding of the ATP competitive inhibitor but still allowing for ATP binding. (2) Mutation of a downstream effector rendering inhibition of an upstream activator ineffective. (3) Loss of feedback control when inhibiting a downstream effector facilitating activation of signaling. (4) The presence of redundant signaling pathways regulating growth

A Network Model for Cell Signaling

The majority of new molecular-targeted therapies are directed against proteins involved in signal transduction [3, 4]. The classical model for signal transduction is that of a signaling pathway consisting of many compartmentalized, hierarchical, and independent proteins. Although it has long been recognized that connections between multiple pathways exist, the understanding of this crosstalk is relatively limited, as many studies designed to analyze these connections do not consider the dynamic, quantitative, or iterative nature of the cell's signaling system [5]. Most research focuses on describing the detail complexity of particular aspects of the total system; for example, how a given kinase cascade relays a growth control signal. However, it is the dynamic complexity, how the detail complexity from a multitude of pathways interacts in time and space, that regulates biologic processes, including carcinogenesis. This concept is supported by data demonstrating that extracellular signals are transmitted through a network of proteins rather than through cross-talk between hierarchical signaling pathways [5–8]. This network model is not at the exclusion of canonical signaling pathways that likely make many of the significant connections within the signaling network.

Additional data in support of a signaling network in cancer come from studies suggesting that cancer cells acquire multiple mutations during the process of cancer development that are necessary for full malignancy [9]. Wide scale sequencing efforts for breast and colorectal cancer genomes projected that there are 81 and 105 mutant genes, respectively [10]. Of these, an average of 14 and 20, respectively, are causative. Interestingly, signal transduction and transcriptional machinery components are common functional categories that are mutated in these cancers. This work has been further supported by more recent sequencing studies of human cancers [11]. A similar story has emerged thus far from The Cancer Genome Atlas; one example is in glioma where sequencing of 206 tumors uncovered dsyregulation in RB, p53, and RTK signaling including ERBB3, RAS, and PI3K [12]. These cancer genome sequencing studies suggest that many mutations are needed to undermine the robust wild-type cell signaling network and give rise to cancer.

Given the multitude of causal mutations in cancer, it is surprising that any one molecular-targeted agent would have any effect. The "oncogene addiction" model for cancer speculates that the many genetic changes during cancer development generate a fragile system that is vulnerable to the stress caused by one perturbation – the inhibition of a causal oncogene [13]. Sharma et al. presented experimental evidence suggesting that the pro-apoptotic outcome of oncogene inhibition results from coordinated differences in the decay of pro-apoptotic and pro-survival/pro-proliferation signals [14]. The phenomenon of oncogene addiction is well documented in multiple mouse tumor models and cancer cell lines [15]. The clinical effectiveness of imatinib, which targets the BCR/ABL fusion protein in chronic myelogenous leukemia (CML), implies that leukemia cells are addicted to the ABL oncogene [16]. Initial responses of other molecular-targeted therapies in patient subsets that are defined by a particular molecular signature are also consistent with the oncogene addiction model; for example, trastuzumab in ERBB2 positive breast cancer. Further evidence for oncogene addiction is seen in the discovery of resistance mutations following treatment with molecular-targeted therapies that are kinase inhibitors [1, 17, 18]. Unfortunately, the clinical reality is that patient responses to most molecular-targeted therapeutics are not universal and are not long lasting [19]. The oncogene addiction model postulates that the clinical ineffectiveness of these therapies is due to tumor cells having the ability to mutate around their addiction, known in this model as oncogenic escape or "addiction switching" [13, 20]. Oncogenic escape or addiction switching are inherent in the signaling network model. The dynamic complexity of the cell signaling network accounts for (1) the functional redundancy in the robust cancer system generating intrinsic resistance and (2) the feedback control generating acquired resistance to molecular-targeted agents. It is the functional redundancy and the feedback control that contributes to the robustness of cancer as a system. The concept of a signaling network is critical to the development of effective molecular-targeted therapeutics as it suggests why inhibition of a single component of a canonical pathway is insufficient to have dramatic effects for the treatment of cancer. Moreover, the signaling network model illustrates how difficult it is to empirically develop effective combinatorial therapies and suggests that finding such fragilities in the cancer system will require an in-depth understanding of the dynamics of the cell signaling network in tumor cells.

There is a concept in Systems Theory termed highly optimized tolerance (HOT), which suggests that robust systems tend to be fragile to unexpected perturbations; resistance to a broad range of perturbations is paid for with extreme sensitivity to seemingly innocuous perturbations [21, 22]. In the context of cancer, HOT theory postulates that identifying fragile loci and therapies that can target these points should lead to more efficacious treatments. This is akin to oncogene addiction but does not require that the fragile loci be a driving mutation. When considering HOT theory and the cell signaling network, fragile loci may exist that are not yet identified.

Systems Theory also suggests another possibility; targeting multiple nodes within the cell signaling network could create a fragile state and thus a more efficacious treatment, especially if the combinations of molecular-targeted agents used have independent selective pressures [22]. These combinations would effectively reduce tumor heterogeneity (as well as heterogeneity within the cell signaling network) and the corresponding robust state, thereby overcoming the limited effectiveness of molecular targeted agents.

Redundant Signaling Pathways

There is a high frequency of receptor tyrosine kinase (RTK) expression and activation in human cancers [23]. RTKs are critical regulators of signaling pathways that regulate diverse cellular functions including growth, survival, differentiation, and motility. Consequently, molecular targeted therapies directed at RTKs have been a major focus and represent the majority of FDA approved molecular targeted therapies to date [19]. Different families of RTKs are activated concurrently through redundant inputs that effectively maintain downstream signaling when any single RTK is inhibited. In nonsmall cell lung carcinoma (NSCLC) there is elevated epidermal growth factor receptor (EGFR) expression, making the EGFR an attractive therapeutic target [24]. However, while EGFR activity is necessary for a response to RTK inhibitors targeting the EGFR, expression of the EGFR does not predict therapeutic response. It is the presence of an activating EGFR mutation or gene amplification that predicts a clinical response to EGFR inhibitors [25–27]. Unfortunately for this subset of patients, the clinical response is not durable. The majority of NSCLC patients are not responsive to EGFR inhibitors or inhibitors that target other RTKs. The simplest explanation is that there are redundant signaling pathways regulating cancer cell growth and survival, and that inhibition of any one pathway is insufficient for a biological effect. Consistent with this, studies have found the expression of many different RTK families at both the mRNA and protein level in primary NSCLC tumors [28, 29]. This would suggest that combinations of RTK inhibitors might be necessary for effective inhibition of NSCLC growth. One study has shown that combinations of EGFR and fibroblast growth factor receptor (FGFR) inhibitors resulted in synergistic growth inhibition [30].

Activation of multiple RTK families is also common in glioblastoma multiforme (GBM). Analysis of GBM cell lines, xenografts, and primary patient tumors showed concurrent activation of multiple RTKs including EGFR, ERBB3, PDGFRA, MET, RET, MST1R, and CSF1R [31]. In this study, expression of a dominant negative EGFR did not alter PI3K activity, suggesting redundant RTK activation of PI3K. The authors go on to show that combinations of RTK inhibitors, such as erlotinib targeting the EGFR and SU11274 targeting MET, were required to disrupt PI3K association with GAB1 as well as downstream AKT and S6 phosphorylation. The erlotinib and SU11274 combination effectively inhibited adherent and anchorage-independent growth. Similar observations were made when RNAi was used to inhibit either MET or PDGFRA expression; knockdown of either MET or PDGFRA conferred sensitivity to EGFR inhibition [31]. These studies are consistent with concomitant activation of multiple RTKs limiting cancer dependency on any one RTK, thereby rendering tumors refractory to a single molecular targeted therapy. Combinations of either multiple RTK inhibitors, or molecular targeted therapies with activity against multiple RTKs could more effectively inhibit downstream intracellular signaling and tumor cell growth and survival.

While redundancy in RTK signaling results in intrinsic resistance to any single RTK inhibitor, another mechanism of intrinsic resistance is the presence of a constitutively active mutation in a signaling protein downstream of the targeted protein. This is essentially an epistasis phenomenon, where there is a regulatory hierarchy such that inhibition of the "upstream" component has no effect since there is mutational activation of the "downstream" component, even when the upstream component is overexpressed and activated. This is an oversimplified argument given what we know now about the cell signaling network (discussed earlier) and feedback loops within the signaling network (discussed later). However, there is clinical evidence for mutational activation of downstream pathway components that render RTK inhibitors ineffective [32, 33].

For both lung and colon carcinoma the presence of KRAS mutations is an important predictive factor for determining which patients will respond to EGFR inhibitors [32, 33]. In lung carcinoma, there was a perfect association with KRAS mutations and resistance to EGFR inhibitors; none of the KRAS mutant tumors responded to either gefitinib or erlotinib [32]. As observed in other studies, EGFR mutations were highly predictive of response to EGFR inhibitors. Similar observations were made in colorectal cancer examining KRAS mutational status [33, 34]. In one study, the KRAS mutational status of 394 patients, half of whom were on the EGFR inhibitor cetuximab and half on best supportive care, was examined [33]. Essentially equivalent numbers of KRAS mutations were found in the two groups.

Cetuximab was effective only in patients with wild-type KRAS where it was associated with improved overall and progression free survival. For patients with a mutant KRAS, there was no difference in overall or progression free survival between cetuximab treatment and best supportive care. Collectively, these studies suggest that the clinical decisions to treat patients with lung and colorectal cancer would be improved by mutational profiling of KRAS and EGFR, since the effectiveness of EGFR inhibitors is limited in the presence of mutational activated KRAS and show a response, albeit limited, in patients with EGFR mutations.

Compensatory Signaling Pathways

Upregulation of Alternative Signaling Pathways

Treatment with molecular targeted agents can lead to the activation of alternative signaling pathways that result in resistance. Resistance to RTK inhibitors often correlates with reactivation of the PI3K-AKT signaling pathway. Gefitinib resistant lung cancer cells were generated by exposure to increasing concentrations of gefitinib [35]. Genome-wide copy number analyses and mRNA expression profiling of the parental and resistant lung cancer cell lines identified MET amplification correlating with gefitinib resistance. Amplification of MET led to MET association with and activation of ERBB3, which in turn reactivated PI3K-AKT signaling. In the gefitinib resistance cells, treatment with either an EGFR or MET inhibitor alone had no effect on cell viability. However, the combination of EGFR and MET inhibitors resulted in cell death. While this resistance mechanism was uncovered using an experimental model, it appears to function in patients who have developed resistance to gefitinib; 22% of lung cancer patients who developed gefitinib resistance had MET gene amplification [35]. In two patients with pre- and postgefitinib treatment paired tumor samples, only the posttreatment sample showed MET amplification, consistent with MET amplification being a compensatory response to EGFR inhibition as opposed to a redundant signaling pathway. It also suggests that MET amplification is a driver of gefitinib resistance. This is further supported by a study using array-based comparative genomics to examine differences in untreated patients or those patients with acquired resistance to either gefitinib or erlotinib [36]. In this analysis, 21% of patients with acquired resistance had MET amplification in contrast to only 3% of untreated patients having amplification of MET.

In other examples of gefitinib resistance in lung cancer models there was an increase in PI3K-AKT signaling [37]. Again, cancer cell lines were exposed to increasing concentrations of gefitinib (lung cancer and HNSCC) or the anti-EGFR antibody therapy, cetuximab (lung cancer), until clinically relevant doses and resistant cell lines emerged. In the resistant cell lines gefitinib continued to inhibit EGFR and EGFR-ERBB3 dimerization as well as activation of downstream ERK signaling. However, under these conditions PI3K-AKT signaling persisted. Gene expression analysis identified decreases in IGFBP3 and/or IGFBP4 expression depending on the specific model of RTK inhibitor resistance. These IGF binding proteins inhibit IGF activation of the IGFR [38]. The decrease in IGFBP expression in the gefitinib and cetuximab resistant cell lines facilitates IGFR signaling to PI3K-AKT [37]. Subsequent combined inhibition of IGFR and EGFR inhibited PI3K-AKT signaling and cell growth in the resistant cells, whereas inhibition of IGFR alone was insufficient. Furthermore, when IGFBP3 was added back to resistant cells, sensitivity to gefitinib was restored, suggesting IGFR signaling as causal in gefitinib resistance.

Collectively, these studies suggest that molecular profiling of patient tumors that have failed molecular targeted therapies could identify mechanisms of resistance and subsequent effective second line therapies. From a systems perspective, the continual targeting of a central pathway such as PI3K-AKT signaling, even when different activators of PI3K-AKT are being targeted, will likely not provide durable clinical responses. There is clearly strong selective pressure for reactivation of the PI3K-AKT signaling pathway and multiple mechanisms to achieve it. Sequential or concurrent treatments of inhibitors can effectively prevent resistance in experimental models. It is not yet known whether such treatments effectively reduce heterogeneity of the cell signaling network and induce a fragile state in patients; however, the lack of independent selective pressures suggests that a fragile state will not be achieved.

Interestingly, the mechanism of resistance to RTK inhibitors is not restricted to compensatory signaling of PI3K-AKT triggered by upregulation of additional RTKs [39]. Short-term treatment of breast cancer cell lines with lapatinib led to an increase in estrogen receptor (ER) dependent cell growth. In this system, increases in the Forkhead transcription factor family member, FOXO3, and caveolin-1 enhanced ER transcriptional activity. This resulted in a switch from ERBB2 dependent regulation of survivin, an important anti-apoptotic regulator, to ER dependent regulation of survivin. Combining lapatinib with the ER antagonist ICI 182.780 abrogated acquired lapatinib resistance. Importantly, lapatinib treatment enhanced the expression of ER-regulated gene products in a rare subset of patients with ERBB2 and ER positive breast cancers suggesting that this mechanism of resistance may be clinically important.

One intriguing example of compensatory signaling in response to EGFR inhibition was observed in a breast cancer system [40]. Gefitinib treatment of breast cancer cells in vitro and in vivo led to a shift in the equilibrium state of ERBB3 phosphorylation and downstream activation of AKT. In cultured cells this increase in ERBB3 phosphorylation was due to increased ERBB3 membrane association and possibly the downregulation of ERBB3 phosphatase activity. Inhibition of EGFR and ERBB2 signaling results in a decrease in AKT activity and subsequent membrane localization of ERBB3. It appears that the loss of negative feedback from AKT may trigger this relocalization since gefitinib treatment does not trigger ERBB3 phosphorylation in the presence of a constitutively active AKT. Feedback control is a major regulator of the cell signaling network. How perturbations in feedback control result in resistance to molecular targeted therapies are discussed below.

Loss of Feedback Control

In normal and cancer cells, activation of the cell signaling network is regulated by feedback control. Molecular targeted therapeutics can disrupt feedback signaling pathways and attenuate the therapeutic response. A fundamental understanding of the intricacies of the cell signaling network is required to design effective therapies that do not trigger unintended consequences. The best examples described to date on how loss of feedback control drives resistance to molecular targeted therapies centers around the PI3K-AKT signaling pathway (Fig. 2.2). In the canonical PI3K pathway, ligand activation of RTKs (e.g., IGFR) leads to activation of PI3K through adapter proteins such as IRS1 [41]. Alternatively, PI3K can be activated through a direct interaction with activated EGFR or RAS. This results in the production of phosphorylated phosphoinositides (e.g., PIP3) and membrane recruitment of phosphoinositide-dependent kinase 1 (PDK1) and AKT. Once at the membrane, AKT is fully activated by PDK1 and mTORC2. Activated AKT then phosphory-lates multiple substrates resulting in the activation of mTORC1 by inhibiting nega-tive regulators of mTORC1 activity. Elevated mTORC1 activity has been observed in multiple cancers [42]. The downstream positioning of mTORC1 in the PI3K pathway, its activation state in cancer, along with the availability of a natural prod-uct inhibitor, rapamycin, quickly led to a focus on mTORC1 as a therapeutic target.

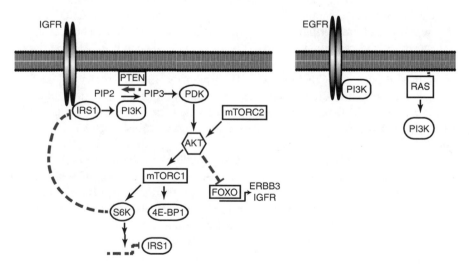

Fig. 2.2 The PI3K – AKT signaling pathway. Positive signals are represented by black arrows. Negative signals are represented by red dashed lines with squared ends. PI3K can be activated by RTKs and small GTPases. PI3K signals to S6K, which inhibits IRS1 through both phosphoryla-tion and transcriptional down regulation. AKT inhibits FOXO, which positively regulates RTK transcription. Inhibition of mTOR with Rapamycin alleviates the negative regulation of IRS1 further stimulating PI3K-AKT signaling. Inhibition of AKT relieves the negative regulation of FOXO resulting in the up regulation of RTKs, including ERBB3 and IGFR

mTORC1 inhibitors, including rapamycin and its derivatives, have shown robust activity in model systems. However, the clinical trial results with mTORC1 inhibitors have been more modest than predicted [42]. The mechanism of resistance to mTORC1 inhibitors is a subject of major therapeutic significance.

Studies have shown that while inhibiting mTORC1 activity in cancer cells effectively suppressed the phosphorylation of downstream effectors such as p70S6K and 4E-BP1, it increased the phosphorylation and activation of AKT. A feedback loop between PI3K, mTORC1, and IRS1 was first described in adipocytes [43]. In this study, two structurally unrelated PI3K inhibitors and rapamycin inhibited insulin-induced phosphorylation and degradation of IRS1; however, MEK inhibition had no effect on IRS1. Interestingly, rapamycin could block the insulin triggered IRS1 phosphorylation and degradation even in the presence of a constitutively active PI3K, placing mTORC1 feedback to IRS1 downstream of PI3K.

Mechanistic details of this feedback loop were uncovered in mouse embryo fibroblasts where tuberous sclerosis 2 (TSC2) was identified as a critical regulator of PI3K signaling [44]. TCS2 suppresses S6K, both an effector and negative regulator of PI3K signaling. S6K transcriptionally represses IRS1 and phosphorylates IRS1 protein on S302, which inhibits its association with activated insulin receptors. S6K also phosphorylates IRS1 on S1101 and loss of this phosphorylation enhances insulin signaling and AKT activation [45].

The clinical implications of this feedback loop are crucial for understanding how inhibitors of PI3K-AKT signaling can be used most effectively in the clinic. In an in vivo cancer model, mice heterozygous for TSC2 develop tumors with alterations in the mTORC1-IRS1-AKT feedback loop and this is accelerated by the loss of PTEN [46, 47]. More importantly, in human cancer biopsies, pharmacological inhibition of mTORC1 leads to AKT activation [48–50]. mTORC1 inhibition induces IRS1 expression and abrogates feedback inhibition, resulting in AKT activation in patient tumors treated with rapamycin or RAD001, a rapamycin derivative. Similar observations were made in breast and prostate cancer cell lines [48]. Inhibition of IGFR blocks rapamycin induced AKT activation thereby sensitizing cancer cells to mTORC1 inhibition. These data suggest that in cancer cells with mTORC1 activation, the feedback loop downregulates RTK signaling. Inhibition of mTORC1 blocks the negative feedback to IRS1, resulting in activation of AKT and attenuation of the growth inhibition by rapamycin. Combination therapy inhibiting both mTORC1 and the IGFR receptor results in additive inhibition of growth in vitro [48].

Similar observations were made in another study using lung carcinoma cells where rapamycin inhibition of mTORC1 activated survival signaling, which attenuated the therapeutic response [51]. Rapamycin effectively inhibited S6K and 4E-BP1 phosphorylation, which are indicative of mTORC1 inhibition; however, rapamycin also increased AKT and eIF4E phosphorylation. Concurrent treatment with a PI3K inhibitor blocked the rapamycin induced activation of AKT and eIF4E and enhanced inhibition of growth and colony formation of lung cancer cells. Collectively, these studies suggest that an increase in AKT activity attenuates the effect of mTORC1 inhibition and facilitates cancer cell growth and survival. Only upon discovery of this mTORC1-IRS1-AKT feedback control system could effective combinatorial treatments be determined; inhibition of IGFR-1 in breast and prostate cancer cell lines and of PI3K in lung cancer cell lines sensitized cells to mTOR inhibition [48, 51].

The advent of polypharmacology, the focus on multitarget drugs, has led to compounds that inhibit both PI3K and mTOR, thereby inhibiting both the PI3K-AKT signaling pathway and the mTORC1-IRS1-AKT feedback loop [52]. Screening a panel of isoform-selective PI3K inhibitors against genetically diverse glioma cell lines identified PI-103 as the most effective inhibitor of growth. The potent growth suppressive activity of PI-103 was due to its ability to inhibit both PI3K and mTORC1, resulting in maximal inhibition of AKT. The combinatorial inhibition of PI3K and mTORC1 by PI-103 was efficacious against glioma xenografts. This is consistent with the studies described above and further suggests that inhibition of PI3K and mTORC1 would be effective in treating cancer driven by aberrant PI3K-AKT signaling. Similar observations have been made with a dual PI3K and mTOR targeted therapeutic in clinical trial, NVP-BEZ235 [53].

The direct role of AKT in the feedback from RTK signaling was recently examined. In multiple cancer cell lines, an allosteric AKT inhibitor induced both the expression and phosphorylation of a subset of RTKs, including ERBB3, IGFR, and Insulin receptor [54]. This results in an increase in ERBB2-ERBB3 heterodimers and increased ERBB3 phosphorylation. The increase in RTK mRNA expression is dependent on the Forkhead transcription factors (FOXO1/3/4) that are negatively regulated by AKT. Inhibition of AKT facilitates activation of FOXO, leading to upregulation of RTKs. This too, results in an increase in ERBB2-ERBB3 heterodimers and increased ERBB3 phosphorylation. Blockade of AKT can thus lead to an increase in RTK signaling, reducing therapeutic benefit. Combined inhibition of ERBB and AKT signaling in two experimental models led to partial tumor regression. Thus, PI3K-AKT signaling is regulated by both FOXO and mTORC1 feedback loops and co-targeting RTKs and AKT can effectively inhibit tumor cell growth. This is further evidence that a thorough understanding of signaling pathways facilitates the design of more efficacious drug combinations.

While the best described alterations in feedback control to date have been observed in the PI3K signaling cascade, recent insights into feedback controls of the RAS-ERK signaling cascade are beginning to impact how inhibitors of this pathway can be used in the clinic (Fig. 2.3). RAS-ERK signaling is a central regulator of growth factor induced cell proliferation and survival [55]. Activation of RAS leads to signaling along several RAS effector pathways, the best studied of which are RAF, PI3K, and RALGDS. The RAS-RAF-MEK-ERK signaling pathway is constitutively activated in cancer through multiple mechanisms, including activating mutations in RAS, RAF, and MEK, loss of the tumor suppressor NF1 (a RAS GTPase), and upstream activation of receptor kinases through mutation, amplification, or ligand activation [55].

Feedback loops in the RAS signaling pathway are thematically similar to those that occur in PI3K signaling. Sprouty (SPRY) and MAP kinase phosphatase (MKP) are proteins that are transcriptionally upregulated by ERK [56, 57]. SPRY binds to GRB2 and prevents GRB2 and SOS1 from interacting with and activating RAS. Additionally, SPRY can directly interact with RAF and prevent RAF activation of

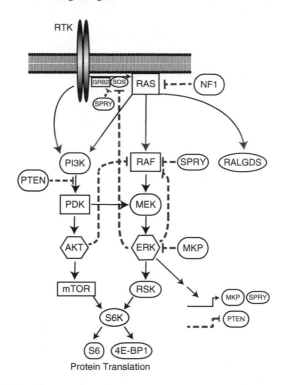

Fig. 2.3 The RAS signaling pathway. Shown are the RAS-ERK signaling pathway and PI3K-AKT cross talk with RAS-ERK signaling. Positive signals are represented by black arrows. Negative signals are represented by red dashed lines with squared ends. SPRY and MKP are negative regulators of RAS-ERK signaling. When MEK is inhibited, the negative feedback from ERK to SOS and ERK to RAF is lost, leading to an up regulation of RAS and RAF activity

MEK. MKP is an ERK phosphatase that dephosphorylates and inactivates ERK. Moreover, ERK itself directly phosphorylates SOS and RAF on inhibitory residues [58, 59]. Thus, there are both transcriptional and posttranslational feedback loops in the RAS-ERK signaling pathway. When ERK activity is blocked by MEK inhibition, the loss of feedback inhibition increases both RAF and MEK phosphorylation [59, 60]. Additionally, MEK inhibition activates EGFR signaling through the loss of ERK feedback to SOS [61]. Thus, inhibition of RAF and MEK can have unintended consequences on upstream signaling.

Several different strategies for inhibiting the RAS-ERK signaling pathway have been explored [62]. The most efficacious to date target RAF. Recent research has revealed insights on how selective RAF inhibitors can be most effectively used in the clinic (Fig. 2.4). Three recent studies demonstrate that while selective BRAF inhibitors effectively inhibit the growth and signaling in mutant BRAF tumors, these inhibitors can also activate CRAF through the formation of RAF dimers [63–65]. Moreover, this phenomenon is potentiated in the presence of mutationally active RAS. These observations have shed critical mechanistic insight into the clinical performance of RAF and MEK inhibitors and are facilitating patient selection

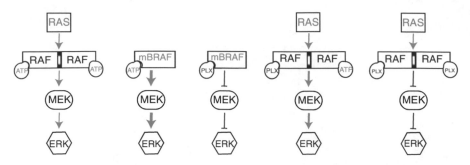

Fig. 2.4 The effects of RAF inhibitors on wild-type and mutant cells. In normal cells RAS-ERK signaling regulates cell growth. Positive signals are represented by green arrows. Negative signals are represented by red lines with squared ends. RAF inhibitors, such as PLX4032 (PLX), effectively inhibit signaling in BRAF mutant cells. However, in the presence of a active RAS low doses of RAF inhibitors leads to activation of RAF via transactivation where the catalytic activity of one dimer partner bound to PLX is inhibited and the wild-type partner bound to ATP is activated by transactivation. High doses of RAF inhibitors effectively inhibit RAF signaling independent of RAF mutational status

for the clinical use of drugs targeting the RAF-MEK-ERK pathway. There is considerable excitement over the recent clinical success of PLX4032, a selective RAF inhibitor, for the treatment of melanoma [66]. PLX4032 caused potent inhibition of signaling and proliferation in mutant BRAF melanoma, with a response rate of 78% by response evaluation criteria in solid tumors (RECIST). What is particularly surprising about the efficacy of PLX4032 is that it contrasts with the lack of clinical efficacy observed with MEK inhibitors. The selective MEK inhibitor, PD325901, had minimal clinical activity in melanoma patients; only 3 patients had RECIST responses and the drug was not pursed further due to neurological toxicity [67, 68]. If MEK is the major RAF effector in cancer cells, then how does inhibition of these two kinases yield such disparate clinical results? The answer may reside with three studies exploring how the inhibition of RAF can lead to the activation of MEK in cells harboring a KRAS mutation [63–65].

The report by Heidorn et al. demonstrated that the selective BRAF inhibitor, 885-A, could bind to wild-type BRAF in mutant KRAS cells, promote the formation of BRAF-CRAF dimers, and facilitate CRAF activation [65]. This study also demonstrated that kinase dead BRAF can similarly form BRAF-CRAF dimers and facilitate MEK activation in the presence of mutant KRAS. This observation that the kinase dead BRAF behaves similarly to the small molecule inhibited mutant BRAF provides an explanation for the apparent paradox of why kinase dead BRAF mutants are found in melanoma, especially since upward of 70% of melanomas carry an activating mutation of BRAF [69].

The report by Hatzivassiliou et al. focused on determining the mechanism of action for two distinct selective BRAF inhibitors, PLX4720 (a compound similar to PLX4032) and GDC-0879 [64]. This group found that GDC-0879 activated MEK in mutant RAS cells through promotion of RAF dimers, including BRAF-CRAF,

BRAF-ARAF, and CRAF-CRAF dimers. Through crystal structure analysis they found that drug binding caused a conformational change in RAF that promotes dimer formation. Interestingly, PLX4720 inhibits BRAF-CRAF dimer formation while still activating MEK signaling. The data reported in this study suggest that PLX4720 induces an alternative conformational change in BRAF that compromises BRAF dimer formation and activated MEK by promoting CRAF homodimer formation.

Further evidence for CRAF homodimer formation in response to PLX4720 in mutant RAS cells comes from Poulikakos et al [63]. Using a series of both gatekeeper and dimerization mutants, they demonstrated that transactivation of RAF dimers is responsible for MEK activation by RAF inhibitors. Importantly, MEK was activated in cells where RAS was activated by upstream oncogenes, including ERBB2. Thus, RAS need not be mutationally activated to facilitate MEK activation by RAF inhibitors. Activated RAS promotes RAF homo- and heterodimer formation, explaining the enhanced ability of RAF inhibitors to activate MEK in cells with active RAS. In cells carrying a mutant BRAF, RAS activity is typically low and transactivation of RAF dimers is not required for activation of MEK. Thus, RAF inhibitors are selectively effective at inhibiting mutant BRAF cells. Low doses of pan RAF inhibitors, including Sorafenib, could also activate MEK signaling. The mechanistic explanation for this is that at low doses of ATP-competitive inhibitors, activation of RAF occurs via transactivation where the catalytic activity of one dimer partner is inhibited and the partner is activated by transactivation. At high doses, the catalytic activity of both partners is inhibited, thus preventing signal transduction to MEK.

Collectively, these studies provide significant insight into the clinical observations with RAF and MEK inhibitors [63–65]. While the excitement over the clinical success of PLX4032 is justified, there are some potential concerns about the long-term treatment of patients with a drug that activates RAF-MEK-ERK signaling in normal tissues. A subset of patients on PLX4032 developed keratoacanthomas and squamous cell carcinomas, possibly due to activation of MEK [66]. Hatziassiliou et al. observed hyperactivation of ERK and hyperproliferation in the skin of mice treated with GDC-0879 consistent with activated ERK signaling driving skin malignancies in patients [64]. The prevalence of RAS mutations in squamous cell carcinoma and the presence of RAS mutations in actinic keratosis are also consistent with active RAS facilitating pathway activation in cells with wild-type BRAF [63]. This suggests caution in the long-term management of patients treated with selective RAF inhibitors, especially in patients where exposure to environmental carcinogens may be higher – either through lifestyle choices or vocation.

These studies also suggest why RAF inhibition may be more effective clinically than MEK inhibition. RAF inhibitors selectively inhibit RAF signaling in cells carrying mutationally activated BRAF and do not inhibit RAF in normal tissues [63, 64]. In fact, the RAF inhibitors may activate ERK in normal tissue. This provides a greater therapeutic window allowing for administration of high doses of RAF inhibitors that effectively inhibit mutant BRAF in tumor cells [63]. This contrasts with MEK inhibitors that inhibit ERK activity in both cancer and normal tissues; any therapeutic activity is derived from the tumor dependence on ERK over normal tissues. Although we must keep in mind that PLX4032 is selective for mutant BRAF over the other RAF proteins; this may contribute to or even explain the improved therapeutic for PLX4032 over PD325901. This may be of critical importance since the Poulikakos study demonstrated that low doses of pan-RAF inhibitors are also able to activate MEK through RAF dimer transactivation [63]. This observation raises the additional clinical caveat that selectivity for mutant BRAF, or the mutant form of any oncoprotein for that matter, will be critical for the clinical success of a drug. It also illustrates that suboptimal doses of a molecular targeted therapy may not only be ineffective but also have deleterious effects. Thus, the effective clinical use of these types of therapies may depend on determining pharmacodynamic endpoints in individual patients.

Feedback controls in the RAS-ERK signaling pathway may also impact the effectiveness of RAF (and MEK) inhibitors. In BRAF mutant melanoma, SPRY is unable to interact and inhibit mutant BRAF, however SPRY feedback at the level of RAS is intact as is the negative feedback phosphorylation of SOS by ERK [70]. This intact feedback loop may account for the low RAS activity levels in mutant BRAF cells, which may be important for the clinical efficacy of PLX4032. In support of this, exogenous expression of activated RAS in mutant BRAF cells renders PLX4720 ineffective [63]. This suggests that activation of RAS in mutant BRAF tumors, either by RAS mutation or activation from an upstream activator, could lead to resistance to PLX4720. Similarly, overexpression of CRAF generates resistance to PLX4720 [63]. However, to date neither of these potential mechanisms has been observed clinically.

The Convergence of PI3K-AKT and RAS-ERK Signaling

Considerable evidence exists for the concurrent mutational activation of PI3K-AKT and RAS-ERK signaling pathways in human cancers. These pathways are intricately linked. PI3K is a major RAS effector and PI3K activation by RAS has been studied extensively. PI3K activity is required for RAS mediated tumorigenesis [71]. In addition to direct activation of PI3K by RAS, RAS-ERK signaling can also modulate PI3K signaling through transcriptional regulation. Overexpression of mutant RAS downregulates PTEN expression in an ERK dependent manner [72]. Moreover, PI3K signaling can directly modulate RAF; AKT phosphorylates both CRAF and BRAF on inhibitory sites reducing RAF activity [73, 74]. Additionally, the kinase upstream of AKT, PDK1 (PDPK1), regulates MEK activity by phosphorylating MEK on the canonical RAF sites, Ser222 and Ser226 (Fig. 2.3) [75].

An additional feedback loop linking the RAS-ERK and PI3K-AKT signaling pathway involves the mTORC1. Inhibition of mTORC1 with rapamycin and its analogs in both experimental models and patient samples led to an increase in ERK activity [76]. This increase in ERK activity was dependent upon RAS, MEK, and PI3K. Expression of a dominant negative RAS construct that blocks RAS signaling or pharmacologic inhibition of MEK with UO126 abrogated rapamycin induction of

ERK as did a constitutively active rapamycin-insensitive S6K and pharmacologic inhibition of PI3K. The linkages between these two signaling pathways may explain in part why concurrent mutational activation is often observed and why inhibition of either pathway alone has insufficient effects on tumor growth and survival.

In addition to the feedback linkages between the PI3K-AKT and RAS-ERK signaling pathways, these signaling pathways converge downstream of ERK and AKT. ERK activates RSK, which in turn phosphorylates and activates S6K [77]. S6K phosphorylates several residues on S6 ribosomal protein and activates protein translation. RSK also phosphorylates eIF4B, which enhances its interaction with eIF3 and promotes translation [78]. AKT promotes the activation of the mTORC1 pathway, which activates protein translation through direct phosphorylation of S6K and 4E-BP1. The phosphorylation of 4E-BP1 results in its dissociation from eIF4E and activation of mRNA translation. A study by She et al, further suggests that 4E-BP1 mediates the effects of mutational activated PI3K-AKT and RAS-ERK signaling [79]. Tumors with mutations in both KRAS and PI3K are resistant to inhibition of either AKT or MEK alone. However, these tumors are sensitive to the combinatorial treatment of AKT and MEK inhibitors. As mentioned above, 4E-BP1 is a downstream effector for both AKT and ERK signaling that regulates protein translation through interaction with eIF4E. Concomitant inhibition of AKT and MEK effectively blocks 4E-BP1 phosphorylation leading to inhibition of tumor growth [79]. Blockade of 4E-BP1 directly by RNAi also decreased tumor growth. This work emphasizes the importance of knowing the mutational status of multiple genes and considering the redundancy present in the cell signaling network when choosing therapies, including combinations of molecular targeted agents.

The Rational Design of Effective Drug Combinations

The focus on combinations derived from the PI3K-AKT and RAS-ERK pathways is logical given the research to date, as is combining inhibitors of these pathways with RTK inhibitors. Uncovering feedback loops within these signaling pathways enables the prediction of effective combinations of molecular targeted therapies. Underlying the malignant phenotype is the extensively rewired cell signaling network. Therefore, the key to successfully treating cancer is identifying critical, functional nodes in the aberrant cancer cell signaling network whose inhibition will result in a fragile state leading to system failure. However, the analysis of feedback loops within these signaling pathways to date also suggests that unintended consequences of drug combinations may yet be uncovered which limit therapeutic efficacy. Thus, the challenge remains to functionally identify effective combination therapies.

One unbiased approach to identify effective drug combinations is analogous to synthetic lethal screening used in yeast genetics [80]. Two genes qualify as synthetic lethal if mutation or loss of either one alone is compatible with cell viability; but the simultaneous loss of both genes results in cell death. While the majority of synthetic lethal interactions have been described for loss of function alleles, synthetic lethality also occurs with gain of function genes. One gene may become essential when another gene is mutationally activated or overexpressed, a phenomenon known as synthetic dose lethality [80]. This concept can be applied to developing cancer therapies – identifying genes that are synthetic lethal with oncogenes or tumor suppressor genes could be effective therapeutic targets. The therapeutic window for these drug targets should also be greater since in cancer one partner of the synthetic lethal pair is generated from an oncogenic or tumor suppressor mutation. Disruption of the pathway containing the second partner in the synthetic lethal pair will kill the cancer cells. However, in normal cells the function of that pathway is intact and will remain unaffected.

This concept of synthetic lethality may underlie clinical observations that are consistent with oncogene addition; CML, which responds well to gleevec, carries mutations in addition to the BCR/ABL fusion. Furthermore, EGFR mutant NSCLC that are initially responsive to gefitinib also carry mutations in addition to EGFR. Tumors may be responding to therapies targeting early mutations in cancer development and progression since subsequent mutations carry a selective advantage in the context of the preceding transforming mutations. These later mutations then may be deleterious in the absence of the earlier mutations. Thus, inhibiting gene targets that are altered early in cancer development may uncover synthetic lethal relationships with genes that are mutated late in cancer progression. This model may also help explain how mutant BRAF is such an excellent target in melanoma, even though mutations in BRAF are an early event found in premalignant nevi [81]. Inhibition of BRAF may be effective initially due to synthetic lethal relationships that are present in frank melanoma carrying additional oncogenic and tumor suppressor mutations.

Unbiased chemical and genetic screens can be used to uncover synthetic lethal relationships. Using RNAi to perform genetic screens, three studies identified STK33, PLK1, and TBK1 as synthetic lethal partners with mutant KRAS [82–84]. Scholl et al targeted approximately 1,000 genes across eight cell lines with half of those cell lines carrying an activating mutation in KRAS as well as normal human fibroblasts and immortalized human mammary epithelial cells [83]. The shRNAs targeted protein kinases, phosphatases, and known cancer related genes. Analysis of shRNAs that caused growth inhibition selective to cell lines harboring a mutant KRAS resulted is a small list of candidate synthetic lethal partners with STK33 ranked as the top hit. Subsequent experiments confirmed the synthetic lethal association of KRAS and STK33. Intriguingly the relationship was specific to KRAS; neither HRAS nor NRAS are synthetic lethal with STK33.

Using a pooled shRNA approach, Luo et al targeted over 30,000 unique transcripts in two isogenic cell lines with one carrying a mutant KRAS and the other a wild-type KRAS [84]. From both the initial screen and subsequent analysis, including experiments using a second isogenic pair of cell lines, a list of 77 genes with a synthetic lethal relationship with KRAS were ultimately identified. Computational analysis suggested that mutant KRAS cells have an increased dependency on genes regulating the proteasome and the mitotic machinery. This led to preferential killing of KRAS mutant cells by drugs that target the mitotic machinery including a preclinical PLK1 inhibitor or a proteasome inhibitor (bortezomib). This effect was specific to mutant KRAS as analysis of isogenic lines with and without an activating PI3K mutation showed the opposite effect; PI3K mutants were less sensitive to mitotic machinery inhibitors.

Barbie et al used a meta-analysis of RNAi screens targeting protein kinases, phosphatases, and cancer related genes in 19 cell lines to identify mutant KRAS synthetic lethal partners [82]. They identified TBK1, which is a noncanonical IKB kinase as the top ranked KRAS synthetic lethal partner. In follow up studies, apoptosis was induced when TKB1 was suppressed in cancer cell lines where mutant KRAS is a driver gene. Mechanistic analysis revealed that TKB1 activated NFkB survival signals involving REL and BCLXL. Interestingly, REL as well as STK33 and PLK1 were identified in this study but fell below the cutoff in secondary analysis. Collectively, these studies establish the paradigm for rationally identifying combinatorial targets for inhibiting cancer growth. Validation of this approach will come as inhibitors of these synthetic lethal partners for mutant KRAS cancers are evaluated in the clinic.

It is plausible that these synthetic lethal partners are the fragile nodes within the cell signaling network predicted from HOT theory. Inhibition of these single nodes generates cytotoxicity that is dependent on the aberrant cell signaling network in the cancer cells. This is consistent with the system robustness, driven by mutational activated RAS signaling, being paid for with fragile nodes such as STK33, PLK1, and TKB1. However, the plasticity of the cell signaling network will likely facilitate resistance. STK33, PLK1, and TKB1 may be fragile nodes in cancer cells, but it is not yet determined if these are fragile nodes for the cancer system. Consistent with this concern is the clinical data, which thus far suggests that the response to single agent molecular targeted therapies is not durable. Thus, it remains likely that drug combinations will still be required. While the clinical effectiveness of these synthetic lethal targets is not yet known, it would be interesting to test if combinations of STK33, PLK1, and TKB1 inhibition are more effective and less likely to give rise to resistance than inhibition of any one synthetic lethal partner in KRAS mutant cancer.

The general paradigm used to date for identifying combinations of molecular targeted agents has relied on our understanding of the cell signaling network. This has led to the preclinical development of drug combinations targeting members of the RAS-ERK, PI3K-AKT, and RTK signaling pathways that have been selected empirically. The synthetic lethal approach has functionally identified targets that conceptually align with combination therapy; inhibition of the synthetic lethal partner is dependent upon combination with the activating oncogene. Another unbiased approach not yet published would be screening for drug or RNAi combinations that display synthetic lethality measured by synergistic growth inhibition. The hope is that the confluence of studies focused on particular subsets of the cell signaling network (e.g., PI3K-AKT and RAS-ERK) and the unbiased screening methods being employed will yield new and effective drug combinations for preclinical development and clinical trials.

Acknowledgments I would like to thank Dr. Neal Rosen for helpful discussions and input on the subject and Dr. Debra McMahon for critically reading the manuscript.

References

1. Gorre ME, Mohammed M, Ellwood K, Hsu N, et al. Clinical resistance to STI-571 cancer therapy caused by BCR-ABL gene mutation or amplification. Science. 2001;293 (5531):876–80.
2. Cortot AB, Janne PA (n.d.). Resistance to targeted therapies as a result of mutation(s) in the target. In: Mechanisms of resistance to molecular targeted therapies. In Press, Springer.
3. Johnson KA, Brown PH. Drug development for cancer chemoprevention: focus on molecular targets. Semin Oncol. 2010;37(4):345–58.
4. Nelson AL, Dhimolea E, Reichert JM. Development trends for human monoclonal antibody therapeutics. Nat Rev Drug Discov. 2010;9(10):767–74.
5. Friedman A, Perrimon N. Genetic screening for signal transduction in the era of network biology. Cell. 2007;128:225–31.
6. Giot L, Bader JS, Brouwer C, Chaudhuri A, et al. A protein interaction map of Drosophila melanogaster. Science. 2003;302:1727–36.
7. Krogan NJ, Hughes TR. Signals and systems. Genome Biol. 2006;7:313.
8. Natarajan M, Lin KM, Hsueh RC, Sternweis PC, Ranganathan R. A global analysis of cross-talk in a mammalian cellular signalling network. Nat Cell Biol. 2006;8:571–80.
9. Vogelstein B, Kinzler KW. Cancer genes and the pathways they control. Nat Med. 2004;10:789–99.
10. Sjoblom T, Jones S, Wood LD, Parsons DW, et al. The consensus coding sequences of human breast and colorectal cancers. Science. 2006;314:268–74.
11. Kan Z, Jaiswal BS, Stinson J, Janakiraman V, et al. Diverse somatic mutation patterns and pathway alterations in human cancers. Nature. 2010;466(7308):869–73.
12. Cancer Genome Atlas Research Network. Comprehensive genomic characterization defines human glioblastoma genes and core pathways. Nature. 2008;455(7216):1061–8.
13. Weinstein IB. Cancer. Addiction to oncogenes – the Achilles heal of cancer. Science. 2002;297:63–4.
14. Sharma SV, Gajowniczek P, Way IP, Lee DY, et al. A common signaling cascade may underlie "addiction" to the Src, BCR-ABL, and EGF receptor oncogenes. Cancer Cell. 2006;10:425–35.
15. Weinstein IB, Joe AK. Mechanisms of disease: Oncogene addiction – a rationale for molecular targeting in cancer therapy. Nat Clin Pract Oncol. 2006;3:448–57.
16. Sawyers CL. Making progress through molecular attacks on cancer. Cold Spring Harb Symp Quant Biol. 2005;70:479–82.
17. Tamborini E, Bonadiman L, Greco A, Albertini V, et al. A new mutation in the KIT ATP pocket causes acquired resistance to imatinib in a gastrointestinal stromal tumor patient. Gastroenterology. 2004;127(1):294–9.
18. Chen LL, Trent JC, Wu EF, Fuller GN, et al. A missense mutation in KIT kinase domain 1 correlates with imatinib resistance in gastrointestinal stromal tumors. Cancer Res. 2004;64(17):5913–9.
19. Ellis LM, Hicklin DJ. Resistance to targeted therapies: refining anticancer therapy in the era of molecular oncology. Clin Cancer Res. 2009;15:7471–8.
20. Sharma, SV, Settleman J. Oncogene addiction: setting the stage for molecularly targeted cancer therapy. Genes Dev. 2007;21:3214–31.
21. Weinberg GM. An introduction to general systems thinking. New York: Dorset House; 2001.
22. Kitano H. Cancer as a robust system: implications for anticancer therapy. Nat Rev Cancer. 2004;4:227–35.
23. Blume-Jensen P, Hunter T. Oncogenic kinase signalling. Nature. 2001;411(6835):355–65.
24. Yarden Y, Sliwkowski MX. Untangling the ErbB signalling network. Nat Rev Mol Cell Biol. 2001;2(2):127–37.

25. Paez J Guillermo, Jänne PA, Lee JC, Tracy S, et al. EGFR mutations in lung cancer: correlation with clinical response to gefitinib therapy. Science. 2004;304(5676):1497–500.
26. Cappuzzo F, Varella-Garcia M, Shigematsu H, Domenichini I, et al. Increased HER2 gene copy number is associated with response to gefitinib therapy in epidermal growth factor receptor-positive non-small-cell lung cancer patients. J Clin Oncol. 2005;23(22):5007–18.
27. Lynch TJ, Bell DW, Sordella R, Gurubhagavatula S, et al. Activating mutations in the epidermal growth factor receptor underlying responsiveness of non-small-cell lung cancer to gefitinib. N Engl J Med. 2004;350(21):2129–39.
28. Rikova K, Guo A, Zeng Q, Possemato A, et al. Global survey of phosphotyrosine signaling identifies oncogenic kinases in lung cancer. Cell. 2007;131(6):1190–203.
29. Müller-Tidow C, Diederichs S, Bulk E, Pohle T, et al. Identification of metastasis-associated receptor tyrosine kinases in non-small cell lung cancer. Cancer Res. 2005;65(5):1778–82.
30. Fischer H, Taylor N, Allerstorfer S, Grusch M, et al. Fibroblast growth factor receptor-mediated signals contribute to the malignant phenotype of non-small cell lung cancer cells: therapeutic implications and synergism with epidermal growth factor receptor inhibition. Mol Cancer Ther. 2008;7(10):3408–19.
31. Stommel JM, Kimmelman AC, Ying H, Nabioullin R, et al. Coactivation of receptor tyrosine kinases affects the response of tumor cells to targeted therapies. Science. 2007;318(5848): 287–90.
32. Pao W, Wang TY, Riely GJ, Miller VA, et al. KRAS mutations and primary resistance of lung adenocarcinomas to gefitinib or erlotinib. PLoS Med. 2005;2(1):e17.
33. Karapetis CS, Khambata-Ford S, Jonker DJ, O'Callaghan CJ, et al. K-ras mutations and benefit from cetuximab in advanced colorectal cancer. N Engl J Med. 2008;359(17):1757–65.
34. Amado RG, Wolf M, Peeters M, Van Cutsem E, et al. Wild-type KRAS is required for panitumumab efficacy in patients with metastatic colorectal cancer. J Clin Oncol. 2008;26(10):1626–34.
35. Engelman JA, Zejnullahu K, Mitsudomi T, Song Y, et al. MET amplification leads to gefitinib resistance in lung cancer by activating ERBB3 signaling. Science. 2007; 316(5827):1039–43.
36. Bean J, Brennan C, Shih J-Y, Riely G, et al. MET amplification occurs with or without T790M mutations in EGFR mutant lung tumors with acquired resistance to gefitinib or erlotinib. Proc Natl Acad Sci USA. 2007;104(52):20932–7.
37. Guix M, Faber AC, Wang SE, Olivares MG, et al. Acquired resistance to EGFR tyrosine kinase inhibitors in cancer cells is mediated by loss of IGF-binding proteins. J Clin Invest. 2008;118(7):2609–19.
38. Pollak M. Insulin and insulin-like growth factor signalling in neoplasia. Nat Rev Cancer. 2008;8(12):915–28.
39. Xia W, Bacus S, Hegde P, Husain I, et al. A model of acquired autoresistance to a potent ErbB2 tyrosine kinase inhibitor and a therapeutic strategy to prevent its onset in breast cancer. Proc Natl Acad Sci USA. 2006;103(20):7795–800.
40. Sergina NV, Rausch M, Wang D, Blair J, et al. Escape from HER-family tyrosine kinase inhibitor therapy by the kinase-inactive HER3. Nature. 2007;445(7126):437–41.
41. Engelman JA. Targeting PI3K signalling in cancer: opportunities, challenges and limitations. Nat Rev Cancer. 2009;9(8):550–62.
42. Meric-Bernstam, Funda and Gonzalez-Angulo, Ana Maria. Targeting the mTOR signaling network for cancer therapy. J Clin Oncol. 2009;27(13):2278–87.
43. Haruta T, Uno T, Kawahara J, Takano A, et al. A rapamycin-sensitive pathway down-regulates insulin signaling via phosphorylation and proteasomal degradation of insulin receptor substrate-1. Mol Endocrinol. 2000;14(6):783–94.
44. Harrington LS, Findlay GM, Gray A, Tolkacheva T, et al. The TSC1–2 tumor suppressor controls insulin-PI3K signaling via regulation of IRS proteins. J Cell Biol. 2004;166(2):213–23.
45. Tremblay F, Brûlé S, Hee Um S, Li Y, et al. Identification of IRS-1 Ser-1101 as a target of S6K1 in nutrient- and obesity-induced insulin resistance. Proc Natl Acad Sci USA. 2007;104(35):14056–61.

46. Ma L, Teruya-Feldstein J, Behrendt N, Chen Z, et al. Genetic analysis of Pten and Tsc2 functional interactions in the mouse reveals asymmetrical haploinsufficiency in tumor suppression. Genes Dev. 2005;19(15):1779–86.
47. Manning BD, Logsdon M Nicole, Lipovsky AI, Abbott D, et al. Feedback inhibition of Akt signaling limits the growth of tumors lacking Tsc2. Genes Dev. 2005;19(15):1773–8.
48. O'Reilly KE, Rojo F, She QB, Solit D, et al. mTOR inhibition induces upstream receptor tyrosine kinase signaling and activates Akt. Cancer Res. 2006;66:1500–8.
49. Cloughesy TF, Yoshimoto K, Nghiemphu P, Brown K, et al. Antitumor activity of rapamycin in a Phase I trial for patients with recurrent PTEN-deficient glioblastoma. PLoS Med. 2008;5(1):e8.
50. Tabernero J, Rojo F, Calvo E, Burris H, et al. Dose- and schedule-dependent inhibition of the mammalian target of rapamycin pathway with everolimus: a phase I tumor pharmacodynamic study in patients with advanced solid tumors. J Clin Oncol. 2008;26(10):1603–10.
51. Sun SY, Rosenberg LM, Wang X, Zhou Z, et al. Activation of Akt and eIF4E survival pathways by rapamycin-mediated mammalian target of rapamycin inhibition. Cancer Res. 2005;65:7052–8.
52. Fan Qi-Wen, Knight ZA, Goldenberg DD, Yu W, et al. A dual PI3 kinase/mTOR inhibitor reveals emergent efficacy in glioma. Cancer Cell. 2006;9(5):341–9.
53. Maira S-M, Stauffer F, Brueggen J, Furet P, et al. Identification and characterization of NVP-BEZ235, a new orally available dual phosphatidylinositol 3-kinase/mammalian target of rapamycin inhibitor with potent in vivo antitumor activity. Mol Cancer Ther. 2008;7(7):1851–63.
54. Chandarlapaty S, Sawai A, Scaltriti M, Rodrik-Outmezguine V, et al. AKT inhibition relieves feedback suppression of receptor tyrosine kinase expression and activity. Cancer Cell. 2011;19:58–71.
55. Schubbert S, Shannon K, Bollag G. Hyperactive Ras in developmental disorders and cancer. Nat Rev Cancer. 2007;7(4):295–308.
56. Kim HJ, Bar-Sagi D. Modulation of signalling by Sprouty: a developing story. Nat Rev Mol Cell Biol. 2004;5(6):441–50.
57. Keyse SM. Dual-specificity MAP kinase phosphatases (MKPs) and cancer. Cancer Metastasis Rev. 2008;27(2):253–61.
58. Cherniack AD, Klarlund JK, Czech MP. Phosphorylation of the Ras nucleotide exchange factor son of sevenless by mitogen-activated protein kinase. J Biol Chem. 1994;269(7):4717–20.
59. Dougherty MK, Muller J, Ritt DA, Zhou M, et al. Regulation of Raf-1 by direct feedback phosphorylation. Mol Cell. 2005;17:215–24.
60. Friday BB, Yu C, Dy GK, Smith PD, et al. BRAF V600E disrupts AZD6244-induced abrogation of negative feedback pathways between extracellular signal-regulated kinase and Raf proteins. Cancer Res. 2008;68(15):6145–53.
61. Mirzoeva OK, Das D, Heiser LM, Bhattacharya S, et al. Basal subtype and MAPK/ERK kinase (MEK)-phosphoinositide 3-kinase feedback signaling determine susceptibility of breast cancer cells to MEK inhibition. Cancer Res. 2009;69(2):565–72.
62. Pratilas CA, Solit DB. Targeting the mitogen-activated protein kinase pathway: physiological feedback and drug response. Clin Cancer Res. 2010;16(13):3329–34.
63. Poulikakos PI, Zhang C, Bollag G, Shokat KM, Rosen N. RAF inhibitors transactivate RAF dimers and ERK signalling in cells with wild-type BRAF. Nature. 2010;464(7287):427–30.
64. Hatzivassiliou G, Song K, Yen I, Brandhuber BJ, et al. RAF inhibitors prime wild-type RAF to activate the MAPK pathway and enhance growth. Nature. 2010;464(7287):431–5.
65. Heidorn SJ, Milagre C, Whittaker S, Nourry A, et al. Kinase-dead BRAF and oncogenic RAS cooperate to drive tumor progression through CRAF. Cell. 2010;140(2):209–21.
66. Flaherty KT, Puzanov I, Kim KB, Ribas A, et al. Inhibition of mutated, activated BRAF in metastatic melanoma. N Engl J Med. 2010;363(9):809–19.
67. Haura EB, Ricart AD, Larson TG, Stella PJ, et al. A phase II study of PD-0325901, an oral MEK inhibitor, in previously treated patients with advanced non-small cell lung cancer. Clin Cancer Res. 2010;16(8):2450–7.

68. Lorusso PM, Adjei AA, Varterasian M, Gadgeel S, et al. Phase I and pharmacodynamic study of the oral MEK inhibitor CI-1040 in patients with advanced malignancies. J Clin Oncol. 2005;23:5281–93.
69. Davies H, Bignell GR, Cox C, Stephens P, et al. Mutations of the BRAF gene in human cancer. Nature. 2002;417:949–54.
70. Tsavachidou D, Coleman ML, Athanasiadis G, Li S, et al. SPRY2 is an inhibitor of the ras/extracellular signal-regulated kinase pathway in melanocytes and melanoma cells with wild-type BRAF but not with the V599E mutant. Cancer Res. 2004;64(16):5556–9.
71. Gupta S, Ramjaun AR, Haiko P, Wang Y, et al. Binding of ras to phosphoinositide 3-kinase p110alpha is required for ras-driven tumorigenesis in mice. Cell. 2007;129(5):957–68.
72. Vasudevan KM, Burikhanov R, Goswami A, Rangnekar VM. Suppression of PTEN expression is essential for antiapoptosis and cellular transformation by oncogenic Ras. Cancer Res. 2007;67(21):10343–50.
73. Guan KL, Figueroa C, Brtva TR, Zhu T, et al. Negative regulation of the serine/threonine kinase B-Raf by Akt. J Biol Chem. 2000;275(35):27354–9.
74. Zimmermann S, Moelling K. Phosphorylation and regulation of Raf by Akt (protein kinase B). Science. 1999;286(5445):1741–4.
75. Sato S, Fujita N, Tsuruo T. Involvement of 3-phosphoinositide-dependent protein kinase-1 in the MEK/MAPK signal transduction pathway. J Biol Chem. 2004;279(32):33759–67.
76. Carracedo A, Ma L, Teruya-Feldstein J, Rojo F, et al. Inhibition of mTORC1 leads to MAPK pathway activation through a PI3K-dependent feedback loop in human cancer. J Clin Invest. 2008;118(9):3065–74.
77. Roux PP, Shahbazian D, Vu H, Holz MK, et al. RAS/ERK signaling promotes site-specific ribosomal protein S6 phosphorylation via RSK and stimulates cap-dependent translation. J Biol Chem. 2007;282(19):14056–64.
78. Shahbazian D, Roux PP, Mieulet V, Cohen MS, et al. The mTOR/PI3K and MAPK pathways converge on eIF4B to control its phosphorylation and activity. EMBO J. 2006;25(12):2781–91.
79. She Q-B, Halilovic E, Ye Q, Zhen W, et al. 4E-BP1 is a key effector of the oncogenic activation of the AKT and ERK signaling pathways that integrates their function in tumors. Cancer Cell. 2010;18(1):39–51.
80. Kaelin WG. The concept of synthetic lethality in the context of anticancer therapy. Nat Rev Cancer. 2005;5:689–98.
81. Pollock PM, Harper UL, Hansen KS, Yudt LM, et al. High frequency of BRAF mutations in nevi. Nat Genet. 2003;33(1):19–20.
82. Barbie DA, Tamayo P, Boehm JS, Kim So Young, et al. Systematic RNA interference reveals that oncogenic KRAS-driven cancers require TBK1. Nature. 2009;462(7269):108–12.
83. Scholl C, Fröhling S, Dunn IF, Schinzel AC, et al. Synthetic lethal interaction between oncogenic KRAS dependency and STK33 suppression in human cancer cells. Cell. 2009;137(5):821–34.
84. Luo J, Emanuele MJ, Li D, Creighton CJ, et al. A genome-wide RNAi screen identifies multiple synthetic lethal interactions with the Ras oncogene. Cell. 2009;137(5):835–48.

Chapter 3
Cancer Signaling Network Analysis by Quantitative Mass Spectrometry

Jason R. Neil and Forest M. White

Keywords Mass spectrometry • Posttranslational modification • Proteomics • Phosphoproteomics • Global analysis • Spectrum • Peptide • Matrix-assisted laser desorption ionization • Electrospray ionization • High-performance liquid chromatography • Fractionation • Enrichment • Collision-activated dissociation • Ion trap • Electron capture dissociation • Electron transfer dissociation • Validation • Quadrupole time-of-flight • SILAC • iTRAQ • Multiple reaction monitoring • Amino acid residue • Immunoaffinity purification • Immobilized metal affinity chromatography • Metal oxide affinity chromatography • Strong cation exchange chromatography • Label-free quantification • Metabolic labeling • Stable isotope • Chemical modification • Spectral counting

Abbreviations

ESI	Electrospray ionization
IMAC	Immobilized metal affinity chromatography
LC-MS/MS	Liquid chromatography tandem mass spectrometry
MALDI	Matrix-assisted laser desorption ionization
MOAC	Metal oxide affinity chromatography
SCX	Strong cation exchange
SILAC	Stable isotope labeling by amino acids in cell culture

F.M. White (✉)
Department of Biological Engineering, Massachusetts Institute of Technology,
Cambridge, MA, USA
e-mail: fwhite@mit.edu

D. Gioeli (ed.), *Targeted Therapies: Mechanisms of Resistance,*
Molecular and Translational Medicine, DOI 10.1007/978-1-60761-478-4_3,
© Springer Science+Business Media, LLC 2011

Introduction

The analysis of global cell signaling networks by mass spectrometry (MS) is a recent technological advance in the field of proteomic research and represents a valuable method for the discovery of cancer biomarkers and the investigation of molecular mechanisms underlying the resistance to targeted therapies in human malignancies [1, 2]. Cell signaling networks governing the response to molecularly targeted therapeutics are comprised of a vast array of protein kinases (~500 kinases encoded by human genome), phosphatases, and numerous other enzymes whose activity is affected or influenced by a diversity of protein posttranslational modifications (PTMs) (e.g., phosphorylation, acetylation, ubiquitination, methylation, glycosylation, and oxidation) [3–5]. These amino acid modifications alter signaling network activity by changing protein architecture, function, trafficking, and turnover. The range of diversity and dynamic changes in protein modification results in a nearly endless possibility of network regulatory mechanisms. To navigate within this vast landscape, a priori knowledge of a particular signaling pathway has often dictated how we pursue and identify cancer promoting cell signaling pathways. However, MS-based analysis of protein PTMs is not dependent on this type of knowledge, and has therefore enabled unbiased interrogation of cell signaling networks and identification of previously unknown protein behavior.

Phosphorylation at serine, threonine, and tyrosine residues governs changes in protein structure, catalytic activity (e.g., phosphorylation of kinase activation loop), and intermolecular interactions (e.g., SH2 domain interaction with phosphorylated tyrosine amino acid residues). Information flows through a network of kinases and phosphatases to facilitate changes in cellular behavior [6]. While early conceptual structures of signal transduction systems were linear and unidirectional, current research supports a much more elaborate interconnected multidirectional signaling network capable of evolving under different cellular contexts. The complexity of such systems is exemplified by the signaling networks regulating cellular transformation, cancer progression, and therapeutic resistance. In fact, although many cancer therapeutic targets are key nodes within well-described signal transduction pathways (e.g., EGFR, HER2, and BCR-Abl), monotherapies targeting these nodes have generally (with the exception of BCR-Abl) exhibited poor efficacy, even in cancers overexpressing activated forms of these kinases. Our current understanding of how signaling networks evolve during cancer progression and therapeutic resistance is sorely lacking. Unfortunately, the dependence on common molecular biology research methods for the identification of therapeutic targets may be strategically flawed, as it is almost impossible to analyze emergent behaviors with reductionist techniques. However, several methods have recently been developed to enable quantitative network-level analysis of these complex biological systems, with MS-based proteomic technologies at the forefront.

The advancement of MS instrumentation and development of methods for the analysis of protein phosphorylation have enabled large-scale coverage of the phosphoproteome. This data, when coupled with concurrent MS-based research on protein–protein interactions, high-throughput identification of protein kinase substrates, and bioinformatics, has enabled system-wide characterization of cell signaling networks governing cancer cell behavior [7–12]. However, to date much of the effort in the MS-based phosphoproteomics field has been focused on method development toward more extensive cataloging of phosphorylation sites. As such, the derivation of biologically significant information, including insights into regulation of signal transduction, governance of cell decision processes, and response/ resistance to therapeutics from these phosphoproteomic data sets, has lagged behind. Given careful technical consideration and experimental design with a biological focus such limitations can be overcome. In this chapter, we will discuss recent developments in MS technologies and phosphoproteomic research methods that are currently available in the field for identifying and evaluating dynamic changes in cell signaling networks by MS and their potential to uncover mechanisms of therapeutic resistance.

Advantages and Limitations of MS-Based Cell Signaling Network Analysis

The choice of currently available methods for the analysis of cell signaling network phosphorylation events is distinguishable by the varying levels of throughput, multiplexing, network coverage, and analytical sample requirements [13]. While there is no "one size fits all" optimal analytical method, MS offers the potential for unbiased, discovery-based analysis of signaling networks, including novel or poorly characterized proteins and phosphorylation sites. However, this benefit in network coverage comes at the cost of throughput and sample requirements: MS-based analyses cannot match the throughput of array-based or fluorescence-based methodologies, and are constrained by starting sample and preparation time requirements (e.g., microgram to milligram of protein requiring hours or days to prepare). Despite these limitations, MS-based phosphoproteomics offers particular advantages in the analysis of therapeutic compounds for specificity and efficacy. Traditionally, these assays have been performed in an in vitro format (e.g., kinase assays with recombinant protein) and consequently have considerable potential for false-positive and false-negative error, as the protein concentration and binding conditions are poorly matched to physiological conditions, and the full cellular context is not considered. Although more limited in throughput, related in vivo analyses (in cell culture or in animal models) with large-scale network coverage can now be performed using MS-based interrogation and have the benefit of providing a biological context where network component expression, interaction, and activity remain intact. Furthermore, MS-analysis of in vivo therapeutic effects offers the potential to discover unexpected off-target effects, since MS is not dependent on antibodies recognizing specific proteins or phosphorylation sites where the identification and characterization of a novel protein phosphorylation site(s) would not be possible.

While significant information and understanding has come from genomic and expression-based analyses of genes governing cell behavior, it is well established that such information only captures a fraction of the network regulatory events occurring at the protein level [14]. MS-based phosphoproteomics, on the other hand, provides a direct measure of these network regulatory events, including accurate, site-specific, dynamic, and temporal quantification of protein phosphorylation and an increasing depth of network coverage with subsequent studies [15, 16]. Despite these clear benefits, it is worth noting that information acquired from global proteomic analyses of signaling networks can be massive and easily overwhelming. The proper sorting and statistical analysis of such information require computational tools, yet dependence on these tools can be problematic as MS-based identifications may yield false-positives (e.g., identification of the wrong peptide and/or phosphorylation site) and false-negatives (e.g., a peptide is not identified because an entry does not exist for it in a protein database) [17]. Furthermore, depending on the instrument and method of analysis, the identification of phosphorylated proteins and their error rates can vary [18]. Therefore careful scrutiny is advised when interpreting published data without also considering the methods used for identifying and validating phosphorylated proteins.

With each of these caveats in place, it is worth noting that with the proper screening for false-positives and validation of MS/MS spectra, MS-based phosphoproteomics can be applied to identify and quantify (see below) hundreds, if not thousands, of phosphorylation sites in any given biological sample. While the throughput may be limited and the sample requirements significant, this technology offers the potential for unprecedented insight into complex signaling networks governing response and resistance mechanisms to classical and novel therapeutic agents.

Fundamentals of Phosphopeptide Analysis and Identification

The analysis of protein phosphorylation by MS has been routinely performed at the peptide level as measurement of intact proteins is much more difficult, with significant potential for error (e.g., inability to measure large/hydrophobic proteins and error resulting from multiple PTMs). Trypsin-mediated proteolysis at the C-terminus of lysine and arginine residues typically generates peptide fragments of 6–20 amino acids in length. These peptides are amenable to MS analysis and phosphorylation site assignment due to their molecular weight distribution (e.g., 700–3,500 Da) and charge state (e.g., +2 to +4 or +5, depending on the number of basic residues and ionization conditions). As trypsin-mediated digestion of phosphorylated proteins may preclude the identification of certain phosphorylation sites due to the peptide size (i.e., those that are too small for accurate identification or too large to be analyzed by MS), alternative or complementary strategies utilizing other enzyme (e.g., chymotrypsin or Glu-C) or chemical (e.g., cyanogen bromide) digestion techniques can provide overlapping peptide sequence and phosphorylation site information.

Analysis of peptides by MS requires that they be vaporized and ionized (e.g., protonated), allowing the MS instrument to control and separate molecules by mass and charge (i.e., each distinct peptide is assigned a mass to charge ratio, m/z) within an electromagnetic field. Two principle ionization methods exist for the generation and introduction of charged biomolecules into the MS. These are matrix-assisted laser desorption ionization (MALDI), in which a sample embedded in a chemical matrix is ionized by a laser, and electrospray ionization (ESI), in which peptides in solution are ionized during desolvation of charged droplets (i.e., in the presence of a high voltage potential difference between the solution and the mass spectrometer) [19–22]. Phosphopeptides are typically singly charged when generated using MALDI and multiply charged (e.g., 2–5 protons) when generated using ESI. While techniques for MALDI-based analysis of phosphopeptides have previously been employed, the majority of MS-based phosphopeptide detection methods utilize ESI instrumentation [23]. One particular advantage of ESI-based analysis is the direct coupling of the ESI source with front end separation of phosphopeptides by high-performance liquid chromatography (HPLC), thereby enabling tandem multi-dimensional separation techniques for improved signaling network coverage, as described in the following section [22, 24].

When a population of peptides is injected into the MS analyzer, the relative abundance and charge state of individual ions are recorded. Current instrumentation provides sufficient resolution to distinguish peptide isotopic peaks within the MS spectrum (e.g., due to natural abundance of ^{13}C, ^{15}N, ^{2}H, and ^{18}O) and enables determination of peptide charge state [25]. For example, a peptide of 1,200 Da with three protons (i.e., +3 charge state) would appear at 401 m/z in the MS spectrum, and would have isotopic peaks separated by 0.33 m/z. In data-dependant analysis, selection and fragmentation of the most abundant ions in the full-scan mass spectrum (e.g., usually 1–10 precursor ions) is performed to generate MS/MS spectra from which sequence information may be obtained. With respect to complex biological samples, fractionation and enrichment methods for phosphorylated proteins/peptides improve detection and selection of precursor ions that would otherwise be obscured by abundant nonphosphorylated peptides. Fragmentation of peptides can be performed through a variety of processes. The most common occurs through collision-activated dissociation (CAD), where peptides are fragmented following transfer of kinetic energy due to collision with an inert gas (e.g., helium) [26]. Fragmentation along the peptide backbone, as described by the "mobile proton model," results in fragment ions (e.g., y and b ions) from which sequence information and phosphorylation site identification can be derived. The labile nature of the phosphate group on phosphopeptides often results in the loss of H_3PO_4 (from phosphoserine and phosphothreonine) or HPO_3 (typically from phosphotyrosine) during CAD, diminished peptide fragmentation, and inadequate sequence information [27]. Observation of this neutral loss is instrument-dependent (e.g., typical of ion trap instruments) and more common with phosphoserine and phosphothreonine-containing peptides [28]. Fragmentation strategies targeting peptides exhibiting neutral loss have been developed and exhibit different degrees of success [29, 30]. Electron-mediated methods for peptide fragmentation, such as electron capture dissociation (ECD) and electron transfer dissociation (ETD), represent recently developed techniques where fragmentation leaves peptide PTMs intact and improves phosphorylation site identification [31].

The pattern of ions generated in the MS/MS spectrum is dependent on the fragmentation method (e.g., CAD MS/MS spectra tend to feature b-ions [fragments containing the N-terminus] and y-ions [fragments containing the C-terminus], while ETD spectra primarily feature c-ions [fragments containing the N-terminus] and z-ions [fragments containing the C-terminus]), but both methods provide a unique series of ions from which the peptide sequence may be determined. In the MS/MS spectrum, the mass of the corresponding amino acid and the fragment charge state determines the difference between two adjacent fragment ion peaks (e.g., b_3 and b_4 ions); phosphorylation sites are represented by an addition of 79.97 Da to the mass of serine, threonine, or tyrosine. A variety of search engines (e.g., SEQUEST and MASCOT) are available that utilize mass and fragmentation information to identify phosphorylated peptides and corresponding proteins [32, 33]. As some peptides are common to a family of proteins (e.g., the phosphopeptide LIEDNEpYTAR can originate from multiple Src-family kinases, including Src, Fyn, Yes, or Lck), analysis and validation of phosphopeptide data may require additional methods of identification. Depending on the source of the sample analyzed (e.g., epithelial cell vs. lymphocyte), narrowing the possible list of target proteins may be straightforward. Prefractionation of protein samples by one-dimensional (1D) or two-dimensional (2D) gel electrophoresis prior to MS analysis provides an additional mechanism of protein identification where peptides can be matched to proteins of a particular mass or mass and pI region.

False-positive identifications are among the primary concerns for MS-based proteomics and phosphoproteomics. For protein identification, the false-positive rate can be decreased by excluding "one-hit-wonders," proteins identified by a single peptide which often have a greater false-positive rate compared to proteins identified by multiple peptides. Unfortunately, the issue is more complicated for phosphoproteomics, as the goal is to identify both the phosphorylation site and the protein. Most phosphorylation sites are "one-hit-wonders" by nature, as they are represented by a single phosphopeptide in the biological sample. Phosphorylated proteins may be represented by multiple peptides, but only if there are multiple sites on the protein. In either case, errors in phosphorylation site assignment and peptide identification can occur when using a search engine, and thus confirmation to conclusively identify the phosphorylation site should involve manual and/or computational validation methods [17, 34, 35]. Briefly, manual validation of identified phosphopeptides provides confirmation of possible contaminating precursor ions within the MS spectrum (i.e., those that could be fragmented and contaminate the MS/MS spectrum) and assignment of MS/MS fragment ions providing accurate peptide sequence and phosphorylation site identification [34]. Additional validation of peptide fragmentation patterns can also be achieved through MS/MS analysis of a recombinant peptide or traditional molecular biology techniques (e.g., kinase assay). A detailed explanation of manual peptide sequencing and validation of phosphorylation site assignment is beyond the scope of this chapter and readers are referred to other sources for this information [25, 34, 36].

Instrumentation Selection for Phosphoproteomic Analysis

To date, phosphoproteomic studies have utilized a variety of MS platforms. These analyzers can be grouped into scanning and ion-beam (e.g., triple quadrupole, quadrupole/TOF) or trapping mass spectrometers (e.g., quadrupole ion trap). Differences in sensitivity, resolution, scanning speed, and mass accuracy characterize each platform. While a full description of each instrument, including advantages and limitations of each platform, is beyond the scope of this chapter, here we will provide a brief overview of "discovery" and "monitoring" experiments that may be performed with each instrument.

For most applications, including analysis of cancer signaling networks and the effects of drug treatment, the initial MS experiment is "discovery" based, with the goal of identifying and possibly quantifying proteins and phosphorylation sites in a particular set of samples. Discovery mode experiments are data-dependent analyses (see above) and may be performed on almost any type of mass spectrometer, although currently the most popular instruments for this application are ion trap instruments (e.g., the Thermo LTQ-Orbitrap) and quadrupole time-of-flight instruments (e.g., ABI QSTAR or Agilent Q-TOF) [37]. These experiments may be coupled with stable isotope labeling (see below) for quantification in either the full scan mass spectrum (i.e., with stable isotope labeling by amino acids in cell culture (SILAC)) or the MS/MS spectrum (i.e., with isobaric tagging for relative and absolute quantification (iTRAQ)). Regardless of the quantification method, data-dependent, discovery mode experiments are fairly unbiased and therefore offer the ability to identify novel components in the network. Unfortunately, discovery mode experiments are notoriously irreproducible, as peak selection is performed automatically when ions pass a given abundance threshold, leading to significant variability in the timing and abundance of each peak selected for MS/MS analysis, especially in complex mixtures [38].

Once the components of the network have been defined by discovery-mode experiments, monitoring or quantification of signaling nodes can be performed by multiple reaction monitoring (MRM) on a triple quadrupole mass spectrometer [39]. In this experiment, phosphorylated peptides representing selected nodes in the network are specifically targeted by isolation in the first quadrupole, fragmentation in the second quadrupole, and monitoring of specific fragment ions (transitions) in the third quadrupole. By monitoring only a couple of fragment ions (instead of acquiring the full MS/MS spectrum), it is possible to increase acquisition time for the selected fragments, thereby significantly improving the detection limit without sacrificing scan speed. Since the same transitions are monitored repeatedly during the chromatographic elution of the peptide, multiple quantitative measurements are averaged, providing much better overall quantification compared to discovery mode experiments. In addition, the linear dynamic range for this approach tends to be much greater than for discovery mode experiments, due to differences in the mass analyzers and detector. The primary limitations of MRM analysis are false-positive quantification (in complex mixtures there is a strong possibility of contamination due to nominally isobaric precursor ions with similar transitions, and it is difficult to ascertain the level of contamination in absence of a full scan mass spectrum) and the lack of discovery potential, as only those proteins and phosphorylation sites that are monitored will be detected.

Methods of Phosphopeptide Separation and Enrichment

Approximately 30% of all cellular proteins may be phosphorylated at any given time in the mammalian cell, a condition that is cell and context dependent [1, 40]. The observation of a specific phosphorylated protein may be exceptionally rare, with only a few copies of the protein per cell, or common when the protein is abundantly expressed and highly phosphorylated. The ability to observe specific phosphorylation events is often dependent on enrichment and fractionation strategies (Fig. 3.1) due to a variety of factors: (1) Nonphosphorylated peptides tend to ionize preferentially relative to phosphorylated peptides, (2) the phosphoproteome is a small fraction of the proteome, (3) the relative abundance of phosphorylated amino acids residues within cellular proteins is considerably different (pSer (~90%), pThr (~10%), and pTyr (≤0.05)), and (4) abundant phosphorylation sites may not be altered by cellular perturbation (i.e., those not associated with a signaling network) while phosphopeptides that are of low abundance (e.g., pTyr) may exhibit significant changes under the same conditions, therefore necessitating enrichment of specific peptides within the phosphopeptide pool. Depending on the overall goal of the application, multiple fractionation and isolation strategies have been developed, at a variety of stages in the sample preparation process. Briefly, these enrichment strategies include immunoaffinity purification, immobilized metal affinity chromatography (IMAC), metal oxide affinity chromatography (MOAC), and strong cation exchange (SCX) chromatography. It is worth noting that a number of studies have included cellular or subcellular fractionation strategies prior to peptide liquid chromatography tandem mass spectrometry (LC-MS/MS) analysis to answer specific network signaling and biological questions. Such approaches have included cell sorting (e.g., for stem cell populations) and separation of cytoskeletal, mitochondrial, or nuclear compartments for proteomic analysis [41–44]. Often such strategies require significant starting material and therefore may not be amenable to all phosphoproteomic studies. Current phosphopeptide enrichment strategies for proteomic studies are detailed below.

Immunoaffinity Enrichment

Prior to enzymatic digestion, enrichment of phosphorylated proteins from cell lysate can be performed using a pan-phosphospecific (e.g., anti-phosphotyrosine, independent of surrounding amino acid sequence), motif specific (e.g., anti-phospho-Akt substrate), or phosphorylation site-specific antibody [45–47].

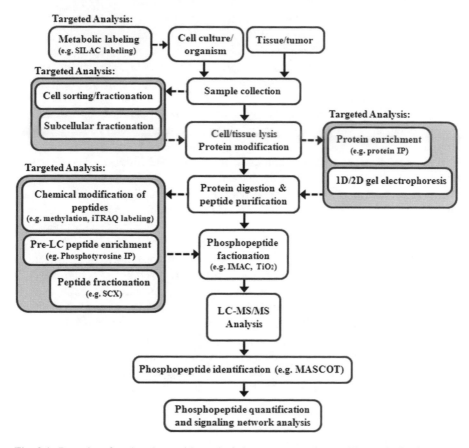

Fig. 3.1 Procedure for phosphopeptide analysis by mass spectrometry. The analysis of cell signaling by MS phosphopeptide quantification requires an experimental method that enriches phosphorylated from nonphosphorylated peptide species while providing the option to fractionate the sample at a variety of stages to simplify the analysis. The goal of MS-based signaling analysis is to accurately discern changes reflective of network activity. A core method characteristic of most studies has involved sample preparation, protein digestion, peptide purification, and basic phosphopeptide enrichment strategies. However, evolution of this method has included various techniques to improved "targeted" analyses of signaling network activity. These approaches occur at different stages of the core process. They include metabolic labeling of proteins (e.g., stable isotope labeling by amino acids in cell culture (SILAC) labeling), cell sorting, subcellular fractionation, protein enrichment, stable isotopic peptide labeling (e.g., isobaric tagging for relative and absolute quantification (iTRAQ) labeling), peptide immunoprecipitation, and peptide fractionation strategies prior to phosphopeptide separation

Immunoprecipitation of phosphorylated classes of proteins is typically followed by 1D or 2D SDS-PAGE separation of immunopurified proteins. While additional protein information (e.g., molecular size and pI) is obtained, sample detection (i.e., staining of proteins on 2D gels favors highly abundant proteins) and isolation of peptides from gels can be challenging [48, 49]. Current protocols utilizing this strategy often use 1D SDS-PAGE separation, cut the gel into multiple (10–20) segments, and analyze all sections of the gel separation (this technique is typically referred to as GeLC/MS). Accurate identification of proteins is achieved (e.g., multiple peptides for a single protein are sequenced by MS/MS), but phosphorylated peptides are often obscured by the abundance of nonphosphorylated peptides within the preparation [50].

To address this issue and specifically enrich for phosphorylated peptides, immunoaffinity enrichment may be performed at the peptide level following digestion of proteins in solution. Successful applications of this method have made use of pan-specific anti-phosphotyrosine antibodies (e.g., 4G10, Millipore; pTyr100, Cell Signaling Technology; and PT-66, Sigma-Aldrich) [16, 51]. While subtle differences in antigen recognition between similar phosphospecific antibodies exist, utilization of multiple antibodies for the purification of phosphopeptides has been a common practice to avoid potential peptide sequence bias [39]. Antibodies against phosphorylated serine and threonine residues are less commonly used, potentially due to weaker affinity or decreased specificity relative to anti-phosphotyrosine antibodies. Motif-specific antibody enrichment may also be performed at the peptide level as demonstrated by the recent profiling of phosphopeptides following DNA damage utilizing an ATM/ATR motif-specific antibody (pS-Q/pT-Q motif) [52]. In many cases, coupling immunoaffinity enrichment of either phosphorylated proteins or peptides to a second stage of enrichment (e.g., IMAC, MOAC, SCX) and/or fractionation (e.g., reverse phase chromatography) has been required to simplify the sample (i.e., by decreasing the level of nonspecifically retained nonphosphorylated peptides and separating peptides of differing hydrophobicity) prior to MS analyses.

Metal Affinity Phosphopeptide Enrichment

Enrichment of phosphorylated peptides is often achieved through interaction with metal matrices. Affinity-based IMAC enrichment of phosphopeptides occurs through the interaction of peptides to immobilized metal ions (e.g., Fe^{3+}, Zn^{2+}, and Ga^{3+}) [53, 54]. Similarly, MOAC-based strategies utilize solid or coated metal beads (e.g., titanium, zirconium, and aluminum oxides) to enrich phosphorylated peptides [55–57]. In either method, the electrostatic interaction of negatively charged phosphopeptides with the positively charged metal resin forms a chelation complex that enables retention of phosphorylated peptides and separation from nonphosphorylated peptides. Elution of bound phosphopeptides from the resin can be achieved through the use of a solution containing chelating agents (e.g., EDTA and EGTA), high pH, or inorganic phosphate [58, 59]. Collection of phosphopeptides either in solution or with a C-18 trapping column after enrichment is followed by LC-MS/MS analysis and peptide identification. Recent comparisons of both strategies demonstrate that differences in efficiency, phosphopeptide specificity, and nonspecific interaction can occur in these methods [18]; complementary analysis with multiple methods may be necessary for complete coverage of the phosphoproteome.

Both IMAC and MOAC enrichment of phosphorylated peptides tend to suffer from nonspecific interaction and retention of acidic peptides (e.g., those containing carboxyl groups). Methods for limiting nonspecific interaction prior to or during the enrichment method include (1) loading of peptides at low pH, (2) chemical modification (e.g., methyl-esterification) of carboxyl groups, and (3) use of 2,5-dihydroxybenzoic acid and/or (4) phthalic acid [18, 27, 55]. Each of these techniques has associated benefits and limitations, a full description is beyond the scope of this chapter.

SCX Phosphopeptide Enrichment

SCX-based peptide enrichment is facilitated by the interaction of positively charged amino acids and N-terminal amino groups of peptides with a negatively charged resin. Under acidic conditions, tryptic peptides tend to have at least a +2 charge state in solution (basic C-terminal amino acid + N-terminal amino group), while phosphorylated tryptic peptides have either neutral or +1 charge state, and therefore display lower affinity for the SCX resin. As such, phosphopeptides elute from the SCX resin at lower salt concentration compared to nonphosphorylated peptides, enabling some separation of phosphorylated and nonphosphorylated peptides. Since the actual charge state in solution varies significantly with peptide sequence, SCX is not sufficient for phosphopeptide enrichment as a standalone method. However, the combination of SCX-based enrichment with IMAC or MOAC enrichment has led to the identification of numerous phosphorylated peptides from complex samples [44, 60, 61].

Quantification of Peptide Phosphorylation

Identification of activated signaling networks by MS-based phosphoproteomics requires relative or absolute quantification of protein phosphorylation sites across multiple cellular stimulation conditions. Multiple quantification strategies have been developed for proteomics and extended to phosphoproteomics, including SILAC, iTRAQ (Applied Biosystems), and label-free quantification strategies [62, 63]. Each method is characterized by different analytical advantages and limitations, which are discussed below in the context of selected examples where the technique has been applied to assess the activity of signaling networks.

Quantification of Phosphopeptides Through Metabolic Labeling

The SILAC quantification method is based on the metabolic incorporation of specific isotope-labeled essential amino acids (e.g., isotopically labeled arginine and/or lysine) into cellular proteins as they are synthesized by cells in culture [62]. As such, a given protein expressed in different samples differs by the cumulative mass of stable isotope-labeled amino acids. Peptides from each stable isotope-labeled sample are represented as separate ion species in the full scan mass spectrum, with the mass difference representing the mass of the stable isotope labeling (Fig. 3.2). Alterations in phosphopeptide intensity in the full scan mass spectrum correlate with changes in their relative abundance and differences in network activity. Since samples can be mixed immediately after cell lysis, slight differences in sample handling do not contribute to quantification error. However, SILAC requires specially prepared cell culture media, successive rounds of cell doubling to ensure near-complete (~99.9%) labeling of all cellular proteins, and only a limited number of possible conditions can be compared within a single MS analysis. At present this strategy can be used for the simultaneous comparison of three cell culture samples (i.e., "light," "medium," and "heavy" labeling conditions). Utilizing this strategy, Pan et al. [64] were able to demonstrate the proportion (~10%) of phosphorylated peptides that were sensitive to U0126 or SB202190 MAPK inhibitors in EGF-stimulated HeLa cells or dasatanib (a Src-family kinase and Abl-family kinase inhibitor) in K562 leukemia cells. A recent SILAC-based phosphoproteomic investigation of differences in network activity governed by mutant EGFR (L858R or ΔE746-A750), previously described to mediate sensitivity to tyrosine kinase inhibitor therapy in lung cancer, identified increased phosphorylation in many known (e.g., Mig-6) and novel (e.g., PTRF) EGFR network components compared to cells expressing wtEGFR [65]. More recently, quantitative identification of differentially expressed proteins in cancer stem cell populations in two breast cancer cell lines (MCF7 and MDA-MB-231 cells) was performed using SILAC labeling and cell sorting [41]. Swaney et al. [66] combined the use of two MS/MS sequencing technologies (CAD and ETD) for the identification of 11,995 phosphorylation sites in the H1 stem cell line, five of which were found on transcription factors critical to stem cell pluripotency. Finally, the application of this quantification method has been successfully used for the global analysis of signaling networks in two different cell lines that were combined for short-term coculture [67]. It is worth noting that SILAC has been extended to model organisms, including mice and *Arabidopsis thaliana* [68, 69]. Future studies will hopefully use these models to quantify tumor-associated cell signaling in tissue in hopes of better defining responses to cancer therapy.

Quantification of Phosphopeptides Through Chemical Modification

Numerous methodologies have been developed for the chemical modification of peptides to incorporate stable isotope labels for quantification. At present, many of these have not been tested (i.e., beyond representative peptides) or are not feasible (i.e., chemical modification of nonphosphorylated residues [e.g., cysteine] occurring

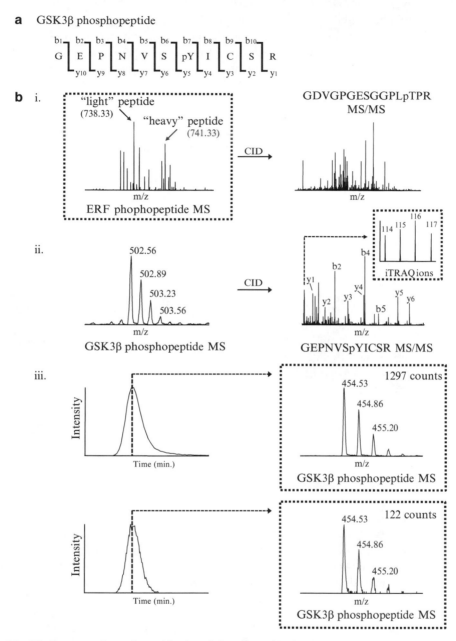

Fig. 3.2 Fragmentation and quantification of phosphopeptide abundance by MS. (**a**) Fragmentation of a representative GSK3β phosphopeptides generates N-terminal "b" and C-terminal "y" ion species representative of sequential amino sections and hence identification of sequence and phosphorylation site assignment. (**b**) Three strategies for the quantification of phosphopeptide levels by MS are based on (i) metabolic labeling of peptides (e.g., SILAC), providing quantification in the full scan mass spectrum, (ii) chemical tagging of peptides after digestion (e.g., iTRAQ labeling), providing quantification in the MS/MS spectrum, and (iii) label-free quantification, in which chromatographic elution profiles are quantified between separate analyses

on a small fraction of peptides) for global phosphoproteomic quantification. However, chemical modification of common amino acids or peptide C- or N-termini is readily applicable to quantitative phosphoproteomics. In fact, iTRAQ-based stable isotope labeling has been successfully applied to a variety of proteomic and phosphoproteomic analyses [15, 70, 71]. The iTRAQ tagging reagent (supplied as either four or eight different isobaric chemical tags) is an amine-reactive molecule capable of modifying free amines found on unmodified lysine and N-terminal peptide amino acid residues [63]. Comparison of multiple samples is performed by separately labeling peptides from each sample with a different isobaric tag followed by pooling, enrichment or fractionation, and analysis by LC-MS/MS. Since the physical properties of the various tags are identical, the retention time (on reversed-phase or ion-exchange resins) is identical for peptides with different tags. The tags are also isobaric, such that a single ion species is detected in the full scan mass spectrum, with a signal level representing the integrated signal from each tagged peptide. Quantification of iTRAQ-labeled peptides occurs in the MS/MS spectrum, as fragmentation of iTRAQ-labeled peptides produces reporter ions at specific m/z values (e.g., reporter ions at 114.11, 115.11, 116.11, and 117.11 m/z for the 4-plex iTRAQ reagent) (Fig. 3.2). Since peptide labeling is performed post-cell lysis, this quantification strategy is generally applicable to almost any biological sample. However, implementation of chemical tagging strategies for peptide quantification requires additional sample handling, providing the potential for quantification errors due to differential digestion or sample handling. Accurate reporting of relative changes in phosphopeptide abundance necessitates normalization of iTRAQ reporter ion values with those from control or housekeeping proteins to account for sample loss or sources of variation.

iTRAQ chemical modification for the quantification of temporal dynamics of tyrosine phosphorylation following EGF stimulation of human mammary epithelial cells led to the identification and quantification of 78 tyrosine phosphorylated sites on 58 proteins within the EGFR network [15]. Further characterization of the ErbB network in a subsequent study identified greater signaling complexity and many additional proteins within the network [51]. Recently, Huang et al. [16] utilized iTRAQ peptide tagging for the quantification of EGFRvIII-driven glioblastoma cell signaling networks and the identification of c-Met transactivation as a mechanism for sensitivity to EGFR kinase inhibitors. Application of this quantification strategy is often averaged over multiple discovery-mode MS analyses but has been successfully implemented in targeted MRM-based investigations [39]. The versatility of the iTRAQ reagent is exemplified by a recent study by Bantscheff et al. [72] where it was used to characterize binding constants for kinases and purine-binding proteins targeted by inhibitors of Abl and Src in a kinobead pulldown. Chemical peptide tagging strategies for the quantification of signaling networks in clinical tumor samples have been the natural progression of this technology for assessing cancer therapeutic strategies. At present, these MS-based analyses have focused on the quantification of putative nonphosphopeptide biomarkers using iTRAQ and the recently developed mTRAQ where quantification for this reagent is performed using MRM [73, 74]. Data acquired from these representative studies is often

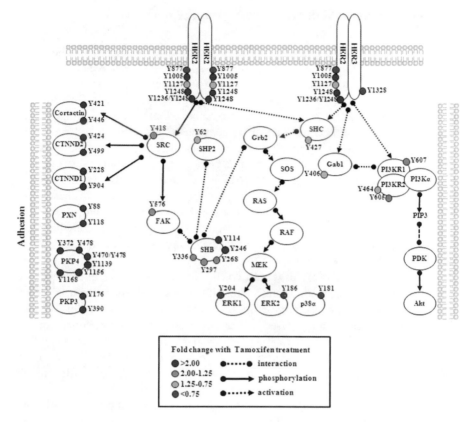

Fig. 3.3 EGFR phosphorylation network signaling diagram. Presentation of quantitative changes in protein phosphorylation can be displayed in the context of known protein interactions and signaling cascades. In this representative experiment, HER2-overexpressing ER+ breast cancer cells are treated with or without tamoxifen for 9 days followed by phosphopeptide quantification using the iTRAQ reagent. Relative changes in protein phosphorylation are compared to those from untreated cells (data courtesy of H. Saito-Benz)

tabulated for each phosphopeptide or displayed in a heat map or signaling network diagram where relative changes in phosphorylation and downstream effects are more effectively communicated (Fig. 3.3).

Additional methods for chemical modification of peptides to incorporate stable isotope labels for interrogation of global phosphoproteomic networks will undoubtedly continue to develop. The upper limit of peptide tagging chemistry will likely be dictated by the size of the molecule, the effect it has on peptide chromatography, and the ease of MS fragmentation. At present, the 8-plex iTRAQ reagent is the limit for sample multiplexing but future developments may expand this technology to allow additional multiplexing for more complex analysis of cell signaling network dynamics.

Label-Free Quantification of Phosphopeptides

Quantification of protein phosphorylation by metabolic or chemical labeling of peptides requires different culture conditions or additional sample handling and can be cost prohibitive, especially for the analysis of potentially hundreds of samples for clinical proteomics. To address these concerns, label-free quantification has emerged as an alternative strategy for quantitative proteomics. Label-free quantification can be performed using either full scan or tandem mass spectra. With full scan mass spectra, peptide intensity (typically the area under the chromatographic peak) for each phosphopeptide of interest is compared across two or more analyses (Fig. 3.2). Alternately, the number of replicate MS/MS spectra in each analysis can be used to roughly approximate the abundance of the phosphorylated peptide across each condition. This "spectral counting" method is not nearly as accurate as either label-free quantification of MS signal level or stable isotope labeling, and is not applicable to low-level peptides or phosphopeptides. In fact, a comparison of spectral counting to metabolic stable isotope labeling led to the finding that spectral counting was less sensitive at detecting changes less than twofold [75]. In general, label-free quantification is limited by error associated with differences in sample preparation and run-to-run variation (e.g., differences in chromatography and instrument sensitivity), although quantification based on comparison of phosphopeptide spectra between experiments using internal peptide standards (i.e., for absolute quantification of a small number of peptides) can provide fairly accurate data. Since run-to-run variation in elution can result in alteration in chromatographic profiles, highly reproducible sample handling, fractionation, and LC-MS are required.

In a recent comparison of ATM/ATR phosphorylated substrates following UV-induced DNA damage, quantification was performed by both label-free and SILAC analysis [52]. Comparison of the two data sets reveals that the quantification results from label-free analysis were much greater compared to stable isotope-labeled quantification. Without an orthogonal validation experiment (e.g., western blot), it is difficult to determine which labeling scheme was accurate in this study, but the general consensus in the field is that stable isotope strategies, when correctly implemented, are more accurate and provide decreased sample-to-sample variance. While significant effort has been put into developing software for label-free analysis of changes in peptide abundance, the utilization of this method for phosphopeptide analysis should be questioned when experimental and biological replicates are low and often a single phosphopeptide per protein is observed.

Future of Expectations for MS-Based Analysis of Cell Signaling Networks

The goal of global analyses of cell signaling networks is to identify key components within pathways that regulate biological response to perturbation (e.g., response to cancer therapy). A significant amount of information on phosphorylation-based signaling networks has been obtained, but the relevance of many phosphorylation sites gathered in these studies to cell and cancer biology needs to be validated. Understanding the regulatory mechanisms behind many signaling networks will not solely be provided by phosphoproteomic studies but will require the integration of this information with studies investigating other PTMs (e.g., ubiquitination, acetylation, etc.) and quantification of downstream biological phenotypic response. Global analysis of ubiquitin modifications of cellular peptides is capable of providing information on protein turnover and protein interaction through the identification of changes in abundance and characterization of ubiquitin chain topology [76]. Recently, global analysis by MS of peptide acetylation was performed using antibody-based acetyl-lysine peptide enrichment to demonstrate dynamic changes in response to a deacetylase inhibitor [77]. As the role of these and other protein modifications in the regulation and function of cell signaling networks represents new areas of global proteomic investigation, future studies will have great potential to offer new insight into cancer therapeutic strategies.

Future improvements to MS-based phosphoproteomic methods will reduce sample preparation and analysis time as well as increase multiplexing of analytical samples. Likewise, as MS instrumentation continues to provide greater sensitivity and resolution, future studies will benefit from greater depth and coverage of network signaling information.

Significant quantities of protein phosphorylation data are being generated by MS-based phosphoproteomics, driving a need for improved bioinformatics and computational modeling tools to integrate this information into signaling networks. When this information is coupled to orthogonal assays such as quantitative kinase activity assays and quantitative phenotypic assays measuring, for instance, proliferation, migration, or apoptosis, it is possible to derive biological insight into network activity as well as formulation of testable hypotheses [13, 51, 78]. Application of these strategies to quantify cancer cell signaling networks and their response to therapeutic treatment will provide significant additional insight into new therapeutic strategies, including novel combinatorial drug targets.

Acknowledgments We thank Amanda Del Rosario and other members of the White laboratory for helpful discussions regarding the contents of this chapter. This work was supported by a Genetech Postdoctoral Fellowship (to J.R.N.) and by National Cancer Institute (NCI) Grants R01-CA118705 (to F.M.W.).

References

1. Nita-Lazar A, Saito-Benz H, White FM. Quantitative phosphoproteomics by mass spectrometry: past, present, and future. Proteomics. 2008;8(21):4433–43.
2. Koomen JM, Haura EB, Bepler G, et al. Proteomic contributions to personalized cancer care. Mol Cell Proteomics. 2008;7(10):1780–94.
3. Manning G, Whyte DB, Martinez R, Hunter T, Sudarsanam S. The protein kinase complement of the human genome. Science. 2002;298(5600):1912–34.

4. Walsh CT, Garneau-Tsodikova S, Gatto Jr GJ. Protein posttranslational modifications: the chemistry of proteome diversifications. Angew Chem Int Ed Engl. 2005;44(45):7342–72.

5. Witze ES, Old WM, Resing KA, Ahn NG. Mapping protein post-translational modifications with mass spectrometry. Nat Methods. 2007;4(10):798–806.

6. Pawson T, Kofler M. Kinome signaling through regulated protein-protein interactions in normal and cancer cells. Curr Opin Cell Biol. 2009;21(2):147–53.

7. Blagoev B, Kratchmarova I, Ong SE, Nielsen M, Foster LJ, Mann M. A proteomics strategy to elucidate functional protein-protein interactions applied to EGF signaling. Nat Biotechnol. 2003;21(3):315–8.

8. Schulze WX, Deng L, Mann M. Phosphotyrosine interactome of the ErbB-receptor kinase family. Mol Syst Biol. 2005;1:2005.0008.

9. Jones RB, Gordus A, Krall JA, MacBeath G. A quantitative protein interaction network for the ErbB receptors using protein microarrays. Nature. 2006;439(7073):168–74.

10. Blethrow JD, Glavy JS, Morgan DO, Shokat KM. Covalent capture of kinase-specific phosphopeptides reveals Cdk1-cyclin B substrates. Proc Natl Acad Sci USA. 2008;105(5):1442–7.

11. Kaushansky A, Gordus A, Budnik BA, Lane WS, Rush J, MacBeath G. System-wide investigation of ErbB4 reveals 19 sites of Tyr phosphorylation that are unusually selective in their recruitment properties. Chem Biol. 2008;15(8):808–17.

12. Pflieger D, Junger MA, Muller M, et al. Quantitative proteomic analysis of protein complexes: concurrent identification of interactors and their state of phosphorylation. Mol Cell Proteomics. 2008;7(2):326–46.

13. Albeck JG, MacBeath G, White FM, Sorger PK, Lauffenburger DA, Gaudet S. Collecting and organizing systematic sets of protein data. Nat Rev Mol Cell Biol. 2006;7(11):803–12.

14. Tian Q, Stepaniants SB, Mao M, et al. Integrated genomic and proteomic analyses of gene expression in Mammalian cells. Mol Cell Proteomics. 2004;3(10):960–9.

15. Zhang Y, Wolf-Yadlin A, Ross PL, et al. Time-resolved mass spectrometry of tyrosine phosphorylation sites in the epidermal growth factor receptor signaling network reveals dynamic modules. Mol Cell Proteomics. 2005;4(9):1240–50.

16. Huang PH, Mukasa A, Bonavia R, et al. Quantitative analysis of EGFRvIII cellular signaling networks reveals a combinatorial therapeutic strategy for glioblastoma. Proc Natl Acad Sci USA. 2007;104(31):12867–72.

17. Chen Y, Zhang J, Xing G, Zhao Y. Mascot-derived false positive peptide identifications revealed by manual analysis of tandem mass spectra. J Proteome Res. 2009;8(6):3141–7.

18. Bodenmiller B, Mueller LN, Mueller M, Domon B, Aebersold R. Reproducible isolation of distinct, overlapping segments of the phosphoproteome. Nat Methods. 2007;4(3):231–7.

19. Whitehouse CM, Dreyer RN, Yamashita M, Fenn JB. Electrospray interface for liquid chromatographs and mass spectrometers. Anal Chem. 1985;57(3):675–9.

20. Hillenkamp F, Karas M, Beavis RC, Chait BT. Matrix-assisted laser desorption/ionization mass spectrometry of biopolymers. Anal Chem. 1991;63(24):1193A–203.

21. Aebersold R, Mann M. Mass spectrometry-based proteomics. Nature. 2003;422(6928):198–207.

22. Yates JR, Ruse CI, Nakorchevsky A. Proteomics by mass spectrometry: approaches, advances, and applications. Annu Rev Biomed Eng. 2009;11:49–79.

23. Bonenfant D, Schmelzle T, Jacinto E, et al. Quantitation of changes in protein phosphorylation: a simple method based on stable isotope labeling and mass spectrometry. Proc Natl Acad Sci USA. 2003;100(3):880–5.

24. Mitulovic G, Mechtler K. HPLC techniques for proteomics analysis – a short overview of latest developments. Brief Funct Genomic Proteomic. 2006;5(4):249–60.

25. Steen H, Mann M. The ABC's (and XYZ's) of peptide sequencing. Nat Rev Mol Cell Biol. 2004;5(9):699–711.

26. Hunt DF, Buko AM, Ballard JM, Shabanowitz J, Giordani AB. Sequence analysis of polypeptides by collision activated dissociation on a triple quadrupole mass spectrometer. Biomed Mass Spectrom. 1981;8(9):397–408.

27. Ficarro SB, McCleland ML, Stukenberg PT, et al. Phosphoproteome analysis by mass spectrometry and its application to *Saccharomyces cerevisiae*. Nat Biotechnol. 2002; 20(3):301–5.
28. Schmelzle K, White FM. Phosphoproteomic approaches to elucidate cellular signaling networks. Curr Opin Biotechnol. 2006;17(4):406–14.
29. Schroeder MJ, Shabanowitz J, Schwartz JC, Hunt DF, Coon JJ. A neutral loss activation method for improved phosphopeptide sequence analysis by quadrupole ion trap mass spectrometry. Anal Chem. 2004;76(13):3590–8.
30. Villen J, Beausoleil SA, Gygi SP. Evaluation of the utility of neutral-loss-dependent MS3 strategies in large-scale phosphorylation analysis. Proteomics. 2008;8(21):4444–52.
31. Zubarev RA, Horn DM, Fridriksson EK, et al. Electron capture dissociation for structural characterization of multiply charged protein cations. Anal Chem. 2000;72(3):563–73.
32. Ducret A, Van Oostveen I, Eng JK, Yates III JR, Aebersold R. High throughput protein characterization by automated reverse-phase chromatography/electrospray tandem mass spectrometry. Protein Sci. 1998;7(3):706–19.
33. Perkins DN, Pappin DJ, Creasy DM, Cottrell JS. Probability-based protein identification by searching sequence databases using mass spectrometry data. Electrophoresis. 1999;20(18): 3551–67.
34. Nichols AM, White FM. Manual validation of peptide sequence and sites of tyrosine phosphorylation from MS/MS spectra. Methods Mol Biol. 2009;492:143–60.
35. Nesvizhskii AI, Vitek O, Aebersold R. Analysis and validation of proteomic data generated by tandem mass spectrometry. Nat Methods. 2007;4(10):787–97.
36. Hunt DF, Yates III JR, Shabanowitz J, Winston S, Hauer CR. Protein sequencing by tandem mass spectrometry. Proc Natl Acad Sci USA. 1986;83(17):6233–7.
37. Hoffmann Ed, Stroobant V. Mass spectrometry: principles and applications. 3rd ed. Chichester, England: Wiley; 2007.
38. Elias JE, Haas W, Faherty BK, Gygi SP. Comparative evaluation of mass spectrometry platforms used in large-scale proteomics investigations. Nat Methods. 2005;2(9):667–75.
39. Wolf-Yadlin A, Hautaniemi S, Lauffenburger DA, White FM. Multiple reaction monitoring for robust quantitative proteomic analysis of cellular signaling networks. Proc Natl Acad Sci USA. 2007;104(14):5860–5.
40. Hunter T. The Croonian Lecture 1997. The phosphorylation of proteins on tyrosine: its role in cell growth and disease. Philos Trans R Soc Lond B Biol Sci. 1998;353(1368):583–605.
41. Steiniger SC, Coppinger JA, Kruger JA, Yates III J, Janda KD. Quantitative mass spectrometry identifies drug targets in cancer stem cell-containing side population. Stem Cells. 2008;26(12):3037–46.
42. Todorovic V, Desai BV, Eigenheer RA, et al. Detection of differentially expressed basal cell proteins by mass spectrometry. Mol Cell Proteomics. 2010;9(2):351–61.
43. Forner F, Kumar C, Luber CA, Fromme T, Klingenspor M, Mann M. Proteome differences between brown and white fat mitochondria reveal specialized metabolic functions. Cell Metab. 2009;10(4):324–35.
44. Olsen JV, Blagoev B, Gnad F, et al. Global, in vivo, and site-specific phosphorylation dynamics in signaling networks. Cell. 2006;127(3):635–48.
45. Amanchy R, Kalume DE, Iwahori A, Zhong J, Pandey A. Phosphoproteome analysis of HeLa cells using stable isotope labeling with amino acids in cell culture (SILAC). J Proteome Res. 2005;4(5):1661–71.
46. Matsuoka S, Ballif BA, Smogorzewska A, et al. ATM and ATR substrate analysis reveals extensive protein networks responsive to DNA damage. Science. 2007;316(5828):1160–6.
47. Konishi H, Namikawa K, Shikata K, Kobatake Y, Tachibana T, Kiyama H. Identification of peripherin as a Akt substrate in neurons. J Biol Chem. 2007;282(32):23491–9.
48. Gygi SP, Corthals GL, Zhang Y, Rochon Y, Aebersold R. Evaluation of two-dimensional gel electrophoresis-based proteome analysis technology. Proc Natl Acad Sci USA. 2000;97(17): 9390–5.
49. Granvogl B, Ploscher M, Eichacker LA. Sample preparation by in-gel digestion for mass spectrometry-based proteomics. Anal Bioanal Chem. 2007;389(4):991–1002.

50. Blagoev B, Ong SE, Kratchmarova I, Mann M. Temporal analysis of phosphotyrosine-dependent signaling networks by quantitative proteomics. Nat Biotechnol. 2004;22(9): 1139–45.
51. Wolf-Yadlin A, Kumar N, Zhang Y, et al. Effects of HER2 overexpression on cell signaling networks governing proliferation and migration. Mol Syst Biol. 2006;2:54.
52. Stokes MP, Rush J, Macneill J, et al. Profiling of UV-induced ATM/ATR signaling pathways. Proc Natl Acad Sci USA. 2007;104(50):19855–60.
53. Porath J, Carlsson J, Olsson I, Belfrage G. Metal chelate affinity chromatography, a new approach to protein fractionation. Nature. 1975;258(5536):598–9.
54. Andersson L, Porath J. Isolation of phosphoproteins by immobilized metal (Fe3+) affinity chromatography. Anal Biochem. 1986;154(1):250–4.
55. Larsen MR, Thingholm TE, Jensen ON, Roepstorff P, Jorgensen TJ. Highly selective enrichment of phosphorylated peptides from peptide mixtures using titanium dioxide microcolumns. Mol Cell Proteomics. 2005;4(7):873–86.
56. Kweon HK, Hakansson K. Selective zirconium dioxide-based enrichment of phosphorylated peptides for mass spectrometric analysis. Anal Chem. 2006;78(6):1743–9.
57. Wolschin F, Wienkoop S, Weckwerth W. Enrichment of phosphorylated proteins and peptides from complex mixtures using metal oxide/hydroxide affinity chromatography (MOAC). Proteomics. 2005;5(17):4389–97.
58. Zhang Y, Wolf-Yadlin A, White FM. Quantitative proteomic analysis of phosphotyrosine-mediated cellular signaling networks. Methods Mol Biol. 2007;359:203–12.
59. Collins MO, Yu L, Husi H, Blackstock WP, Choudhary JS, Grant SG. Robust enrichment of phosphorylated species in complex mixtures by sequential protein and peptide metal-affinity chromatography and analysis by tandem mass spectrometry. Sci STKE. 2005;2005(298):pl6.
60. Villen J, Beausoleil SA, Gerber SA, Gygi SP. Large-scale phosphorylation analysis of mouse liver. Proc Natl Acad Sci USA. 2007;104(5):1488–93.
61. Villen J, Gygi SP. The SCX/IMAC enrichment approach for global phosphorylation analysis by mass spectrometry. Nat Protoc. 2008;3(10):1630–8.
62. Ong SE, Blagoev B, Kratchmarova I, et al. Stable isotope labeling by amino acids in cell culture, SILAC, as a simple and accurate approach to expression proteomics. Mol Cell Proteomics. 2002;1(5):376–86.
63. Ross PL, Huang YN, Marchese JN, et al. Multiplexed protein quantitation in *Saccharomyces cerevisiae* using amine-reactive isobaric tagging reagents. Mol Cell Proteomics. 2004;3(12):1154–69.
64. Pan C, Kumar C, Bohl S, Klingmueller U, Mann M. Comparative proteomic phenotyping of cell lines and primary cells to assess preservation of cell type-specific functions. Mol Cell Proteomics. 2009;8(3):443–50.
65. Guha U, Chaerkady R, Marimuthu A, et al. Comparisons of tyrosine phosphorylated proteins in cells expressing lung cancer-specific alleles of EGFR and KRAS. Proc Natl Acad Sci USA. 2008;105(37):14112–7.
66. Swaney DL, Wenger CD, Thomson JA, Coon JJ. Human embryonic stem cell phosphoproteome revealed by electron transfer dissociation tandem mass spectrometry. Proc Natl Acad Sci USA. 2009;106(4):995–1000.
67. Jorgensen C, Sherman A, Chen GI, et al. Cell-specific information processing in segregating populations of Eph receptor ephrin-expressing cells. Science. 2009;326(5959):1502–9.
68. Kruger M, Moser M, Ussar S, et al. SILAC mouse for quantitative proteomics uncovers kindlin-3 as an essential factor for red blood cell function. Cell. 2008;134(2):353–64.
69. Gruhler A, Schulze WX, Matthiesen R, Mann M, Jensen ON. Stable isotope labeling of *Arabidopsis thaliana* cells and quantitative proteomics by mass spectrometry. Mol Cell Proteomics. 2005;4(11):1697–709.
70. Kim JE, White FM. Quantitative analysis of phosphotyrosine signaling networks triggered by CD3 and CD28 costimulation in Jurkat cells. J Immunol. 2006;176(5):2833–43.
71. Schmelzle K, Kane S, Gridley S, Lienhard GE, White FM. Temporal dynamics of tyrosine phosphorylation in insulin signaling. Diabetes. 2006;55(8):2171–9.

72. Bantscheff M, Eberhard D, Abraham Y, et al. Quantitative chemical proteomics reveals mechanisms of action of clinical ABL kinase inhibitors. Nat Biotechnol. 2007;25(9): 1035–44.
73. DeSouza LV, Grigull J, Ghanny S, et al. Endometrial carcinoma biomarker discovery and verification using differentially tagged clinical samples with multidimensional liquid chromatography and tandem mass spectrometry. Mol Cell Proteomics. 2007;6(7):1170–82.
74. DeSouza LV, Romaschin AD, Colgan TJ, Siu KW. Absolute quantification of potential cancer markers in clinical tissue homogenates using multiple reaction monitoring on a hybrid triple quadrupole/linear ion trap tandem mass spectrometer. Anal Chem. 2009;81(9):3462–70.
75. Hendrickson EL, Xia Q, Wang T, Leigh JA, Hackett M. Comparison of spectral counting and metabolic stable isotope labeling for use with quantitative microbial proteomics. Analyst. 2006;131(12):1335–41.
76. Meierhofer D, Wang X, Huang L, Kaiser P. Quantitative analysis of global ubiquitination in HeLa cells by mass spectrometry. J Proteome Res. 2008;7(10):4566–76.
77. Choudhary C, Kumar C, Gnad F, et al. Lysine acetylation targets protein complexes and co-regulates major cellular functions. Science. 2009;325(5942):834–40.
78. Janes KA, Lauffenburger DA. A biological approach to computational models of proteomic networks. Curr Opin Chem Biol. 2006;10(1):73–80.

Chapter 4
Development and Implementation of Array Technologies for Proteomics: Clinical Implications and Applications

Julia D. Wulfkuhle, Menawar Khalil, Joseph C. Watson, Lance A. Liotta, and Emanuel F. Petricoin III

Keywords Tissue microarray • Protein microarrays • Forward-phase protein microarray • Reverse-phase protein microarray • Personalized medicine • Cancer • Proteomics • Targeted therapeutics • Therapeutic resistance

Introduction

In practice, physicians have been utilizing personalized therapeutic strategies for their cancer patients for years, taking into consideration a myriad of underpinning individual attributes for each patient when they consider treatment options. In the past, morphological parameters such as tumor size, degree of tumor cell differentiation, nodal involvement, cytogenetics, and immunohistochemical (IHC) assessments of protein expression for molecules such as EGFR and HER2 have played an important role in therapeutic decision-making. However, these determinants do not truly begin to address the molecular complexity and patient-specific heterogeneity of cancer that can lead to the ultimate success or failure of a targeted therapeutic agent. Based on the explosive growth of knowledge about the basis of cancer coupled with new genomic and proteomic technologies, physicians now have a cadre of molecular-based information to assist them in selecting the most appropriate therapy for their patient. Array-based technologies, providing "-omic" level understanding of tumors at the DNA, RNA, and protein levels, have led to the uncovering of new disease susceptibility genes, therapeutic targets, and expression profiles related to disease outcomes and markers of therapeutic sensitivity and resistance [1, 2]. Indeed, gene expression profiling has shown considerable potential for prognosis of disease outcome [3]. However, transcript profiling alone cannot accurately predict the ongoing protein-based signaling of a tumor cell because gene transcript

J.D. Wulfkuhle (✉)
Center for Applied Proteomics and Molecular Medicine,
George Mason University, Manassas, VA, USA
e-mail: jwulfkuh@gmu.edu

D. Gioeli (ed.), *Targeted Therapies: Mechanisms of Resistance*,
Molecular and Translational Medicine, DOI 10.1007/978-1-60761-478-4_4,
© Springer Science+Business Media, LLC 2011

levels have been found not to correlate significantly with protein expression or the activated/phosphorylated isoforms of the encoded proteins that comprise the signaling networks [4–6].

Analysis of signaling network activation is of critical importance because nearly all current molecular-targeted therapeutics that are either in the development pipeline or FDA-approved (e.g., EGFR inhibitors, mTOR inhibitors, etc.) are directed at modulating protein kinase activity, hence, the proteins themselves are the drug targets. The cellular "circuitry" that represents the activation state of protein signaling networks fluctuates constantly based on the cellular microenvironment and the biological context of the cell itself. Thus, it is crucial that the information basis of pathway activation be rooted in the analysis of actual diseased human tissue to generate data. Molecular approaches that can determine the ongoing signaling activity of protein drug targets will be critical for the realization of patient-tailored therapy.

Identification of patients who will respond to a given targeted therapy will require information, prior to treatment initiation, about which signaling pathways are activated in each patient's cancer, and this information would be generated from a biopsy specimen/surgical sample. However, because there is no PCR-like amplification strategy for proteins, proteomic technologies face significant limitations for measuring low abundance analytes (i.e., phosphorylated signaling proteins) when applied to specimens where only a few thousand cells may be procured, such as tiny biopsy specimens and needle aspirates. Current proteomic methodologies and approaches where many tissue proteins are measured at once, such as two-dimensional polyacrylamide gel electrophoresis, antibody arrays, and mass spectrometry platforms, require tens to hundreds of millions of cells to measure activation states of signaling proteins, which is many more cells than could realistically be procured from a biopsy specimen [7–11]. Conventional ELISA, antibody arrays, flow cytometry-based methods, and suspension bead array technologies can achieve multiplexed quantitative measurements of signaling protein activation/phosphorylation, but these methods are severely limited in their breadth of coverage of the protein signaling circuitry because they require two antibodies recognizing independent epitopes for every analyte measured. Consequently, newer array-based and multiplexed approaches that can measure signaling network activation in very small tissue samples from a patient and can perform broad-scale pathway mapping will be best poised to deliver most effectively the needed predictive, prognostic, and therapy-guiding information to the bedside.

Tissue Microarrays: Potential for Prediction of Therapeutic Response

First described over 20 years ago [12], tissue microarrays (TMAs) represent a technology that can have an important and specialized impact on evaluation of markers for drug resistance in cancer research. A number of reviews describe the methodology and construction of TMAs that will not be detailed here [13–17]. Briefly, TMAs assemble cores from tens to hundreds of tissue specimens into a single block and provide a simplified means to semiquantitatively analyze DNA, RNA, or protein endpoints in many samples simultaneously [18]. Most commonly used with formalin-fixed, paraffin-embedded tissues, sectioning of a TMA block results in each sample being represented as a 0.6–2 mm diameter spot dubbed a "histospot," within a gridded array. TMA technology has also been adapted to frozen tissues [19], needle biopsies [20] as well as adherent and suspension cultured cells [21, 22].

It is in the multiplexed IHC assessment of biomarkers in tissues where the strengths and drawbacks of TMAs are most obvious [23]. Traditional IHC analyses of large study sets of tumors require a time investment of weeks to months in processing and evaluation by a pathologist. TMAs create a much more efficient workflow in that if the pathologist is involved in prospective identification of tumor-rich areas from samples for inclusion in the array, evaluation of IHC staining can be undertaken by a researcher with minimal training, resulting in a tremendous time savings [23]. Other advantages include: tremendous cost savings in reagents and personnel time, the conservation of tissues with the potential to include cores from a single specimen in large numbers of independent arrays, the significant increase in the number of tumors that can be analyzed in a given cohort from tens to hundreds or even thousands of specimens, and a means to maintain experimental uniformity and reduce batch-to-batch variability in staining and analysis, all of which have a tremendous positive impact on data quality, significance, and reliability in biomarker studies.

Despite the significant advantages TMAs have brought to IHC-based analysis and validation of biomarkers, they are limited by a number of factors. The quality of a TMA is primarily dependent on the quality of the tissues included in the array. Changes and improvements in tissue fixation and storage methods over time that can significantly impact the quality of a TMA assembled from cohorts of tissues collected over long periods of time. Another drawback to TMAs is the short timeline resulting in loss of tissue antigenicity once the TMA is sectioned onto slides, which creates a need to balance maximizing the number of sections obtained from a TMA and minimizing loss of antigenicity due to tissue oxidation [23]. TMAs are also limited by the availability of high-quality, validated antibodies for IHC.

One of the main concerns surrounding the use of TMAs in biomarker validation is tissue heterogeneity and, specifically, that a single core may not adequately assess markers that exhibit heterogeneity among tissues or geographically within a tissue specimen. General consensus holds that two small cores adequately represent IHC staining across a whole tissue section in most circumstances [24, 25], however, heterogeneity issues between cores taken at different tissue depths are still a concern, particularly with small in situ lesions. A lack of well-established standards and controls for expression in IHC tests has slowed the development of standardized IHC-based diagnostic tests in general and this is also true for TMAs. Researchers have begun to address this issue by generating TMAs containing cell lines that have a broad range of expression levels for a particular biomarker and can serve as a de facto dilution series reminiscent of an ELISA standard curve [26].

The development of a number of automated analysis systems for TMAs has brought a significant advancement to the field. They allow for quantitative analysis of staining intensity on a continuous scale rather than a nominal scale and eliminate the subjectivity of manual scoring methods. Continuous scale scoring of staining could provide opportunities for developing biologically relevant cut points for biomarkers rather than broader, more arbitrary divisions. Fluorescent detection strategies are particularly amenable to automated analysis in that they provide a much broader dynamic range for quantification and the use of multicolor immunofluorescence allows for discrimination of different tissue and subcellular compartments [23]. Automated systems also allow for accurate storage of data and help to prevent transcriptional errors.

Historically, TMAs have been used to confirm the correlation of various biomarkers with clinical parameters such as survival in a particular cohort of tumors or tumors from clinical trials. As researchers complete more and more of these correlative TMA studies and tissues are collected with these analyses in mind in ongoing and future clinical trials, TMAs can be used to help identify and validate markers that are predictive of drug response and resistance. Indeed, a number of recent studies have begun to identify biomarkers for therapeutic resistance in a number of different types of cancer. Têtu et al. assessed the expression of ten different proteins in advanced stage ovarian cancers whose gene expression was associated with progression-free survival [27]. IHC analysis of TMAs containing 158 ovarian cancer cases revealed that higher expression of MMP1 was associated with a higher risk of progression and high expression of HSP10, which was independently associated with longer progression-free survival [27].

A number of studies have used TMAs to identify potential biomarkers associated with tamoxifen resistance in breast cancer. One study found that patients with ER-positive tumors (90+% ER-positive cells) with greater than 1% phospho-ERK1/2 positive cells did not have improved overall survival compared to untreated patients, but ER+/pERK-negative patients did have improved survival in response to tamoxifen [28]. Another study found an association between VEGF-A expression and tamoxifen resistance in ER+ tumors [29]. In a third study, Tovey et al. analyzed TMAs containing 402 ER+ breast tumors treated with tamoxifen [30]. They found that overexpression of HER1–3 proteins and/or progesterone receptor (PR) status predicted early relapse in ER+, tamoxifen-treated patients in both univariate and multivariate analyses. Interestingly, this prediction was time-sensitive and applied only to the first 3 years of treatment. The authors suggested that ER+/PR-negative tumors or patients with HER1–3 overexpressing tumors may derive benefit from initial treatment with aromatase inhibitors [30].

TMAs provide an excellent means for the high-throughput analysis of biomarkers. As the technology matures over the next several years it is likely that TMA technology will play a significant role in identification and validation of predictive biomarkers for both therapeutic response and resistance.

Protein Microarrays

Protein microarray technology is rapidly becoming a powerful tool for drug discovery, biomarker identification, and signal transduction profiling of cellular material. The power of protein microarrays lies in their ability to provide a "map" of known cellular signaling proteins that generally reflect the state of information flow through protein networks in individual specimens. Identification of critical interactions within these networks is a potential starting point for drug development, characterization of drug resistance mechanisms, and the design of individual therapeutic regimens [31–35]. Protein microarrays allow examination of protein–protein interaction events, such as phosphorylation, in a high-throughput manner and can be used to profile the activity of cellular signaling pathways more directly than is possible with gene arrays [32, 36–42]. Protein microarrays can be used to monitor changes in protein phosphorylation over time, before and after treatment, between disease and nondisease states, and between therapeutic responders and nonresponders.

At a basic level, protein microarrays are comprised of a series of immobilized spots. Each spot contains a homogeneous or heterogeneous "bait" molecule. A spot on the array can display an antibody, a cell or phage lysate, a recombinant protein or peptide, nucleic acids, or glycans [31, 32, 36, 37, 42–48]. The array is queried with either a probe (a labeled ligand or antibody), or an unknown biologic sample (e.g., a serum sample or cell lysate) containing analytes of interest. By directly or indirectly tagging the query molecules with a signal-generating moiety, a pattern of positive and negative spots is generated. For each spot, the intensity of the signal is proportional to the quantity of applied query molecules bound to the bait molecules. A digital image of the spot pattern is collected and then analyzed and interpreted [49]. Protein microarray formats are defined into two major classes, forward-phase arrays (FPAs) and reverse-phase arrays (RPAs), depending on whether the analyte or analytes of interest are captured from solution or bound to the solid phase (Fig. 4.1) [49].

Forward-Phase Arrays

In FPAs, capture molecules are immobilized onto the substratum and act as the bait molecule (Fig. 4.1, top). Each spot contains one type of known analyte: an immobilized protein, fractionated lysate, or other type of bait molecule. In the FPA format, each array is incubated with a single test sample (e.g., a cellular lysate from one treatment condition or a serum sample from disease or control patients), and multiple analytes are measured at once. A number of excellent reviews have summarized the applications and new advances in FPA technology [50–56]. For example, FPAs of human, microbial, or viral recombinant proteins can be used to screen individual serum samples from disease and control subjects to characterize the immune response and identify potential diagnostic markers, and therapeutic or

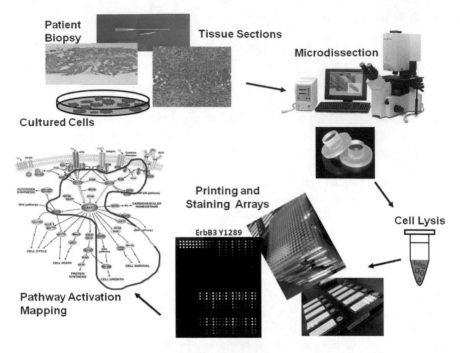

Fig. 4.1 Protein microarray formats. Forward-phase arrays (*top*) immobilize a bait molecule such as an antibody designed to capture specific analytes from a mixture of test sample proteins. The bound analytes are detected by a second sandwich antibody, or by labeling the analyte directly. Reverse-phase arrays immobilize the test sample analytes on the solid phase (*bottom*). An analyte-specific ligand (e.g., antibody; *lower left*) is applied in solution phase. Bound antibodies are detected by secondary tagging and signal amplification (*lower right*)

vaccine targets [52, 53, 57]. The advantage of these arrays is that they provide a means for multiplexed screening of well-defined sets of proteins and/or molecules. This format can be limited, however, by a lack of available ready-made recombinant molecules for spotting. Antibody arrays represent another example of FPAs that have broad applications [50, 52, 54]. Examples of their use in cancer research include identifying serum protein biomarkers for bladder cancer diagnosis and outcome stratification [58], prostate cancer diagnosis [42, 59], and identification of serum proteins for the diagnosis of pancreatic cancer [60]. Antibody arrays have also been used to identify differentially expressed cell surface markers in colon cancer cells [61]. Despite their great potential, the use of antibody arrays is limited due the lack of availability of well-characterized antibodies. A second drawback of antibody arrays lies in the detection methods for bound analytes on the array. Current options include the use of specific antibodies that recognize distinct analyte epitopes from the capture antibodies (similar to a traditional sandwich-type ELISA), or direct labeling of the analyte probe molecules. Both of these methods present distinct technical challenges [50].

Reverse-Phase Arrays

In contrast to the FPA format, the RPA format immobilizes an individual test sample in each array spot, such that an array is comprised of hundreds of different cellular lysates or patient samples (Fig. 4.1, bottom). Though not limited to clinical applications, the RPA format provides the opportunity to screen clinical samples available in very limited quantities, such as biopsy specimens or bone marrow aspirates [36, 62–66]. Since human tissues are composed of hundreds of interacting cell populations, RPAs also provide a unique opportunity for discovering changes in the cellular proteome which reflect the cellular microenvironment [67, 68]. Established technologies such as laser capture microdissection [69] make it possible to isolate pure cell populations from tissue specimens; the resulting protein lysates can then be spotted onto nitrocellulose-coated slides using a robotic arrayer [56] (Fig. 4.2). As many as 100 slides can be printed from a lysate of 5,000 microdissected cells depending on the volume printed per spot. Each array is incubated with one detection protein, such as an antibody, and a single analyte endpoint is measured and compared directly across multiple samples on each slide (Fig. 4.2). The RPA format is capable of highly sensitive analyte detection, with detection limits approaching attogram $(1.0 \times 10^{-18}$ g) amounts of a given protein and the ability to detect variances of less than 10% [66, 70]. This level of sensitivity, which is higher than bead arrays or ELISA, means that RPAs can be used to measure low abundance analytes such as phosphorylated protein isoforms from a spotted lysate representing less than 10 cell equivalents [36]. This is critical if the starting input material is only a few hundred cells from a biopsy specimen. Also, because the RPA technology requires only one antibody for detecting each analyte, it provides a facile method for broad profiling of pathways where hundreds of phospho-specific analytes can be measured from very small tissue specimens, such as needle biopsies, which are routinely procured in a physician's private office or hospital radiology center. These measurements can be used to create portraits illustrating signaling activation from individual tumors or groups of tumors (Fig. 4.2). Alternatively, measurements for a study set of tumors can be subjected to two-way unsupervised hierarchical clustering as a means to identify subgroups of tumors or samples with similar signaling patterns (Fig. 4.3). For example, two-way, unsupervised clustering of a small pilot study set of brain tumors and brain metastases from breast and lung cancers shows the metastatic tumors forming a cluster with several brain tumors that have higher relative levels of signaling than the second subgroup (Fig. 4.3). Subclusters of samples that form in hierarchical clustering can then be tested for statistical associations with clinical or other experimental parameters.

Key technological components of the RPA method offer unique advantages over tissue arrays [71] or antibody arrays [31, 32]. First, the RPA can use denatured lysates, so antigen retrieval and antibody performance issues, which are commonly problematic with tissue arrays and IHC, are minimized. Also, RPAs need only a single specific antibody for detecting each analyte protein and do not require direct tagging of the

Forward Phase Protein Microarray

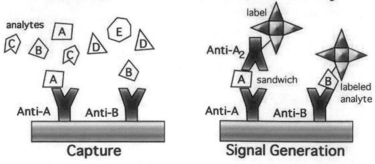

Reverse Phase Protein Microarray

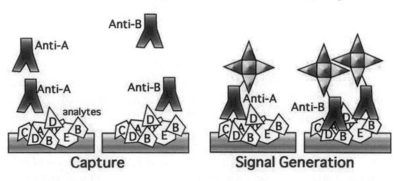

Fig. 4.2 Reverse-phase protein microarray workflow. Clockwise from *top left*: Cultured cells and tissues are prepared and processed for laser capture microdissection (for tissues) or for direct lysis as whole tissue or cell lysates. Following lysate preparation, samples are loaded into 384-well plates for printing onto nitrocellulose-coated slides. Printed arrays are then incubated with a single antibody whose binding is visualized either by fluorimetric (shown) or colorimetric detection strategies. Following image capture and analysis, data for the samples can be visualized by a variety of pathway activation mapping strategies. Pathway diagram reproduced courtesy of Cell Signaling Technology, Inc. (www.cellsignal.com); used with permission

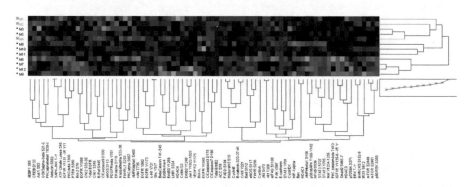

Fig. 4.3 Example of a two-way, unsupervised hierarchical cluster map. A heatmap generated by unsupervised, hierarchical clustering analysis of phosphoproteins from eight GBMs (M3, M5–M7, M9–M12), one recurrent GBM(M8) and three metastases (two from breast [M2, M4]

analyte as a readout for the assay, which allows for better reproducibility, sensitivity, and robustness compared with other techniques [72]. The availability of high-quality, specific antibodies, however, particularly those specific for posttranslational modifications or active states of proteins, is a major limiting factor for the successful implementation of RPA technology [73]. Unlike the probes for gene expression analysis, the probes for protein microarrays (antibodies, aptamers and ligands) cannot be manufactured with predictable affinity and specificity. Antibody specificity must be thoroughly assessed and validated by immunoblot prior to use in any protein array format, and appropriate standards for specificity established. Such standards should include evidence of a single, appropriately sized band in immunoblots using complex biological samples similar to those planned for array analysis, such as cell lines or whole or microdissected tissue samples. Assessment of a phospho-specific antibody should also require evidence of a differential signal between control and treated samples known to possess the pathway or endpoint of interest. These same positive and negative controls can also be printed directly on each array to assess specificity in real-time (Fig. 4.4).

Perhaps the biggest challenge facing the widespread use of the RPA in the clinical laboratory setting is the standardization of each step and process involved in array production, bioinformatic analysis, and ensuring that tissue is processed and handled rapidly and optimally. During printing, each patient sample can be arrayed in multiple dilutions in duplicate or triplicate, either as a serial dilution curve or as an undiluted sample and one or more dilutions of choice (Fig. 4.4a). This representation allows for direct quantitative measurement once antibody dilutions are determined to be in the linear range of detection. Currently, there is limited standardization in the field with regard to methods, analysis, and controls used and also data validation. These issues often prevent productive data comparisons between laboratories and platforms and between experiments separated in time. This is a particularly relevant issue with regard to the analysis of clinical trial specimens by protein arrays, where accrual of samples may occur over extended periods of time and analysis may require the use of multiple arrays to accommodate all samples for a particular study. In addition to the standardization of tissue handling techniques and sample preparation protocols, development of a universal reference standard that could be printed onto every array would allow identification of, and compensation for variations in instrumentation, reagents, samples, and operators in different laboratory settings and across time. Ideally, RPA reference standard(s) would serve as a universal positive control for the staining process and antibody validation and also be incorporated into data analysis. A good quality reference standard should be renewable, reproducible on a large scale, reliable across a broad range of endpoints, and stable over long periods of time. A reference standard should also resemble the test samples as closely as possible [74]. Our group has assessed various types of

---

Fig. 4.3 (continued) and one from lung [M1]). The tumor samples are shown on the vertical axis while the phosphoproteins of interest are shown on the horizontal axis. Relative protein expression levels are designated on a scale where *red* represents high relative levels, *black* corresponds to intermediate levels, and *green* indicates a low level relative to all other samples

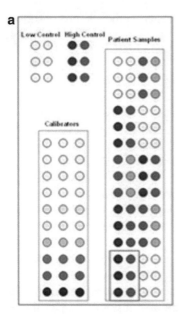

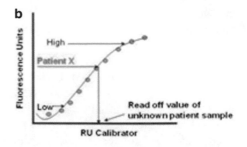

Fig. 4.4 Prototypical reverse-phase protein microarray construction for use as a calibrated assay. (a) In a calibrated assay format, samples would be printed in triplicate and possibly in one or more dilutions. High and low expression controls for endpoints of interest would be printed alongside the calibrator sample which is printed in an extended dilution curve. (b) Example of method for converting sample staining intensities to reference standard units. Intensities for the calibrator dilutions are plotted vs. the assigned standard units and the reference standard unit corresponding to the sample intensity is determined from this curve

source materials for use as a reference standard on our RPA platform. Human tissue extracts, although essentially identical to our test samples, are not renewable or routinely available in large enough quantities for large scale reference standard production. We also found that any particular tissue extract often does not provide reliable signal for all phospho-specific endpoints of interest in our profiling studies. Multiple tissue extracts could be combined into a reference standard to overcome this problem, but this only serves to compound the problems of large scale production and renewability. Phosphopeptides represent an invariant, renewable, scalable, and reproducible source material for a reference standard. Since they are often the immunogen source itself, they bind probe antibodies with high affinity. Peptides can be printed in mixtures on arrays in extended dilution curves and be used to develop a reference calibration curve. One major drawback for the use of peptides as reference standards is cost. One must either purchase available immunogens from antibody vendors which are usually only available as solubilized forms in small volumes, or synthesize individual antigenic phosphopeptides corresponding to each antibody of interest, which could total up to hundreds of individual peptides. Many companies consider the exact sequences of their immunogens for antibodies to be proprietary information, so while an individual investigator can make a reasonable guess regarding the sequence of an immunogen for any particular antibody, there is a significant risk that a synthesized peptide will not bind with the same affinity if the length of the peptide doesn't match and/or the sequence frame selected is shifted from the actual immunogen. A second drawback to the use of peptide based reference standards is that different peptides can have varying solubilities in aqueous buffers, which makes accurate quantification of the amount of an individual peptide present in a mixture such as a reference standard difficult at best. However, phosphopeptides may be an excellent option as high and low controls for a calibrated assay. A third alternative source material suitable for a phosphopeptide reference standard is extracts from a wide variety of treated cell lines that can be purchased commercially. While cell line extracts potentially share the same problems of stability and reproducibility found with tissue extracts, because they are generated repeatedly from a homogeneous source and are subjected to quality control measures prior to release, they will likely demonstrate significantly less batch-to-batch variability than tissue extracts. Also, treated cell lines will also exhibit more predictable and possibly higher levels of phosphorylation for many endpoints than a tissue extract would be expected to. Our group has assembled a set of reference standards composed of treated cell lysates that are printed on all arrays produced in the lab in extended dilution curves and can be used as a calibration curve for conversion of sample intensity values to reference standard units (Fig. 4.4b). For routine clinical implementation, much like how an ELISA is used, each phospho-specific analyte measurement for any experimental sample that falls into the linear range of the calibrator can be converted into reference standard units based on the calibrant and the dilution factor. The use of a universal reference standard on every array produced in a single facility or a number of different laboratories will facilitate normalization and comparison of test samples across time, platforms, studies, and sites. Under CAP/CLIA regulations, technologies that can rapidly assess and measure multiple phosphorylation endpoints, such as the RPA, or even a multiplexed ELISA, will require the development of reference standards, controls and calibrators, as well as measures of proficiency [75].

A number of studies illustrate the utility of RPAs for the analysis of human tissues and demonstrate the potential of this technology to produce valuable information that can be used in therapeutic decision-making [62, 63, 65–67, 76–79]. RPA technology was first described when it was utilized to demonstrate that pro-survival proteins and pathways are activated during prostate cancer progression [36]. RPAs have also been used to study signal pathway activity in primary and metastatic cancer lesions [63, 66, 78, 79]. Cancer is often not diagnosed until the disease has spread to distant sites. Since the tissue microenvironment of the metastatic cancer cell is completely different from that of the primary tumor, there is a distinct possibility that phosphorylation events in the metastatic tumor cells will differ significantly from those of the primary tumor cells. It can be argued that the signaling derangements manifested within the metastatic lesion might be the most appropriate basis for the selection of targeted therapy because the effective treatment of metastatic disease is the key to ultimate response. Preliminary published data support this concept. Analysis of a small set of microdissected, patient-matched primary colorectal cancer lesions and liver metastases suggested that signaling in metastatic hepatic lesions differed considerably from that of the matched primary lesions, but the metastatic lesions showed similar signaling patterns [63]. These observations are consistent with those in a similar study of six primary ovarian tumors and patient-matched omental metastases taken simultaneously at surgery [66]. Signaling profiles in the metastatic tissues were altered dramatically compared to their matched primary counterparts, and partition analysis revealed that increased levels of phospho-c-KIT could distinguish five of the six metastases from the primary lesions. The evidence that metastatic cell signaling is so dissimilar from that of the primary tumor highlights the critical need for patient-tailored therapy that is designed to target the disseminated cells specifically, if improved clinical outcomes are to be achieved. In an alternative approach to the study of metastatic disease, a recent study attempted to identify signaling biomarkers predictive for occult metastasis in colon cancer [78]. Using a set of 34 primary colon cancer tumors from patients presenting with synchronous liver metastases and 18 cases of primary colon cancer that never metastasized, the investigators found that primary tumors from patients with metastases exhibited higher relative activation of EGFR and COX2 signaling pathways. Studies are ongoing to validate this observation in larger tumor study sets including CRC primary tumors from patients who later developed metachronous liver metastasis upon follow-up. If these initial observations are confirmed, clinical trials testing combinations of inhibitors that reduce COX2 and EGFR signaling might be an intriguing consideration for the treatment of patients with predicted occult disease. This study highlights that protein pathway biomarkers could play important roles as prognostic determinants to discern which patients harbor occult metastasis destined to appear later with high probability, and also as therapeutic targets that could be considered for molecular-based treatment strategies to target the occult metastatic tumor cells.

Therapeutic resistance to treatment is another important area where the RPA technology can have significant impact. Indeed, a number of recent studies have used RPA analysis to identify protein markers predictive of therapeutic response or resistance in a number of different types of cancers [80–86]. Studies in ovarian cancer and colon cancer cell lines identified markers involved in nucleotide excision repair that were associated with drug activity of cisplatin and ecteinascidin 743 (Trabectedin) [80]. In studies of melanoma cell lines and patient samples, O'Reilly et al. found that phosphorylation of 4E-BP1 was increased in melanoma cell lines carrying mutations in BRAF and PTEN compared to cells with wild-type RAS/RAF/PTEN and normal melanocytes and was associated with worse overall and post-recurrence survival [81]. The authors hypothesize that targeted inhibition of pathways leading to 4E-BP1 phosphorylation may improve outcome in patients with metastatic melanoma. Studies of 30 breast cancer cell lines found that distinct patterns of signaling were present in groups representing different molecular subtypes of breast cancer that were not obvious from gene expression studies [82]. They found that the activation of signaling modules appeared to occur in a subtype-specific manner and may be useful for prediction of response to phosphatidylinositol-3-kinase (PI3K) and MEK inhibitors in vivo. Interestingly, they found that treatment of basal type cells with MEK inhibitors resulted in increased signaling in PI3K/AKT pathways, which could have implications for treatment response to other therapeutic agents, and emphasizes the value of conducting preclinical in vitro studies to identify off-target effects of therapeutics that could impact combination therapies.

In looking for markers of response and resistance to the PI3K inhibitor, PX-866, Ihle et al. combined cell xenograft studies with RPA analysis [83]. They found that mutations in the genes for PI3K and loss of PTEN activity were sufficient, but not necessary as predictors of sensitivity to PX-866. Mutant, oncogenic Ras was a dominant factor determining resistance to treatment, even in the presence of PI3K mutations. Measurements of phosphorylated AKT S473 as a surrogate for PI3K activity in tumors was not sufficient to predict sensitivity to the drug. They also observed that levels of c-MYC and Cyclin B, which are downstream targets of Ras, were upregulated in PX-866 resistant cell lines in vivo and were also negatively associated with response to the drug.

Drugs targeting the EGFR signaling pathway are some of the most intensely studied in the field of molecular-targeted therapies. A recent study by Havaleshko et al. discussed the development of predictive models for sensitivity to lapatinib, a small-molecule inhibitor of EGFR, in bladder cancer [84]. Using 39 different bladder cancer cell lines, they measured in vitro sensitivity to lapatinib and then developed several predictive models for sensitivity to the agent based on: (1) transcriptome profiling; (2) RPA signaling profiles of EGFR pathway targets; and (3) a combination of transcriptome and RPA data. Their results found that the transcriptome-based model performed better (93–98% accuracy) than the phosphoprotein-based model (54–61% accuracy). A third model combining the transciptome-based model with phospho-EGFR Y1173 RPA data improved the mean predictive accuracy to 98%. They observed that most of the predictive probes in their models did not have clear relationships to the known mechanism of action of the drug and may suggest the existence of novel mechanisms of drug response modulation. The authors noted that only endpoints directly related to EGFR signaling were profiled by RPA in this study and perhaps a broader RPA profiling study including more off-target measurements would improve the phosphoproteomics-based prediction models. In total, all of these studies illustrate the valuable contribution that RPA profiling can make to the identification and validation of drug response-related biomarkers.

Conclusion

The impact of multiplexed, protein array-driven measurements at the bedside has certainly not been felt yet, but a view to the near future reveals just how substantial the effects may be. Instead of a pathology report delineating a list of single measurements of selected analytes such as Ki67, ER, EGFR, and HER2 levels, the molecular pathologist will include information about pathway activation portraits of each tumor specimen. Instead of a molecular characterization of the tumor based solely on histology, or even genomic information (e.g., basal, luminal A, etc., for breast cancer), new classification schemas could arise based on the protein signaling profiles for individual tumors.

In order to maximize the technological advances that have been made in approaches such as the RPA, we will need to turn our attention to generating widespread patient population data focused on cataloging and indexing which pathways are truly activated and driving cancer development and progression from premalignancy through local invasion and metastasis. Moreover, the future of cancer therapy lies in combinatorial therapeutics, and a rationalized approach with a foundation in molecular information will be needed whereby entire signaling cascades and networks can be monitored throughout the course of therapy. Protein array-based profiling provides an ideal means to measure broad ranges of endpoints and assess drug effects on entire signaling pathways and not just the drug target itself, which may be a key to true therapeutic success. Finally, protein array-based approaches for predictive, prognostic and therapy-guiding purposes may have their greatest impact through the identification of aggressive signaling signatures within premalignant and early stage lesions for many types of cancers that can be developed and implemented into screening tests. Combined with continued efforts to identify and monitor protein markers indicative of therapeutic response or resistance, protein array-based technologies are uniquely poised to provide direct functional information for individual patient tumors in time frames which were never before possible and could have a tremendous positive impact on therapeutic decision-making and ultimately on disease outcome.

References

1. Baak JP, Path FR, Hermsen MA, et al. Genomics and proteomics in cancer. Eur J Cancer. 2003;39:1199–215.
2. Segal E, Friedman N, Kaminski N, et al. From signatures to models: understanding cancer using microarrays. Nat Genet. 2005;37(Suppl):S38–45.
3. Brennan DJ, O'Brien SL, Fagan A, et al. Application of DNA microarray technology in determining breast cancer prognosis and therapeutic response. Expert Opin Biol Ther. 2005;5:1069–83.
4. Nishizuka S, Charboneau L, Young L, et al. Proteomic profiling of the NCI-60 cancer cell lines using new high-density reverse-phase lysate microarrays. Proc Natl Acad Sci USA. 2003;100:14229–34.
5. Celis JE, Gromov P. Proteomics in translational cancer research: toward an integrated approach. Cancer Cell. 2003;3:9–15.
6. Hunter T. Signaling – 2000 and beyond. Cell. 2000;100:113–27.
7. Görg A, Weiss W, Dunn MJ. Current two-dimensional electrophoresis technology for proteomics. Proteomics. 2004;4:3665–85.
8. Gygi SP, Rist B, Gerber SA, et al. Quantitative analysis of complex protein mixtures using isotope-coded affinity tags. Nat Biotechnol. 1999;17:994–9.
9. Krutchinsky AN, Kalkum M, Chait BT. Automatic identification of proteins with a MALDI-quadrupole ion trap mass spectrometer. Anal Chem. 2001;73:5066–77.
10. Washburn MP, Wolters D, Yates III JR. Large scale analysis of the yeast proteome by multidimensional protein identification technology. Nat Biotechnol. 2001;19:242–7.

11. Zhou G, Li H, DeCamp D, et al. 2D differential in-gel electrophoresis for the identification of esophageal scans cell cancer-specific protein markers. Mol Cell Proteomics. 2002;1:117–24.
12. Wan WH, Fortuna MB, Furmanski P. A rapid and efficient method for testing immunohistochemical activity of monoclonal antibodies against multiple tissue samples simultaneously. J Immunol Methods. 1987;103:121–9.
13. Voduc D, Kenney C, Nielsen TO. Tissue microarrays in clinical oncology. Semin Radiat Oncol. 2008;18:89–97.
14. van der Vegt B, de Bock GH, Hollema H, et al. Microarray methods to identify factors determining breast cancer progression: Potentials, limitations, and challenges. Crit Rev Oncol Hematol. 2009;70:1–11.
15. Hewitt SM. Design, construction and use of tissue microarrays. Methods Mol Biol. 2004; 264:61–72.
16. Hewitt SM. The application of tissue microarrays in the validation of microarray data. Methods Enzymol. 2006;410:400–15.
17. Dancau AM, Simon R, Mirlacher M, et al. Tissue microarrays. Methods Mol Biol. 2010; 576:49–60.
18. Kononen J, Bubendorf I, Kallioneimi A, et al. Tissue microarrays for high-throughput molecular profiling of tumor specimens. Nat Med. 1998;4:844–7.
19. Schoenberg-Fejzo M, Slamon D. Frozen tumor tissue microarray technology for analysis of tumor RNA, DNA and proteins. Amer J Pathol. 2001;159:1645–50.
20. Datta MW, Kahler A, Macias V, et al. A simple, inexpensive method for the production of tissue microarrays from needle biopsy specimens: examples with prostate tissue. Appl Immunohistochem Mol Morphol. 2005;13:96–103.
21. Li R, Ni J, Bourne PA, et al. Cell culture block array for immunocytochemical study of protein expression in cultured cells. Appl Immunohistochem Mol Morphol. 2005;13:85–90.
22. Montgomery K, Zhao S, van de Rijn M, et al. A novel method for making "tissue" microarrays from small numbers of suspension cells. Appl Immunohistochem Mol Morphol. 2005;13:80–4.
23. Camp RL, Neumeister V, Rimm DL. A decade of tissue microarrays: progress in the discovery and validation of cancer biomarkers. J Clin Oncol. 2008;26:5630–7.
24. Camp RL, Charette LA, Rimm DL. Validation of tissue microarray technology in breast carcinoma. Lab Invest. 2000;80:1943–9.
25. Torhorst J, Bucher C, Kononen J, et al. Tissue microarrays for rapid linking of molecular changes to clinical endpoints. Am J Pathol. 2001;159:2249–56.
26. Chung GG, Zerkowski MP, Ghosh S, et al. Quantitative analysis of estrogen receptor heterogeneity in breast cancer. Lab Invest. 2007;87:662–9.
27. Têtu B, Popa I, Bairati I, et al. Immunohistochemical analysis of possible chemoresistance markers identified by micro-arrays on serous ovarian carcinomas. Mod Pathol. 2008;21: 1002–10.
28. Svensson S, Jirstrom K, Ryden L, et al. ERK phosphorylation is linked to VEGFR2 expression and Ets-2 phosphorylation in breast cancer and is associated with tamoxifen treatment resistance and small tumours with good prognosis. Oncogene. 2005;24:4370–9.
29. Ryden L, Stendahl M, Jonsson H, et al. Tumor-specific VEGF-A and VEGFR2 in postmenopausal breast cancer patients with long-term follow-up. Implication of a link between VEGF pathway and tamoxifen response. Breast Cancer Res Treat. 2005;89:135–43.
30. Tovey S, Dunne B, Witton CJ, et al. Can molecular markers predict when to implement treatment with aromatase inhibitors in invasive breast cancer? Clin Cancer Res. 2005;11:4835–42.
31. Eckel-Passow JE, Hoering A, Therneau TM, et al. Experimental design and analysis of antibody microarrays: applying methods from cDNA arrays. Cancer Res. 2005;65:2985–9.
32. Haab BB. Antibody arrays in cancer research. Mol Cell Proteomics. 2005;4:377–83.
33. Leuking A, Cahill DJ, Mullner S. Protein biochips: a new and versatile platform technology for molecular medicine. Drug Disc Today. 2005;10:789–94.
34. Liotta LA, Kohn E, Petricoin EF. Clinical proteomics: personalized molecular medicine. JAMA. 2001;286:2211–4.

35. Petricoin EF, Zoon KC, Kohn EC, et al. Clinical proteomics: translating benchside promise into bedside reality. Nat Rev Drug Discov. 2002;1:683–95.
36. Paweletz CP, Charboneau L, Bichsel VE, et al. Reverse phase protein microarrays which capture disease progression show activation of pro-survival pathways at the cancer invasion front. Oncogene. 2001;20:1981–9.
37. Zhu H, Snyder M. Protein chip technology. Curr Opin Chem Biol. 2003;7:55–63.
38. Cutler P. Protein arrays: the current state-of-the-art. Proteomics. 2003;3:3–18.
39. Ge H. UPA, a universal protein array system for quantitative detection of protein–protein, protein–DNA, protein–RNA and protein–ligand interactions. Nucleic Acids Res. 2000; 28:e3.
40. Liotta L, Petricoin E. Molecular profiling of human cancer. Nat Rev Genet. 2000;1:48–56.
41. MacBeath G. Protein microarrays and proteomics. Nat Genet. 2002;32(Suppl):526–32.
42. Miller JC, Zhou H, Kwekel J, et al. Antibody microarray profiling of human prostate cancer sera: antibody screening and identification of potential biomarkers. Proteomics. 2003;3: 56–63.
43. Humphery-Smith I, Wischerhoff E, Hashimoto R. Protein arrays for assessment of target selectivity. Drug Discov World. 2002;4:17–27.
44. MacBeath G, Schreiber SL. Printing proteins as microarrays for high-throughput function determination. Science. 2000;289:1760–3.
45. Petach H, Gold L. Dimensionality is the issue: use of photoaptamers in protein microarrays. Curr Opin Biotechnol. 2002;13:309–14.
46. Weng S, Gu K, Hammond PW, et al. Generating addressable protein microarrays with profusion covalent mRNA-protein fusion technology. Proteomics. 2002;2:48–57.
47. Yue T, Haab BB. Microarrays in glycoproteomics research. Clinics Lab Med. 2009;29:15–29.
48. Taylor AD, Hancock WS, Hincapie M, et al. Toward an integrated proteomic and glycomic approach to finding cancer biomarkers. Genome Med. 2009;1:57–66.
49. Liotta LA, Espina V, Mehta AI, et al. Protein microarrays: meeting analytical challenges for clinical applications. Cancer Cell. 2003;3:317–25.
50. Angenendt P. Progress in protein and antibody microarray technology. Drug Disc Today. 2005;10:503–11.
51. LaBaer J, Ramachandran N. Protein microarrays as tools for functional proteomics. Curr Opin Chem Biol. 2005;9:14–9.
52. Hultschig C, Kreutzberger J, Seitz H, et al. Recent advances of protein microarrays. Curr Opin Chem Biol. 2006;10:4–10.
53. Robinson WH. Antigen arrays for antibody profiling. Curr Opin Chem Biol. 2006;10:67–72.
54. Haab BB. Applications of antibody array platforms. Curr Opin Biotechnol. 2006;17:415–21.
55. Kingsmore SF. Multiplexed protein measurement: technologies and applications of protein and antibody arrays. Nat Rev Drug Discov. 2006;5:310–20.
56. Spurrier B, Honkanen P, Holway A, et al. Protein and lysate array technologies in cancer research. Biotechnol Adv. 2008;26:361–9.
57. Madoz-Gurpide J, Kuick R, Wang H, et al. Integral protein microarrays for the identification of lung cancer antigens in sera that induce a humoral immune response. Mol Cell Proteomics. 2008;7:268–81.
58. Sanchez-Carbayo M, Socci ND, Lozano JJ, et al. Profiling bladder cancer using targeted antibody arrays. Am J Pathol. 2006;168:93–103.
59. Shafer MW, Mangold L, Partin AW, et al. Antibody array profiling reveals serum TSP-I as a marker to distinguish benign from malignant prostatic disease. Prostate. 2007;67:255–67.
60. Orchekowski R, Hemelinck D, Li L, et al. Antibody microarray profiling reveals individual and combined serum proteins associated with pancreatic cancer. Cancer Res. 2005;65:11193–202.
61. Ellmark P, Belov L, Huang P, et al. Multiplex detection of surface molecules on colorectal cancers. Proteomics. 2006;6:1791–802.
62. Grubb RL, Calvert VS, Wulfkuhle JD, et al. Signal pathway profiling of prostate cancer using reverse phase protein microarrays. Proteomics. 2003;3:2142–6.

63. Petricoin III EF, Bichsel VE, Calvert VS, et al. Mapping molecular networks using proteomics: a vision for patient-tailored combination therapy. J Clin Oncol. 2005;23:3614–21.
64. Wulfkuhle JD, Aquino JA, Calvert VS, et al. Signal pathway profiling of ovarian cancer from human tissue specimens using reverse-phase protein microarrays. Proteomics. 2003;3:2085–90.
65. Gulmann C, Espina V, Petricoin III E, et al. Proteomic analysis of apoptotic pathways reveals prognostic factors in follicular lymphoma. Clin Cancer Res. 2005;11:5847–55.
66. Sheehan KM, Calvert VS, Kay EW, et al. Use of reverse-phase protein microarrays and reference standard development for molecular network analysis of metastatic ovarian carcinoma. Mol Cell Proteomics. 2005;4:346–55.
67. Sheehan KM, Gulmann C, Eichler GS, et al. Signal pathway profiling of epithelial and stromal compartments of colonic carcinoma reveals epithelial-mesenchymal transition. Oncogene. 2008;27:323–31.
68. Espina V, Wulfkuhle J, Liotta LA. Application of laser capture microdissection and reverse-phase protein microarrays to the molecular profiling of cancer signaling pathway networks in the tissue microenvironment. Clin Lab Med. 2009;29:1–13.
69. Emmert-Buck MR, Bonner RF, Smith PD, et al. Laser capture microdissection. Science. 1996;274:998–1001.
70. Anderson T, Wulfkuhle J, Liotta L, et al. Improved reproducibility of reverse-phase protein microarrays using array microenvironment normalization. Proteomics. 2009;9:5562–6.
71. Giltrane JM, Rimm DL. Technology insight: identification of biomarkers with tissue microarray technology. Nat Clin Pract Oncol. 2005;1:104–11.
72. Espina V, Mehta AI, Winters ME, et al. Protein microarrays: molecular profiling technologies for clinical specimens. Proteomics. 2003;3:2091–100.
73. Wulfkuhle J, Espina V, Liotta L, et al. Genomic and proteomic technologies for individualisation and improvement of cancer treatment. Eur J Cancer. 2004;40:2623–32.
74. Cronin M, Ghosh K, Sistare F, et al. Universal RNA reference materials for gene expression. Clin Chem. 2004;50:1464–71.
75. Wulfkuhle J, Edmiston KH, Liotta LA, et al. Technology insight: pharmacoproteomics for cancer – promises for patient-tailored medicine using protein microarrays. Nat Clin Pract Oncol. 2006;3:256–68.
76. Zha H, Raffeld M, Charboneau L, et al. Similarities of prosurvival signals in Bcl-2-positive and Bcl-2-negative follicular lymphomas identified by reverse phase protein microarray. Lab Invest. 2004;84:235–44.
77. Gulmann C, Sheehan KM, Conroy RM, et al. Quantitative cell signalling analysis reveals down-regulation of MAPK pathway activation in colorectal cancer. J Pathol. 2009;218:514–9.
78. Pierobon M, Calvert V, Belluco C, et al. Multiplexed cell signaling analysis of metastatic and nonmetastatic colorectal cancer reveals COX2-EGFR signaling activation as a potential prognostic pathway biomarker. Clin Colorectal Cancer. 2009;8:110–7.
79. Grubb RL, Deng J, Pinto PA, et al. Pathway biomarker profiling of localized and metastatic human prostate cancer reveal metastatic and prognostic signatures. J Prot Res. 2009;8:3044–54.
80. Stevens EV, Nishizuka S, Antony S, et al. Predicting cisplatin and trabectedin drug sensitivity in ovarian and colon cancers. Mol Cancer Ther. 2008;7:10–8.
81. O'Reilly KE, Warycha M, Davies MA, et al. Phosphorylated 4E-BP1 is associated with poor survival in melanoma. Clin Cancer Res. 2009;15:2872–8.
82. Boyd ZS, Wu QJ, O'Brien C, et al. Proteomic analysis of breast cancer molecular subtypes and biomarkers of response to targeted kinase inhibitors using reverse-phase protein microarrays. Mol Cancer Ther. 2008;7:3695–706.
83. Ihle NT, Lemos R, Wipf P, et al. Mutations in the phosphatidylinositol-3-kinase pathway predict for antitumor activity of the inhibitor PX-866 while oncogenic Ras is a dominant predictor for resistance. Cancer Res. 2009;69:143–50.

84. Havaleshko DM, Smith SC, Cho HJ, et al. Comparison of global versus epidermal growth factor receptor pathway profiling for prediction of lapatinib sensitivity in bladder cancer. Neoplasia. 2009;11:1185–93.
85. Pernas FG, Allen CT, Winters ME, et al. Proteomic signatures of epidermal growth factor receptor and survival signal pathways correspond to gefitinib sensitivity in head and neck cancer. Clin Cancer Res. 2009;15:2361–72.
86. Park ES, Rabinovsky R, Carey M, et al. Integrative analysis of proteomic signatures, mutations, and drug responsiveness in the NCI 60 cancer cell line set. Cancer Res. 2010;9(2): 257–67.

Chapter 5
Using Phosphoflow™ to Study Signaling Events of Subpopulations Resistant to Current Therapies

Omar D. Perez

Keywords Phosphoflow™ • Flow cytometry • Signaling • Minimal residual disease • Biomarker • Patient stratification

Introduction

Cellular processes are underscored by a series of complex and interactive signaling networks, many of which are dependent on phosphorylation or dephosphorylation of key signaling proteins. A variety of these signaling cascades are well established; for example the MAPK kinase family, cell survival pathways (AKT/PI3K), stress response pathways (JNK/p38), and immune cell signaling pathways (STAT pathways, TCR and BCR pathways). The identity of specific kinases, phosphatases, and cellular receptors that are differentially modulated in a disease state has enabled opportunities for the development of targeted agents that are highly selective for the diseased tissues. What is often less well understood is how these common pathway proteins can effectively interact as a network.

Additionally, it less well understood how this network is altered over the course of disease progression. In a nondiseased state, environmental cues such as cytokines, growth factors or other chemical entities may have a consistent network activation and end-result. That is to say, the same input, whether it be agonistic or antagonistic, results in the same output, such as cellular differentiation, gene transcription, or protein activation. However, in a diseased state, the rules of cellular and molecular activation no longer apply. The same environmental cues may have drastically altered cellular responses due to molecular alterations at both the genetic and protein level that occurred because of the disease progression, thereby resulting in perturbed system functions. Furthermore, molecular alterations that arise due to

O.D. Perez (✉)
Preclinical Development, Tocagen, Inc.,
San Diego, CA, USA
e-mail: operez007@gmail.com

D. Gioeli (ed.), *Targeted Therapies: Mechanisms of Resistance*,
Molecular and Translational Medicine, DOI 10.1007/978-1-60761-478-4_5,
© Springer Science+Business Media, LLC 2011

disease progression can also initiate de novo and extensive signal pathway crosstalk that can activate distinct pathways not normally activated.

A primary focus of the molecular understanding of disease pathogenesis is to identify targets for future drug development. Complicating the generation of targeted agents is also the fact that under different environmental conditions, many extracellular receptors activate similar and common pathways to mediate gene transcription. Blocking a specific pathway protein does not necessarily mean the end target of that pathway cascade is completely inhibited. It is possible for an alternative signaling pathway to overcome the inhibition by bypassing the inhibited protein and ultimately reaching the same common downstream effector. Signaling nodes therefore represent the signal pathway gatekeepers to downstream activities. These signaling nodes are intermediate points of pathway communication and serve as both attractive molecular targets and also points of signal bifurcation when unregulated. The loss of drug specificity and nonspecific target effects (i.e., off-target effects) can result because of signal network crosstalk that changes as cellular resistance emerges.

This "genetic plasticity," a hallmark of oncogenesis, oftentimes results in cell populations that become resistant to any given drug agent over time. Drug selection pressures can contribute to the evolution of the cancer in unpredicted ways. The outgrowth of these resistant cellular populations contributes to the heterogeneity of malignancy and presents challenges for treatment. Molecular redundancies in signal transduction pathways can also compensate for targeted therapies, contributing to the propensity for development of resistant cells and their selective outgrowth. Identifying the emergence of these early resistant populations in a manner that is correlated with nonresponse to treatment would be highly beneficial for making informed treatment decisions. Notably, the information can be used to select broad-spectrum or multikinase-targeted therapies instead of narrow spectrum and presumably single target therapies; the hope being that early identification of resistant cellular populations may influence treatment decisions earlier in order to render the best possible outcome for the patient.

The development of resistance to targeted agents as a result of genetic changes or additional mutations to the protein targets themselves is common for many small molecule protein-targeted agents. Similarly, chronic exposure to treatments, such as cell-targeted monoclonal antibodies, can also modify the cellular subset distribution thereby selecting cell subsets for outgrowth. There are at least three different types of targeted therapies: (1) small molecules aimed at specific protein kinases or receptor kinases that effectively interfere with their ATP binding or ATP processing; (2) anti-receptor antibodies that effectively interfere with receptor dimerization, receptor/ligand interactions or receptor activation, and additionally can target cells for antibody-dependent cell cytotoxicity; (3) agents that target oncogenic processes such as angiogenesis or metastasis. The specificity of "targeted treatments" has also grown to include agents such as multi-family kinase inhibitors which are believed to have less resistant emergences, viral treatments, and a number of combinatory agents that collectively can target specific onco-activities [1–4]. All together, the genetic plasticity and heterogeneity of cancer can render targeted and even nontargeted treatments ineffective over time.

This current challenge has fueled the creation of many technologies in the postgenomic and proteomic era to develop molecular diagnostics to identify why certain patients respond to treatment when they do, and more importantly, to identify why certain patients do not respond to treatment. It is the nonresponders that present challenges for treatment paradigms, particularly when there is no rational methodology for trying the next treatment. Unfortunately, combating resistance becomes a trial and error process. Moreover, collection of the molecular data and information for understanding the difference between response vs. nonresponse in particular disease settings has value in that it can be used to model a preliminary hypothesis for predictive and prognostic marker development that can be tested in larger patient cohort populations. The development of many of these molecular diagnostic approaches, notably, companion diagnostics, is quickly gaining precedence as a means to aid in the therapeutic decision-making process. This chapter discusses how intracellular flow cytometry can be used to identify and study signaling events of specific cellular populations that have become resistant to targeted treatments and how this information can be used to guide drug development efforts and ultimately guide treatment decisions.

The Power of Flow Cytometry

It is well understood that autoimmune diseases and cancer are governed by a deregulation of intrinsic cellular signaling systems. The complexity of understanding these signaling pathways in a nondisease context vs. a disease context has been further obscured by molecular redundancy and heterogeneity of patient-derived samples. The heterogeneity of whole blood material from patients can be studied using standard biochemical analyses or even more modern quantitative diagnostic assessments. However, these techniques do not assess the subcellular heterogeneity that can be of significance in trying to identify resistant cell populations. Therefore, a true understanding of the nature of signaling dysfunctions during disease processes in heterogeneous patient samples has not been easily achievable.

This is where flow cytometry has an advantage. Flow cytometry is a powerful tool that immunologists and stem cell biologists have utilized to characterize cellular phenotypes. Surface immunophenotyping is commonly performed for hematological disorders and is required for facilitating the staging of diseases such as leukemias and lymphomas. Intracellular proteins are also stained to identify unique cell populations in certain malignancies. For example, terminal deoxynucleotidyl transferase (TdT) is present in over 90% of acute lymphocytic leukemia [5, 6]. More recently, development of methodology for intracellular staining for phospho-epitopes has allowed the study of signaling events within the native context of the cell [7–10]. Detection of single phospho-epitopes provides information of the presence of a phospho-protein as well as its relative quantity. Detection of multiple phospho-epitopes, particularly of distinct kinase pathways, can simultaneously provide information across pathways, allowing target and nontarget assessments to be made at the same time [11, 12].

A key advantage of flow cytometry is the ability to combine intracellular and extracellular measurements in order to obtain detailed information about kinase activity in immunophenotyped cells and simultaneously correlate cellular function and cell status in defined populations. For example, it has been possible to simultaneously monitor intracellular kinase activation states in highly immunophenotyped cells both in human and in mouse [7, 13–19]. The multiparameter aspect of flow cytometry, coupled with intracellular agents to assess phospho-epitope status allows for subset-specific analyses to be performed from whole blood specimens. Understanding these cell subset-specific signaling differences both as a function of disease progression as well as a function of treatment can be used to diagnose resistant populations. With the routine use of flow cytometry for the diagnosis of hematological malignancies by immunophenotype analyses, creating databases with signaling information from longitudinal sampling can help identify the emergence of early resistant cell populations.

The study of signaling events in primary cells also provides exciting new opportunities for analyses of signal transduction in the context of clinical research. It has been difficult to access samples for in vitro biochemical studies, since many times the cells would require short-term culturing or were obtained in insufficient amounts for protien functional assays. Using flow cytometry, it is possible to access the biochemical signatures directly from blood, with the potential to investigate subset-specific phosphorylation. Identity of these specific phospho-signatures could provide unique tools if correlated to be predictive of disease state. Furthermore, it is also possible to perform pharmacodynamic monitoring of drug treatments or regimens on specific cellular populations. This would be advantageous in directly observing cell-specific targeted treatments, such as the humanization of many monoclonal antibodies directed at specific cell surface antigens or cell-specific effects of small molecule antagonists. A hope is that in this manner, it will be possible to understand the signaling differences in those that respond from those that do not respond to such treatments, and eventually use this information to predict or tailor treatments.

Clinical Applications

There are several key areas in which phosphoflow™ cytometry can be utilized to identify resistant cellular populations. One major application of the technology has been in its application of pharmacodynamic assays to monitor the effects of targeted kinase inhibitors within specific cellular populations. A second major application is in the use of potentiators to initiate signaling for detection of alteration in understood signaling pathways. This means to use short-term stimulants such as cytokines or growth factors to provoke the cells to reveal its inner network workings and use this information as a differentiating aspect to identify unique cellular populations. Thirdly, the combination of potentiation and pharmacodynamic monitoring can elucidate cellular populations defined by their signaling network status rather than by immunophenotype, yielding a promising potential to identify cell subsets that emerge as resistant populations and are commonly associated with minimum residual disease.

Pharmacodynamic Assays

A variety of pharmacodynamic assays have been developed for phosphoflow™ cytometry to initiate the information gathering that is required for resistant population analysis. Chen et al. utilized phosphoflow™ cytometry to evaluate the phosphorylation of Syk (525/526) in B-cell receptor-mediated survival signal in diffuse large B-cell lymphoma (DLBCL) and identified primary DLBCL that were nonresponsive to BCR signaling and insensitive to R406, a specific Syk inhibitor [20]. This data suggests that phosphoflow™ can be used to monitor patient responsiveness to a Syk inhibitor and provide pharmacodynamic data on drug efficacy. Given the cell-specific nature of the Syk inhibitor, phospho-Syk monitoring in distinct cell subpopulations over time may yield valuable information particularly in autoimmune diseases where Syk can be differentially expressed across cell types [21, 22]. Mortarini et al. utilized phosphoflow™ cytometry to assess STAT activation to IL-2 in T lymphocytes from melanoma patient samples [23]. They found that IL-2 induced STAT1 and STAT5 activation was impaired in T lymphocytes from melanoma patient samples at stage III and IV patients but not that of Stages I and II [23]. A decreasing response to IL-2 induced STAT5 activation in melanoma patients could potentially be early signs of disease progression from Stage II to Stage III, warranting a more aggressive course of action. Dahl et al. report the development of a phospho-CCR5 specific flow cytometric pharmacodynamic assay to assess differential responses to ligands and antagonists in T cell subsets [24]. Extending phospho-CCR5 analysis to HIV patient samples may potentially identify subsets of cells more or less susceptible to infection or a potential predictor of antiretroviral therapy resistance. Clearly, in these examples, longitudinal samples and defined clinical cohorts would be required to make predictive assessments of the assays aforementioned; however, they identify a promising application for phospho-specific flow cytometry as a powerful tool to identify these predictive cellular populations.

What is Normal?

A significant attention has been focused on understanding disease or progression of disease. But do we really know what normal primary cell signaling is? This is a rather important topic given that the majority of our knowledge of signal transduction pathways has been derived from in vitro cell systems or murine models or ex vivo culture adaptations of primary cells. Although these are all important, it is rather difficult to extend these conclusions to primary human systems in the absence of a proper investigation or at least verification. As we have come to appreciate that in mouse and human immunology, signaling proteins and homologous proteins can have different functions [25–27]. A mentor once told me that the "absence of evidence is not evidence of absence." When you apply the phosphoflow™ methodologies to primary cell signaling across donors, a clear picture emerges – "normal" is rather difficult to define. Figure 5.1 displays a lineage tree of immune

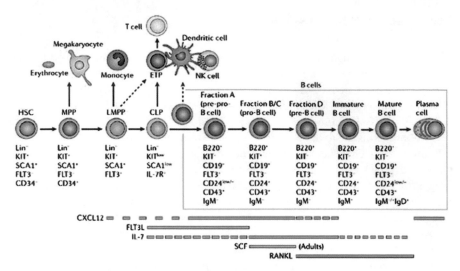

Fig. 5.1 Lineage tree of immune cell development. Hematopoietic stem cells (HSCs) are highly purified as lineage (Lin)⁻B220⁻KIT⁺SCA1⁺ fms-related tyrosine kinase 3 (FLT3)⁻CD34⁻ cells. Lin⁻B220⁻KIT⁺SCA1⁺FLT3⁻CD34⁺ cells are thought to be enriched for nonself-renewing hematopoietic multipotential progenitors (MPPs). Lin⁻B220⁻KIT⁺SCA1⁺FLT3⁺ cells lack erythro-megakaryocytic differentiation potential but retain myeloid-cell, B-cell, and T-cell potential and are termed lymphoid-primed multipotential progenitors (LMPPs). Lin⁻KIT^low^SCA1^low^ interleukin-7 receptor (IL-7R)⁺cells can give rise to B cells and T cells but not myeloid-lineage cells, and are a common lymphoid progenitor (CLP) population. B-cell precursors, consisting of cells that are negative for cell-surface immunoglobulin (Ig) but positive for the B-cell-lineage marker B220 can be divided into four subsets according to their differential expression of a range of cell-surface markers during development. These four subsets are termed fractions A (pre-pro-B cells), B (pro-B cells), and C (pro-B cells), and D (pre-B cells). Immature B cells, which are generated from fraction D cells, exit the bone marrow and reach the spleen, where they mature into peripheral mature B cells and plasma cells. CXC-chemokine ligand 12 (CXCL12) is essential for the generation of pre-pro-B and pro-B cells and for the homing of plasma cells to the bone marrow, but its requirement by LMPPs and CLPs has not been determined. FLT3 ligand (FLT3L) is essential for the generation of CLPs and pre-pro-B cells. IL-7 is essential for the generation of pro-B and pre-B cells but possibly not CLPs or pre-pro-B cells. IL-7 is required for B-cell differentiation potential of CLPs and pre-pro-B cells. Stem-cell factor (SCF) has an essential role in adults from the pro-B-cell stage. Receptor activator of nuclear factor-κB ligand (RANKL) is involved in the generation of pre-B cells and immature B cells. *ETP* early T-cell-lineage progenitor; *NK* natural killer. Reprinted by permission from Macmillan Publishers Ltd.: Nagasawa [58]. Copyright 2006

cell development as we currently understand it. Immune cells are derived from hematopoietic stem cells that undergo a series of cellular differentiation steps that can be identified by surface immunophenotyping. These differentiation steps and expression of the surface markers to detect the stages of development are governed by signal transduction pathways and signaling thresholds [28–32].

When you begin to analyze these distinct compartments in just 20 nondiseased PBMCs from healthy volunteers, there are signaling nodes that present great variability and others that do not present variability under certain stimulatory

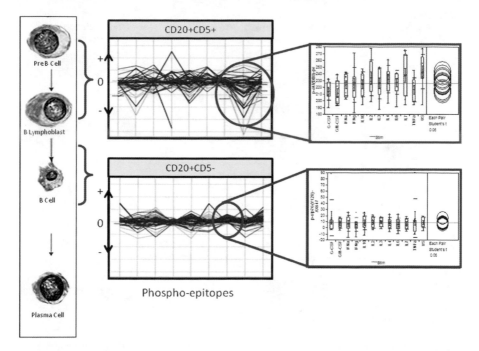

Fig. 5.2 Distinct phosphoprofiles in B-cell subsets. PBMCs from 20 nondiseased individuals were analyzed by phosphoflow™. PBMCs were collected under defined SOPs and stimulated with a broad stimulation panel (GCSF, GMCSF, IFNalpha, IFNgamma, IL-10, IL-2, IL-3, IL-4, IL-6, IL-7, TNFalpha, and vehicle) for 15 min. Cells were gated on CD20 and CD5, and subsequently analyzed for phospho-SLP76(Y128) and phospho-AKT(T308). Data was analyzed in Flowjo for subset determination, exported to SAS for statistical processing of mean fluorescent intensities, then processed in Spotfire software for visual representation of signaling node analysis. B-cell lineage tree (*left*) depicts B-cell developmental stages. *Arrows* indicate what stage of B-cells was analyzed. Phospho-profiles relative to nonstimulated condition is presented as differential line analysis (*middle*). All stimulatory conditions are not presented for visual simplification in the line profile analysis. Expansion of the variability in a particular phospho-signaling node is highlighted (*right*). Whisker plot analysis is displayed, stimulation conditions on the X-axis, phospho-epitope on the Y-axis in mean fluorescent intensity units

conditions (Fig. 5.2). This signaling node variability is cell specific as the immature B cell compartment (CD20+CD5+) exhibits a greater dynamic range in phospho signaling as compared to the mature B cell compartment (CD20+CD5−) within the same PBMC sample. Although standard criteria were employed for healthy donor evaluation, if the PBMC cohorts were expanded, age, gender, over-the-counter medications, or preexisting health conditions could be assessed as potential contributors to the donor heterogeneity. In a disease context, it is interesting to point out that the clonal expansion in chronic lymphatic leukemia (CLL) is the CD20+CD5+ immature B cell compartment [33, 34]. From the nondiseased PBMC profiling, it seems that the signaling heterogeneity in the mature B cell compartment was less variable for a given node across donors than that of the immature B cell

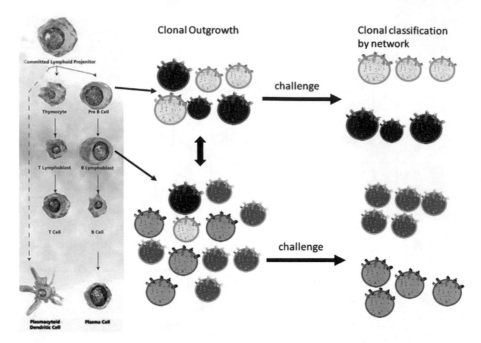

Fig. 5.3 Challenging cells to reveal their inner signaling networks. Illustration depicting the concept of potentiation. Cells are challenged with a variety of conditions to provoke signal processing. Activation of cellular networks stratifies cellular response. Signal-based classification of cell subsets can then be correlated to phenotype or outcome

compartment (Fig. 5.2). The propensity for the immature B cell compartment to be deregulated in a diseased state may be an inherent function of its "plasticity" as the maturation process of B cells results in less signaling heterogeneity when stimulated under defined conditions. The signaling variation appears to follow a theme: young and wild, older and reserved. Importantly, revealing these pathway alterations or signal node potentiation requires cellular provocation with stimulatory or even inhibitory agents. That is to say, using potentiators, cell-based signatures demask themselves (Fig. 5.3). This enables subset stratification based on their signaling profile rather than their phenotype and ultimately, information of which can be integrated with clinical information for correlation to treatment response and outcome. Understanding the developmental pathways of lymphocytes can set a foundation for assessing the potential emergence of resistant populations in diseased states.

Disease States

CML is characterized by the fusion product of BCR and ABL, generating the BCR-ABL protein that leads to uncontrolled cell proliferation and inhibition of cellular apoptotic mechanisms. These deregulated pathways are a driving force for the disease pathogenesis of CML [35]. A targeted tyrosine kinase inhibitor, imatinib mesylate (Gleevac), was one of the first successful targeted therapies developed and is the poster child, if you will, for molecular-targeted therapies because of its great success as first line management for CML [36, 37]. The drug works by binding the active site of the ABL kinase, stabilizing the inactive form of BCR-ABL, and inhibiting phosphorylation and downstream activation. However, over time, subsets of patients have developed resistance to Gleevac as a result of genetic mutations that render the BCR-ABL fusion product less sensitive to Gleevac inhibition. An investigation led by Charles Sawyers and team identified at least 15 mutations in the BCR-ABL gene that caused resistance to Gleevac [38, 39]. Further work assessing mutational status of the BCR-ABL transcript in larger cohorts of resistant populations has identified that many of these acquired mutations do not have anything to do with the drug-binding pocket of Gleevac, but rather affect some tertiary structure or protein confirmation of the BCR-ABL fusion product. The accumulation of these cells that contain these mutated BCR-ABL proteins occurs through a drug selection process where a number of those cells, unaffected by the presence of the drug, grow and survive and ultimately cause relapse. There is a high concordance of Gleevac failure with patient relapse and several of these mutations. The point mutation T315I in the ABL kinase domain appears to confer resistance not only to Gleevac but also to second and third generation drugs [39]. It is worthy to point out that single molecular diagnostics tests cannot detect other mechanisms of drug resistance such as amplification of the BCR-ABL fusion gene. Thus, resistance testing by virtue of cell population analysis may be useful to help guide CML treatment with alternative therapies.

A multiparameter flow cytometric assay can be developed to detect both the total protein content of BCR-ABL as well as the phosphorylation of downstream proteins such as phospho-CRKL and phospho-STAT5. Various groups have developed individual stains for staining BCR-ABL and phospho-CRKL in primary CML cells. Chan et al. have demonstrated that phospho-CRKL flow cytometric staining can be used to monitor phosphorylation pre and posttherapy in CML blasts [40]. Desplat et al. demonstrate that BCR-ABL positive cells can be identified by flow cytometry [41]. Recently, La Rosée reported the phospho-CRKL monitoring of patients with imatinib resistant or intolerant CML or Ph+ ALL treated with nilotinib in an open label dose escalation phase I protocol [42]. This paper demonstrates data supporting serial peripheral blood phospho-CRKL monitoring of patients with treatment as a potential means to establish both effective nilotinib (a secondary BCR-ABL inhibitor) inhibition as well as the potential for detection of BCR-ABL reactivation in nilotinib-resistant patients. With sufficient patient samples, it may be possible to specifically analyze emerging residual leukemic population that correlates with therapy resistance.

Disease Classification Based on Signaling Taxonomy

Acute myeloid leukemia (AML) is a cancer of the blood and bone marrow. AML represents 90% of all adult acute leukemias with an average of 12,000 new cases per year. In AML, common myeloid progenitor stem cells develop abnormally and do not mature into healthy white blood cells. These abnormal cells are called leukemia or blasts. Current methods of diagnosis for AML have been limited to morphological and pathological analysis that has contributed to the inconsistency of disease staging by clinical centers. In the absence of accurate disease staging, treatment decisions become difficult often necessitated multiple rounds of induction therapy. Although advances in treatment paradigms have been reported [43, 44], it is not possible to predict upfront which patients will respond to treatment and when currently treated patients will fail their therapy.

Diagnosis of AML currently suffers from the lack of a standard staging system for accurate classification of the disease. Morphological tests are often used to classify the stages of the disease and therefore suffer from inconsistency and subjectivity across clinical organizations. This makes clinical decisions as to drug treatment difficult and is often attributed to what is referred to as ineffective drug induction, a cycle in which AML patients undergo treatment with drugs until an efficacious drug is found. Given that the majority of the AML population is over 60 years old and that drug discovery efforts have produced nonspecific drugs that only attack rapidly dividing cells and are therefore toxic to many cells in the body, there are large opportunities for development of a molecular-based disease staging system that can facilitate patient treatment and further aid next generation drug discovery efforts.

In 2004, Irish et al. demonstrated that phospho-specific flow cytometric staining is feasible for blood compartment analysis of AML and that it is possible to identify phospho-signatures that correlated with outcome [45]. In this body of work, it was shown that the varied genetic and clinical phenotypes of leukemic tumors are profoundly linked to discernible patterns in phospho-protein signal transduction networks. Leukemic signaling profiles of phospho-protein targets were linked with FLT3 mutations, cytogenetic changes, expression of the cell surface CD15 marker, and response to chemotherapy. With this data, patient-derived signaling phenotypes could be correlated to clinical outcome and resulted in a signal-based methodology for disease classification. Critical to this profiling was the inclusion of the response of signaling networks to environmental cues and not only basal levels of phosphorylation. The observed differences in potential for activation of tumor signaling pathways, combined with the ability to correlate this with clinical outcome, suggested that phospho-specific flow cytometry can be used to predict treatment outcome and the emergence of cellular subsets that were resistant to therapy. Indeed, recent presentations at the American Society of Hematology in 2009 by Nodality Inc., presented data showing that single cell network profiling revealed significant differences in signaling in FLT3 ITD relative to wildtype AML samples across multiple pathways (ASH 2009 poster 1588). Recent work from Nodality Inc. has also demonstrated that intracellular signaling profiles dominant at relapse in AML could be identified in subpopulations of cells present at diagnosis and tested whether intracellular signaling profiles at diagnosis could predict for disease relapse (ASH 2009 poster 397). An "SCF functional signature" was identified and present in early relapse that was undetectable by standard c-kit analysis. These analyses propose that predictive prognostic single network-based signatures can be derived by using phosphoflow™ cytometric analysis.

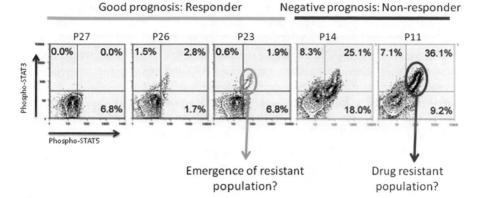

Fig. 5.4 Phosphoflow™ for monitoring drug response and clinical progression. Acute myeloid leukemia patient samples were analyzed by multiparameter phosphoflow™. Different patient responses to GCSF stimulation in CD33+ cells are presented for phospho-STAT3 and phospho-STAT5. Data is from [45]

An exciting discovery from the work by Irish et al. was that when you compared cell-specific signaling of responders vs. nonresponders, a very distinct phospho-defined cell population was present and appeared to expand as a function of disease status (Fig. 5.4). The CD33+ phospho-STAT3/phospho-STAT5 positive induced populations by GCSF stimulation correlated with negative outcome. Granted, the data presented in Fig. 5.4 are not from the exact same patient over time nor are they signaling profiles from longitudinal sampling of the same people. They are in fact different and unrelated individuals, and although no predictive or diagnostic assessment can be made, it did however provide evidence for the possibility of the phosphoflow™ technology to be able to reveal signal-based cell populations that can be linked to treatment response. Moreover, it provided data to begin asking the more complicated questions such as (1) Can we predict patient relapse based on signaling cell populations? (2) Can we utilize such observations to predict who will fail treatment? (3) Can these measurements be used to predict who will fail expensive procedures such as bone marrow transplants? (4) Can this method bring certainty to the uncertainty of the "watch and wait" period so common in myelodysplastic syndromes and other diseases? (5) Can future drug development efforts be aimed at targeting these newly revealed cell populations?

Autoimmune Disease

Multiparameter phosphoflow™ analysis in rheumatoid arthritis (RA) is also yielding novel insights into the current understanding of signal transduction in arthritic lymphocytes. Galligan et al. analyzed PBMCs from healthy, early stage and late stage RA patients and osteoarthritis patients [46]. Fifteen different phospho-epitopes were analyzed in a variety of immune cell compartments. The relative ratio of phospho-AKT to phospho-p38 was observed to correlate with early RA onset [46]. Stratification by drug treatment (anti-TNF inhibitors, steroids, or leflunomide) represented marked reduction in phosphorylation states across cell compartments. Further analysis of the phospho-active cellular subsets identified peripheral blood fibrocytes to correlate with disease severity, suggesting that they could be a potential diagnostic indicator of disease worsening, and if monitored throughout the course of treatment paradigms, a potentially novel source of cells to monitor for RA therapy resistance [47].

From this work, insights to the disturbed signaling of arthritic lymphocytes were observed. For example, it is well established that the p38 kinase is important in arthritic development and has been a target for pharmaceutical development of inhibitory small molecules for the past 15 years [48–50]. Unfortunately, the class of p38 inhibitors has not yielded promising leads for agents that bring benefit to the patient. The development of such agents has encountered unexpected toxicities that many pharmaceutical companies have halted the development of their p38 inhibitor program [51, 52]. Exact reasons why p38 inhibitors have failed as a class are unclear, but it could be due to the molecular redundancies of the p38 kinase family (there are least four isozymes), their ubiquitous presence and function in many cell and tissue compartments in the body, or possibly due to off-target effects of closely related kinases. Despite these shortcomings of the p38 kinase inhibitors, in the phosphoflow™ profiling of PBMCs from RA patients, the ratio of phosphorylated p38 to phosphorylated AKT or phosphorylated JNK was an epitope that was elevated as compared to non-RA and also osteoarthritis samples [46]. Interestingly phospho-STAT3 was also observed to be elevated in certain samples, but more revealing was the concordance between phospho-p38 and phospho-STAT3 double positive cells, a population whose frequency appeared to increase in late state RA samples vs. early RA samples (Fig. 5.5). Again, the data presented in Fig. 5.5 are not from the same patient nor are they longitudinal samples of patients over time or statistically supportive given the cohort sample size. They are in fact distinct and unrelated data sets from the arthritic pool analyzed. However, these observations suggest that if you combined a p38 inhibitor with a STAT3 inhibitor, you could effectively target these cells with doses of a p38 inhibitor that are much lower than the doses needed for the single agent, and hopefully reduce the toxicities that are typically triggered at high doses. Although this is an unconventional approach for classical drug development, the phosphoflow™ approaches can aid in identifying potential drug combinations for the development of multi-targeted therapies that a priori would not have attempted.

Blood as a Surrogate Tissue

An outstanding question for the application of phosphoflow™ cytometry is whether the application can be extended to tissue other than whole blood. It is appreciated that whole blood and peripheral blood mononuclear preparations are easily analyzed

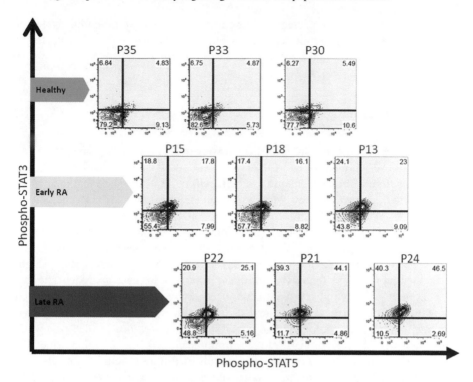

Fig. 5.5 Phosphoflow™ for monitoring emerging signal-based cell populations during disease progression. Early rheumatoid arthritis (early RA) and late rheumatoid arthritis (late RA) patient samples were analyzed by multiparameter phosphoflow™ and compared to nondiseases PBMCs (Healthy). CD3+ T cells were assessed for phospho-p38 and phosphor-STAT3. Percent frequency of populations gated by quadrant is presented. Data is from [46]

using flow cytometry as well as intracellular flow cytometry. However, many of the myeloproliferative diseases, such as AML and CML, initiate their rapid growth of white blood cells in the bone marrow. Sourcing of bone marrow samples for longitudinal sampling, compliance testing, or molecular diagnostics is not as easily obtained vs. whole blood. It would be interesting to compare matched bone marrow and peripheral blood samples under the same potentiated analyses for responsivity of a defined stimulation panel to investigate if blood samples could substitute for bone marrow specimens. The same methodology could be extended to synovial tissue vs. blood for RA, cerebrospinal fluid for CNS diseases, or bronchial lavages for lung or allergy-related disease.

Solid tumors represent a prime opportunity for phosphoflow™ analysis given that many of the targeted therapies developed target pathways intrinsic to solid tumors. A shortcoming of this application is not in the staining methodology but in the sample acquisition protocols and cell preparation procedures. Standard operating protocols for isolation and preservation have not been thoroughly investigated as they have been for blood [9]. This is of particular importance given that tissue biopsy material and subsequent processing can alter the phospho-epitope status of the material. Furthermore, the techniques currently employed to grind up tissue isolates can damage the cell for potentiated cell response assessment.

What to Measure?

It is often remarked that phospho-specific flow cytometric compatible antibodies do not exist for every protein of interest and that one would have to measure an extensive panel before a unique signature can be identified. It is expected that the expansion of multiparameter flow cytometry and the phosphoflow™ technique to simultaneously measure more features per cell, with more upstream stimuli (in isolation or combination), will allow for more relevant mapping of signaling pathways across disease states. While many other approaches for measuring multiple events exist (gene chips, protein chips, microfluidic technologies or high-throughput proteomics), there is a significant difference in these approaches to that of phosphoflow™ cytometry. First, many technologies rely on "averaged" cell populations rather than assessing and differentiation across cellular subsets. At practically every immunological and hematological conference in the last several years, a new cell population of clinical importance is being presented and discussed. Whole blood is comprised of hundreds of different cellular subsets. The "grind them all up" and get an average measurement will never identify cell-specific signatures and will not access compartments such as cancer stem cells that are gaining attention. Second, a static readout of signaling is useful; however, it does not provide a dynamic picture. Ultimately, in the various bodies of work presented in this chapter and others that will be published in the years to come, the data is suggesting that it is the immediate response of signaling networks, at the cell by cell level, that ultimately defines signaling output – whether such output is gene expression or new protein translation. Before we can understand how transcription integrates such signals in normal or diseased cells, we must understand how different cells respond biochemically to stimuli and we must measure these events simultaneously in a fully correlated manner.

Knowledge of intracellular signaling differences among diseases could therefore provide the basis for improved oncogenic and autoimmune classification systems. Importantly, such a classification system would go beyond a simple signature, but could be used to infer mechanism associated with the signature. The work by Irish et al. demonstrated that by surveying phospho-protein responses to cytokine stimulation, in addition to widely studied basal phosphorylation states, we can reveal underlying dysregulated signaling nodes in primary human tumors and enable identification of tumor signaling pathology profiles. It was not necessary to study thousands of phospho-signaling proteins – differences in signaling biology can be revealed by responses of a representative group of signaling nodes to a set of environmental cues when these nodes are queried across a set of diverse tumor networks. Unsupervised clustering of phospho-protein profiles was used to identify patient groups that correlate with prognostic indicators. For AML, these included mutation of the receptor tyrosine kinase FLT3 and resistance to anthracycline containing chemotherapy regimens. This new approach to tumor classification suggests that strategies for therapeutic inhibition of leukemic signal transduction might be effective against tumors with specific phospho-protein biosignatures.

The central hypothesis of these studies was that patients whose tumors share similar mechanisms of signal transduction will respond similarly to a defined tumor cell killing regimen. Underlying this idea is the additional hypothesis that heritable differences among tumors will detectably modify tumor cell signaling networks. Cell enumeration of signaling mechanisms will reveal disease cell heterogeneity and distinguish cell subsets whose presence correlates with disease outcome in oncologies (leukemia and lymphoma) and autoimmune diseases [53]. Grammer et al. have reported application of phospho-epitope assessment in samples from SLE patients and found that SLE samples have elevated levels of internal phosphorylation demonstrating that intracellular signal assessment in patients with autoimmune disease is possible and informative [54]. A long range goal of these projects is to develop a predictive model of clinical outcome based on molecular mechanisms of signaling detected in heterogeneous disease cell populations.

If resources were not limited, disease-specific signaling databases could be constructed and data mined for the development of future drugs or retasking of current drugs. As cell-specific information is obtained from patient populations including the emergence of resistant cell populations in conjunction with drug responsiveness and outcome, pathway-specific virtual drug screening of current targeted therapies may be possible. In this manner, it may be possible to identify novel uses for currently existing drugs. For example, the development of the anti-CD20 monoclonal antibodies to target B cells was originally developed for B-cell lymphomas [55]. However, it was surprising to discover their efficacy in RA patients, a presumed T cell-specific disease [56]. In a similar manner, statin drugs, routinely used for lowering cholesterol, have been discovered to have effects on the TH1 and TH2 lymphocyte development, making them attractive for use in autoimmune diseases such as multiple sclerosis [57]. In the age of cloud computing, flow cytometers around the world may be able to upload cellular analyses for data mining and biomarker discovery. There may one day be a way to match specific drugs or combination of drugs to target resistant cell populations based on a signature profile as a novel way to bring together the personal medicine field with the drug development world.

References

1. Krug M, Hilgeroth A. Recent advances in the development of multi-kinase inhibitors. Mini Rev Med Chem. 2008;8(13):1312–27.
2. Gutierrez ME, Kummar S, Giaccone G. Next generation oncology drug development: opportunities and challenges. Nat Rev Clin Oncol. 2009;6(5):259–65.

3. Rossi A et al. Recent developments of targeted therapies in the treatment of non-small cell lung cancer. Curr Drug Discov Technol. 2009;6(2):91–102.

4. Hersey P et al. Small molecules and targeted therapies in distant metastatic disease. Ann Oncol. 2009;20 Suppl 6:vi35–40.

5. Paietta E et al. Differential expression of terminal transferase (TdT) in acute lymphocytic leukaemia expressing myeloid antigens and TdT positive acute myeloid leukaemia as compared to myeloid antigen negative acute lymphocytic leukaemia. Br J Haematol. 1993;84(3):416–22.

6. Drach J, Gattringer C, Huber H. Combined flow cytometric assessment of cell surface antigens and nuclear TdT for the detection of minimal residual disease in acute leukaemia. Br J Haematol. 1991;77(1):37–42.

7. Perez OD, Nolan GP. Simultaneous measurement of multiple active kinase states using polychromatic flow cytometry. Nat Biotechnol. 2002;20(2):155–62.

8. Perez OD, et al. Multiparameter analysis of intracellular phosphoepitopes in immunophenotyped cell populations by flow cytometry. Curr Protoc Cytom. 2005;Chapter 6:Unit 6.20.

9. Perez OD, Krutzik PO, Nolan GP. Flow cytometric analysis of kinase signaling cascades. Methods Mol Biol. 2004;263:67–94.

10. Krutzik PO et al. Analysis of protein phosphorylation and cellular signaling events by flow cytometry: techniques and clinical applications. Clin Immunol. 2004;110(3):206–21.

11. Krutzik PO et al. High-content single-cell drug screening with phosphospecific flow cytometry. Nat Chem Biol. 2008;4(2):132–42.

12. Perez OD, Nolan GP. Phospho-proteomic immune analysis by flow cytometry: from mechanism to translational medicine at the single-cell level. Immunol Rev. 2006;210:208–28.

13. Perez OD, Mitchell D, Nolan GP. Differential role of ICAM ligands in determination of human memory T cell differentiation. BMC Immunol. 2007;8:2.

14. Perez OD et al. Leukocyte functional antigen 1 lowers T cell activation thresholds and signaling through cytohesin-1 and Jun-activating binding protein 1. Nat Immunol. 2003;4(11):1083–92.

15. Shachaf CM et al. Inhibition of HMGcoA reductase by atorvastatin prevents and reverses MYC-induced lymphomagenesis. Blood. 2007;110(7):2674–84.

16. Hale MB et al. Stage dependent aberrant regulation of cytokine-STAT signaling in murine systemic lupus erythematosus. PLoS One. 2009;4(8):e6756.

17. O'Gorman WE et al. The initial phase of an immune response functions to activate regulatory T cells. J Immunol. 2009;183(1):332–9.

18. Lee AW et al. Single-cell, phosphoepitope-specific analysis demonstrates cell type- and pathway-specific dysregulation of Jak/STAT and MAPK signaling associated with in vivo human immunodeficiency virus type 1 infection. J Virol. 2008;82(7):3702–12.

19. Krutzik PO, Hale MB, Nolan GP. Characterization of the murine immunological signaling network with phosphospecific flow cytometry. J Immunol. 2005;175(4):2366–73.

20. Chen L et al. SYK-dependent tonic B-cell receptor signaling is a rational treatment target in diffuse large B-cell lymphoma. Blood. 2008;111(4):2230–7.

21. Irish JM et al. Kinetics of B cell receptor signaling in human B cell subsets mapped by phosphospecific flow cytometry. J Immunol. 2006;177(3):1581–9.

22. Irish JM et al. Altered B-cell receptor signaling kinetics distinguish human follicular lymphoma B cells from tumor-infiltrating nonmalignant B cells. Blood. 2006;108(9):3135–42.

23. Mortarini R et al. Impaired STAT phosphorylation in T cells from melanoma patients in response to IL-2: association with clinical stage. Clin Cancer Res. 2009;15(12):4085–94.

24. Dahl ME et al. A novel CCR5-specific pharmacodynamic assay in whole blood using phosphoflow cytometry highlights different ligand-dependent responses but similar properties of antagonists in CD8+ and CD4+ T lymphocytes. J Pharmacol Exp Ther. 2008;327(3):926–33.

25. Mestas J, Hughes CC. Of mice and not men: differences between mouse and human immunology. J Immunol. 2004;172(5):2731–8.

26. Buclin T, Spertini F. Type 1 IFNs in human versus mouse. Nat Immunol. 2000;1(4):265.

27. Miggin SM, Kinsella BT. Investigation of the mechanisms of G protein: effector coupling by the human and mouse prostacyclin receptors. Identification of critical species-dependent differences. J Biol Chem. 2002;277(30):27053–64.

28. Soderberg SS, Karlsson G, Karlsson S. Complex and context dependent regulation of hematopoiesis by TGF-beta superfamily signaling. Ann N Y Acad Sci. 2009;1176:55–69.
29. Shizuru JA, Negrin RS, Weissman IL. Hematopoietic stem and progenitor cells: clinical and preclinical regeneration of the hematolymphoid system. Annu Rev Med. 2005;56:509–38.
30. Weissman IL. Developmental switches in the immune system. Cell. 1994;76(2):207–18.
31. Domen J, Weissman IL. Hematopoietic stem cells need two signals to prevent apoptosis; BCL-2 can provide one of these. Kitl/c-Kit signaling the other. J Exp Med. 2000;192(12):1707–18.
32. Kondo M et al. Lymphocyte development from hematopoietic stem cells. Curr Opin Genet Dev. 2001;11(5):520–6.
33. Herishanu Y, Polliack A. Chronic lymphocytic leukemia: a review of some new aspects of the biology, factors influencing prognosis and therapeutic options. Transfus Apher Sci. 2005; 32(1):85–97.
34. Dunphy CH. Comprehensive review of adult acute myelogenous leukemia: cytomorphological, enzyme cytochemical, flow cytometric immunophenotypic, and cytogenetic findings. J Clin Lab Anal. 1999;13(1):19–26.
35. Van Etten RA. Mechanisms of transformation by the BCR-ABL oncogene: new perspectives in the post-imatinib era. Leuk Res. 2004;28 Suppl 1:S21–8.
36. Hochhaus A. First-Line management of CML: a state of the art review. J Natl Compr Canc Netw. 2008;6 Suppl 2:S1–10.
37. Hughes T et al. Monitoring CML patients responding to treatment with tyrosine kinase inhibitors: review and recommendations for harmonizing current methodology for detecting BCR-ABL transcripts and kinase domain mutations and for expressing results. Blood. 2006; 108(1):28–37.
38. Shah NP et al. Multiple BCR-ABL kinase domain mutations confer polyclonal resistance to the tyrosine kinase inhibitor imatinib (STI571) in chronic phase and blast crisis chronic myeloid leukemia. Cancer Cell. 2002;2(2):117–25.
39. Gorre ME et al. Clinical resistance to STI-571 cancer therapy caused by BCR-ABL gene mutation or amplification. Science. 2001;293(5531):876–80.
40. Chan HE et al. Monitoring cell signaling pathways by quantitative flow cytometry. Methods Mol Biol. 2007;378:83–90.
41. Desplat V et al. Rapid detection of phosphotyrosine proteins by flow cytometric analysis in Bcr-Abl-positive cells. Cytometry A. 2004;62(1):35–45.
42. La Rosee P et al. Phospho-CRKL monitoring for the assessment of BCR-ABL activity in imatinib-resistant chronic myeloid leukemia or Ph+ acute lymphoblastic leukemia patients treated with nilotinib. Haematologica. 2008;93(5):765–9.
43. Kuendgen A, Germing U. Emerging treatment strategies for acute myeloid leukemia (AML) in the elderly. Cancer Treat Rev. 2009;35(2):97–120.
44. Fathi AT, Grant S, Karp JE. Exploiting cellular pathways to develop new treatment strategies for AML. Cancer Treat Rev. 2010;36(2):142–50.
45. Irish JM et al. Single cell profiling of potentiated phospho-protein networks in cancer cells. Cell. 2004;118(2):217–28.
46. Galligan CL et al. Multiparameter phospho-flow analysis of lymphocytes in early rheumatoid arthritis: implications for diagnosis and monitoring drug therapy. PLoS One. 2009;4(8):e6703.
47. Galligan CL et al. Fibrocyte activation in rheumatoid arthritis. Rheumatology (Oxford). 2010;49:640–51.
48. Pargellis C, Regan J. Inhibitors of p38 mitogen-activated protein kinase for the treatment of rheumatoid arthritis. Curr Opin Investig Drugs. 2003;4(5):566–71.
49. Campbell J et al. A novel mechanism for TNF-alpha regulation by p38 MAPK: involvement of NF-kappa B with implications for therapy in rheumatoid arthritis. J Immunol. 2004;173(11):6928–37.
50. Redman AM et al. p38 kinase inhibitors for the treatment of arthritis and osteoporosis: thienyl, furyl, and pyrrolyl ureas. Bioorg Med Chem Lett. 2001;11(1):9–12.
51. Noel JK et al. Systematic review to establish the safety profiles for direct and indirect inhibitors of p38 mitogen-activated protein kinases for treatment of cancer. A systematic review of the literature. Med Oncol. 2008;25(3):323–30.

52. Dominguez C, Powers DA, Tamayo N. p38 MAP kinase inhibitors: many are made, but few are chosen. Curr Opin Drug Discov Devel. 2005;8(4):421–30.
53. Perez OD. Appreciating the heterogeneity in autoimmune disease: multiparameter assessment of intracellular signaling mechanisms. Ann N Y Acad Sci. 2005;1062:155–64.
54. Grammer AC et al. Flow cytometric assessment of the signaling status of human B lymphocytes from normal and autoimmune individuals. Arthritis Res Ther. 2004;6(1):28–38.
55. Molina A. A decade of rituximab: improving survival outcomes in non-Hodgkin's lymphoma. Annu Rev Med. 2008;59:237–50.
56. Boumans MJ, Tak PP. Rituximab treatment in rheumatoid arthritis: how does it work? Arthritis Res Ther. 2009;11(6):134.
57. Peng X et al. Immunomodulatory effects of 3-hydroxy-3-methylglutaryl coenzyme-A reductase inhibitors, potential therapy for relapsing remitting multiple sclerosis. J Neuroimmunol. 2006;178(1–2):130–9.
58. Nagasawa T. Microenvironmental niches in the bone marrow required for B-cell development. Nat Rev Immunol. 2006;6(2):107–16.

Chapter 6
Mathematical and Computational Models in Cancer

Sudhir Chowbina, Kevin A. Janes, Shayn M. Peirce, and Jason A. Papin

Keywords Mathematical modeling • Cancer cell signaling • Computation • Metastasis • Multiscale modeling

Introduction

Signal transduction is the process by which cells internally transmit molecular information to respond to changes in their environment [1]. Aberrant cell signaling leads to a variety of diseases such as autoimmunity, diabetes, and cancer. Indeed, deregulated cell signaling underpins all of the "hallmarks" of cancer: (a) self-sufficiency in growth signals; (b) insensitivity to antigrowth signals; (c) evading apoptosis; (d) limitless replicative potential; (e) sustained angiogenesis; and (f) tissue invasion and metastasis [2]. As these hallmarks and others emphasize [3], cancer progression is not just a function of signaling pathways that interact within a single cell, but rather a multiscale problem in which multiple pathways, cells, and tissues play roles in the evolution of the disease [4, 5]. At the subcellular scale, interlinked signaling pathways control cell cycle progression and apoptosis [6]. Feedback loops and compartmentalization of signals generates a tremendous amount of complexity. These subcellular processes lead to multicellular interactions as tumor and host cells interact and support cell proliferation in the tissue. At the macroscopic scale, angiogenesis [7] becomes critical for the continued growth of a tumor and the progression to malignancy [7]. Tumorigenesis requires multiple perturbations at all of these interconnected levels. Because of this complexity, systems approaches become increasingly valuable to tackle such questions as: How do signaling networks disrupt cellular behaviors that promote tumorigenesis?

J.A. Papin (✉)
Department of Biomedical Engineering, University of Virginia,
Charlottesville, VA, USA
e-mail: papin@virginia.edu

D. Gioeli (ed.), *Targeted Therapies: Mechanisms of Resistance*,
Molecular and Translational Medicine, DOI 10.1007/978-1-60761-478-4_6,
© Springer Science+Business Media, LLC 2011

How does the complex interplay between cellular- and tissue-scale dynamics induce invasion and metastasis? What are the molecular determinants that control how cancer cells and tumors will respond to targeted therapies?

A key component of the systems approach is the integration of quantitative experiments with computational modeling. The computational model provides a simplified mathematical description of a complex biological process. It is important to stress this definition of a model in the context of cancer biology because our knowledge of the molecular mechanisms is limited. However, even the known mechanisms of tumorigenesis are complex and intertwined such that computational models can still be valuable to keep track of more variables than we can by intuition. Given that a computational model of cancer will always be an approximation, the question is whether a model's simplification is good enough to make useful predictions that can guide new experiments. Often, new experiments are suggested by predictions from the model. The results from these experiments will support or refute the model prediction, leading to model refinement and new predictions. The iterations of model prediction and testing facilitate experimental design, enable a succinct integration of hypotheses for a given system, and can help to quantify system-level properties of a biological system. Usually, effective interplay between modeling and experiments requires multidisciplinary teams with expertise in physics, molecular biology, computer science, and engineering [8]. However, young scientists trained at this interface can effectively span different disciplines and pursue quantitative systems' questions individually or in small collaborations [9, 10].

In this chapter, we provide an overview of computational models (see Tables 6.1–6.3) [11–22] that have been developed to interrogate cell signaling at the intracellular pathway, whole-cell, and tissue levels (see Fig. 6.1). We focus on insights uniquely afforded by the computational analysis and relate these findings to their therapeutic impact whenever possible. We conclude with comments on future challenges and opportunities that systems biology may face and offer as its application to cancer is expanded.

Table 6.1 Examples of pathway-level models

Biological process	Modeling method	Model focus	References
DNA mutation	Discrete Wright–Fisher process	Somatic evolution of colon cancer	Beerenwinkel et al. [25]
	Differential equations	Reaction kinetics of RAS mutants	Stites et al. [37]
DNA repair	Stochastic/probabilistic approaches	Progression of cell cycle and DNA mismatch repair	Kinsella [33]
Signal transduction and cell cycle	Differential equations	Regulation of apoptosis	Albeck et al. [46]
	Differential equation	The effect of the VEGF-Bcl-2-CXCL8 pathway on tumor progression	Jain and Nor [84]
	Differential equations	The effects of CDK inhibitors	Chassagnole et al. [41]

Table 6.2 Examples of cell-level models

Biological process	Modeling method	Model focus	References
Cell invasion	Cellular automata	The effect of blood flow and variability of red blood cells on cancer cell growth	Alarcon et al. [16]
		Early tumor invasion	Patel et al. [17]
	Cellular potts model coupled with a continuous model	The role of matrix metalloproteinases (MMPs) in cell invasion	Giverso et al. [18]
Cell proliferation	Agent-based model	The cellular patterns arising from cell microenvironment interactions	Mansury et al. [19]
	Partial differential equations	Proliferation and invasion of glioma cells	Szeto et al. [20]
Cell migration	Hybrid partial differential equations and agent-based model	The influence of microenvironment on cell motility	Chen et al. [21] and Walker et al. [22]

Table 6.3 Examples of tissue-level models

Biological process	Modeling method	Model focus	References
Avascular tumor	Partial differential equations	Dimensions of quiescent and necrotic regions of avascular tumors.	Kiran et al. [11]
	Reaction-diffusion model	Nutrient levels and avascular tumor morphology	Ferreira et al. [12]
	Ordinary differential equations	Tumor growth rate and p53 mutation status	Levine et al. [13]
Vascular tumor growth and angiogenesis	Ordinary differential equations	Angiogenesis and the interactions between VEGF receptor and neuropilins	Mac Gabhann and Popel [14]
	Agent-based modeling	Cell proliferative behaviors and microvasculature growth patterns	Peirce et al. [15]

Modeling of Intracellular Processes

Cancer arises from the progressive accumulation of mutations in genes over decades [6]. Mathematical modeling can provide a systematic framework to understand how cancer develops as a result of a slow accumulation of many mutations. One of the earliest examples of cancer modeling was concerned with the hereditary and spontaneous forms of retinoblastoma. Knudson showed that retinoblastoma prevalence and latency was most consistent with a "two-hit" statistical model of carcinogenesis, where two key mutational events were required for tumor formation [23]. The eventual cloning and characterization of the Rb tumor suppressor [24] ultimately validated the model's prediction, as both *RB* alleles must be disrupted for tumors to arise.

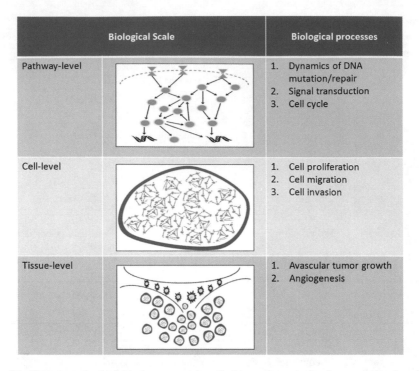

Biological Scale		Biological processes
Pathway-level		1. Dynamics of DNA mutation/repair 2. Signal transduction 3. Cell cycle
Cell-level		1. Cell proliferation 2. Cell migration 3. Cell invasion
Tissue-level		1. Avascular tumor growth 2. Angiogenesis

Fig. 6.1 Representative biological processes described in mathematical and computational models

More recently, Beerenwinkel et al. modeled the intermediate progression of colon adenocarcinoma from 10^6 cells to 10^9 cells simulated over a period of 20 years [25]. A mathematical approach that captures genetic drift in a finite population, called the Wright–Fisher model [26], was used to relate the selective advantage that a mutation confers to the number of cells in a population. The authors analyzed cancer progression as a function of cell population size, the per-gene mutation rate, and the average selective advantage per mutation with the aim of understanding various evolutionary forces on cancer progression. The model suggested that individual mutations only confer a mild selective advantage (~1%) to explain the genetic diversity of tumors sequenced experimentally [27]. This analysis could conceivably be applied to relapsed drug-resistant tumors to gain an estimate of the selective pressures that act on cancer cells upon the addition of targeted anticancer therapies.

The prediction of drug responses or mechanisms of drug resistance is also enabled by mathematical modeling of DNA damage and repair. For example, the status of genetic mutations in the genes *BRCA1*, *BRCA2* [28], *TP53* [29], and *PTEN* [30] significantly affect prognosis and likelihood of adverse reactions to certain therapies in breast cancer. Enderling et al. developed differential equation models representative of breast tumor growth and invasion as a function of mutational status and in the context of breast stem cells [31]. This model enabled a prediction of the relationship between cells that become cancerous and the development stage of the individual (pre- and postpuberty). A rationale for localized radiotherapy was also suggested based on the modeling results.

In normal cells, the accumulation of genetic mutations is inhibited by DNA repair pathways. Mutational deactivation of DNA repair genes is a key aspect of many cancers and leads to genomic instability [32]. DNA repair pathways also influence the efficacy of chemotherapeutics that target DNA replication [33, 34]. Kinsella and coworkers built a computational model to optimize chemotherapy and ionizing radiation (IR) regimens for cancer cells deficient in DNA mismatch repair (MMR) [33, 35, 36]. IR rapidly stops cells from cycling, but chemotherapies such as 5-iododeoxyuridine must be incorporated during DNA synthesis to be effective. A validated computational model could therefore be useful for exploring different treatment protocols to identify one that is cytotoxic for MMR-deficient tumors and tolerated by normal cells with intact DNA repair pathways.

In addition to defects in DNA repair signaling, cancer is also stereotyped by chronic proliferative signaling [2]. One very common oncogene that is strongly linked with proliferation is the small G protein, Ras. Stites et al. built a computational model of Ras activation by guanine exchange factors (GEFs) and Ras inactivation by GTPase activating proteins (GAPs) [37]. The authors used biochemical parameters derived from the literature to construct the model and then challenged it to predict the outcome of Ras mutations that are commonly observed in human tumors. One key observation was that the insensitivity of the mutant Ras allele to the available pool of GAPs could lead to a competitive inhibition of GAP activity on wild-type Ras alleles, thus leading to a further increase in total Ras activation. The authors performed experiments to measure wild-type Ras signal (Ras bound to GTP) and detected an increase in wild-type Ras-bound GTP in cells that also had a mutant Ras allele. They used this model to compare cells with and without various Ras mutations and the model found that drug strategies that target wild-type and mutant Ras-GTP equally may preferentially target cells with an oncogenic Ras mutation.

Mutations in cell division control genes enable cancer cells to evade signals which start and stop the cell cycle [38], and this has been modeled extensively [39]. Each stage of the cell cycle is comprised of multiple signals that coordinate the transition between the different phases of the cell cycle. For example, Qu et al. formulated a model for regulation of the G1-to-S transition. The network controlling the transition from G1-to-S was systematically analyzed with a collection of signaling modules described by differential equations. The importance of multisite phosphorylation for bistability and oscillation within the G1-to-S transition was characterized [40].

Cell-cycle models have also had an impact on drug discovery efforts. Chassagnole et al. used mathematical modeling to simulate and characterize the effect of multitarget kinase inhibitors of CDKs (cyclin dependent kinases). The cytotoxicity of a set of kinase inhibitors based on the in vitro IC_{50} measurement values was simulated. The authors assessed the pharmaceutical value of these inhibitors as anticancer therapeutics [41].

Another key signaling circuit that is often disrupted during cancer is apoptosis [42]. Various groups have modeled the signaling pathways that control programmed cell death in different contexts [43–45]. One particularly interesting result stemmed from the analysis of Albeck et al. [46] toward cytokine-induced apoptosis. A validated computational model [46] enabled the authors to identify perturbations in key inhibitors of apoptosis (IAP) proteins that would disrupt the apoptosis-survival "switch." When treated with apoptotic stimuli, IAP-disrupted cancer cells partially began to execute an apoptotic program, but many did not finish dying and instead survived in a "half dead" state. These damaged-but-viable cells could give rise to genomic instability and revealed an IAP phenotype that would have been otherwise overlooked without the aid of a computational model (Table 6.1).

Modeling at the Whole-Cell Level

Deregulated intracellular pathways lead to changes in the behavior of individual cancer cells. However, solid tumors are a heterogeneous collection of cells with dramatically different capacities to proliferate, stimulate host responses, and metastasize [47, 48]. The cell behavior and dynamics of tumor populations and subpopulations thus represents another scale at which computational models can contribute.

Early cancers arise from a cell of origin and the developing tumor mass can be reasonably approximated as a spheroid. Stein et. al employed a continuum-modeling approach to the growth pattern and dispersion of glioblastoma "spheroids" [49]. Model predictions were partially validated experimentally as different tumor cell lines with different genetic backgrounds showed different dispersion rates. To capture intratumor heterogeneity, a multiscale model was recently developed to characterize the necrotic regions of vascularized tumors [50]. This model accounted for the effects of glucose, oxygen, and pH changes to predict the size and metabolism of the necrotic core of EMT6/Ro spheroids in mouse mammary carcinoma cells.

Computational modeling of very early tumors can help to bridge the gap between the first cell-transformation event and a full-blown tumor that is diagnosed clinically. Mansury et. al developed an agent-based model of tumor cells that captured microscopic and multicellular patterns of cell–cell and cell microenvironment interactions in early avascular glioblastoma multiforme (GBM). These analyses suggested that invasiveness was the critical factor in spatial expansion of the tumor rather than the proliferative cell phenotype [19]. A major challenge with these models, however, is the general lack of clinical data on cancers that are below the current diagnostic sensitivity.

For more advanced cancers, cell migration and invasion become increasingly important as the tumor builds the capacity to metastasize. Models have been developed which aim to simulate the migratory and invasive properties of the cell to understand cancer progression [51]. For example, in ovarian cancer, a Cellular Potts model (grid-based 3D multiscale mathematical model) was used to simulate transmesothelial migration [18]. The results demonstrated agreement with experiments indicating that transmesothelial migration is regulated by the crosstalk between cell–cell and cell–matrix adhesion molecules such as matrix metalloproteinases (MMPs).

In the case of brain cancer, Szeto et al. built a reaction-diffusion model to assess glioma tumors in situ [20]. They combined their efforts with advanced imaging techniques to extract key cellular rates of proliferation and invasion given the measured hypoxic volume of the tumor. Computational modeling can thus be combined with state-of-the-art measurement technologies to extract additional information from tumor observations.

A critical component of cancer cell invasion is deregulated cell motility, and cell migration is an area where much computational work has been done [52]. An agent-based model of cancer cell migration within a tumor microenvironment can yield insights into underlying factors of cell migration [21]. This model incorporated three factors: chemoattraction, haptotactic permission, and biomechanical resistance, known to influence cell migration. By varying these three parameters, Chen et al. characterized the net migration landscape of the modeled tumor. The authors quantified the role of these parameters in increasing the effectiveness of cell migration, which could prioritize which cellular behaviors would be most effective to target in the design of new therapies. This work provides a clear example of how multiple cell-level parameters, which would be difficult to keep track of simultaneously in a developing tumor, can readily be incorporated in a computational framework (Table 6.2).

Modeling Cancer at the Tissue Level

Elucidating the inherent and intricate behavior of tumor growth is a major challenge in tumor biology. Mathematical and computational modeling has been adopted to understand tumor proliferation and invasive growth patterns at different phases of avascular tumor growth [11, 53–55]. Levine et al. published a mathematical model which predicted the onset of avascular tumor growth among cells with a p53 mutation as a function of cell population density. This model was comprised of ordinary differential equations that described a tumor cell population in its microenvironment accounting for the kinetics of cell metabolism. Additional simulations showed that a p53 mutation with strong intensity or occurring over a long duration or involving large number of cells leads to aberrant and uncontrolled avascular tumor growth [13]. In an effort to describe tumor morphology after onset of an avascular tumor, a reaction-diffusion growth model was developed by Ferreira et al. The model was capable of reproducing primary avascular tumor morphologies. The model incorporated mathematical expressions for proliferating and dying cells with nutrient diffusion constraints to indicate that papillary tumor morphology was caused by a competition for nutrients between normal and cancer cells [12]. These two models captured the onset of an avascular tumor and the subsequent changes in morphology as a function of nutrient constraints.

Nutrient starvation induces a "switch" in tumors that promotes the recruitment of a dedicated blood supply [56]. This complex process in which existing microvessels generate new blood vessels is called angiogenesis. This vessel growth results in the delivery of additional nutrients and oxygen to the hypoxic cells, thereby feeding a tumor that otherwise would be largely necrotic. Angiogenesis occurs as a function of a complex interplay between proliferation, migration, cell–cell adhesion and various biochemical signals. Models capturing this process fall into two broad categories: cell-based discrete models and continuum models [57, 58].

In order to understand the temporal transition between avascular and vascular tumor growth, Hogea et al. developed a computational model using partial differential equations (PDEs). The model accounted for interactions between the tumor and its surrounding tissue. Based on the nutrient levels, the model predicted the transition from the avascular to vascular phase, and it highlighted the differences in tumor boundaries in different vascularization regimes [59].

Mac Gabhann and Popel developed a computational model that included VEGF, its receptors, and neuropilin-1, a nonsignaling coreceptor for VEGF, with the aim of describing the function of VEGF receptors in angiogenesis under the influence of various stimuli. The model was used to evaluate three different treatment strategies in which VEGF signaling is inhibited via neuropilin manipulation: (1) blockade of neuropilin-1 expression, (2) inhibition of VEGF-neuropilin-1 binding, and (3) inhibition of VEGF-R/neuropilin-1 coupling. Specifically, the model predicted that blocking VEGF-R/neuropilin coupling could be the most effective therapeutic strategy. Thus, the model assisted in the design of experimental studies and specific therapies [14].

Recently experiments have provided support for the importance of vasculogenesis in tumor vascularization [60]. In short, vasculogenesis is the development of new blood vessels where none exist and angiogenesis is the formation of new vessels as sprouts from existing vessels. Komarov et. al developed an ODE-based model to test the hypothesis that angiogenesis-driven development of tumors is distinct from vasculogenesis-driven tumor development. The model predicted the growth of tumor mass and the level of endothelial progenitor cells (EPCs) as a function of the two vascularization mechanisms. The authors demonstrated that when a tumor growth is supported by angiogenesis, its mass grows as a function of time cubed (t^3). In contrast, if the tumor growth is supported through vasculogenesis, then tumors grow as a linear function of time. Further experiments were proposed to help discriminate between angiogenesis and vasculogenesis as drivers of tumor development [61]. Such models can be extended further to investigate possible therapeutic strategies that target specific endothelial cell populations, growth factors, and other components specific to angiogenic and vaculogenic mechanisms [62].

Tumor angiogenesis is initiated by activated endothelial cells that migrate from the locally permeabilized vasculature [56]. Discrete modeling approaches, such as agent-based modeling (ABM), are well suited to tracking the behavior of these individual cells at the tissue level. ABMs integrate simple sets of rules to investigate high-level patterns emerging from cell–cell interactions and tumor microenvironment interactions [63, 64]. Angiogenesis has been modeled to study the impact of growth factors on microvascular remodeling. Peirce et al. built an ABM to predict microvascular network remodeling in response to VEGF. The ABM enabled the characterization of a functional module of different growth signals and cell–cell contact signals responsible for the vascular growth [15]. As another example, Athale et al. modeled the effects of EGFR protein expression and cell interactions as an ABM and predicted that cell proliferation and migration phenotypes of brain cancer cells can be discerned solely as a function of the activity of EGFR [65]. These examples illustrate the predictive power of cell-level models as tools for identifying key growth factors driving tissue-level phenomena and consequently as a means for predicting viable drug targets (Table 6.3).

Integrating Across Scales

Multiscale analyses integrate models across spatial and temporal scales [15, 66, 67]. These models typically describe global phenotypes (e.g., angiogenesis in response to low oxygen) as functions of intracellular pathway activity (e.g., activation of a transcription factor). The integration of molecular level processes that coordinate feedback and drive tissue-level physiology may be powerful tools to unravel the dynamics of tumor formation and may help to identify drug targets that could have an effect on tumor physiology.

While mathematical models at subcellular, cellular, and tissue scales can provide mechanistic detail and generate insight into the underlying biological process, a key goal of systems-based approaches involves integrating across these spatial and temporal scales. Some cell variables must be treated continuously and other variables need to be represented discretely. Therefore, the development of "multiscale" models, which capture molecular-, cellular-, and tissue-level processes, is an active area of research. Models which integrate agent-based models with PDEs or other continuous approaches, for example, may provide insight into complex properties of biological systems [68].

There have been recent developments of multiscale modeling that are used to analyze avascular multicellular tumors [69, 70]. Jiang et. al developed a model which accounted for proliferation, adhesion, viability, nutrients, waste, as well as growth promoter and inhibitor concentrations. This multiscale model used Monte Carlo methods, Boolean networks, and reaction-diffusion equations to model avascular tumor growth at cellular, subcellular, and extracellular scales, respectively. The model simulations agreed with in vitro observations of morphology, size, and cell cycle stage over a 20 day period [69]. Moreover, the authors' model allowed them to predict the required effective diffusivity of promoters and inhibitors of proliferation that were compatible with experimental observations. One could envision how this model could be revised to include the effect of targeted proliferation inhibitors that have larger effective diffusivities, such as small-molecule drugs.

Multiscale modeling has also been used to study tumor evolution toward invasion and metastasis. Anderson et al. built a hybrid model that combined: (1) PDEs for oxygen diffusion and extracellular matrix proteins, (2) ABMs for single cell behaviors in the evolving tumor, and (3) an iterative mutation step that changed each cell's behavioral traits over time depending on the local microenvironment [71].

The model predicted that harsher microenvironmental conditions would lead to the evolution of more-aggressive cancers, because of the selection for a small number of invasive clones in the overall tumor. Conversely, conditions that more uniformly favored the growth of all cancer cells led to tumors with more benign morphologies and cleaner tumor margins. These types of models could become increasingly relevant as our ability to measure the tumor microenvironment improves.

The Role of Mathematical Modeling in the Development of Therapeutic Strategies

There is evidence that tumor growth can be inhibited [72, 73] or accelerated [74, 75] by targeted drugs, but identifying appropriate biomarkers is vital for assessing the efficacy of such therapeutics [76]. As an example, the activation of alternative proangiogenic pathways in response to antiangiogenic agents may play a role in the development of resistance to such therapeutic strategies [77]. Antiangiogenic agents, for example, are known to cause a reduction in tumor vessel permeability and interstitial fluid pressure resulting in vessel normalization. Mathematical models using transport equations have been used to understand how the transport properties of vessel walls influence tumor interstitial fluid pressure and interstitial fluid velocity [78]. The authors concluded that vascular normalization could be achieved by blocking different forms of VEGF receptors. Therefore, the identification of potential biomarkers and the evaluation of alternative drug targets in response to resistance represent areas in which mathematical models may play an important role in the development of therapeutic strategies.

As mentioned, acquired resistance is one reason for the failure of anticancer therapy. This resistance can be reduced by optimizing drug dosage regimes, an area in which mathematical modeling can also play a key role [79]. Pharmacokinetic models that simulate the distribution of anticancer drugs [80] can also help evaluate the effectiveness of combination therapies [81]. A mathematical and computational modeling strategy to understand the interaction between the microenvironment and cancer cells enabling quantitative predictions of which pathways are disrupted due to therapies [82] may also be very valuable to overcome challenges in the effective implementation of anticancer therapies.

Concluding Remarks

Although many of the fundamental biochemical reactions and cellular properties contributing to cancer have been well described, there is an increasing appreciation for the interconnectivity, complexity, and heterogeneity of the underlying biology, necessitating new approaches to integrate and analyze vast collections of data. As mathematical and computational modeling efforts begin to capture many of the fundamental hallmarks of cancer, such analyses may facilitate in the prevention, diagnosis, and treatment of this complex disease.

A mathematical and computational model can provide a new perspective on a biological system of interest and help to generate testable predictions. For example, as the dynamics of a cancer cell in its tissue context and in consideration of its underlying signaling pathways are captured and quantitatively analyzed by mathematical models, predictions can be made regarding mechanisms of resistance and ideal drug targets, which can then be pursued experimentally. Therefore, mathematical models may be important in the development of targeted therapies [83]. Furthermore, computational models may be effective in enabling the exploration of complex parameters (e.g., varying adhesion forces between cells or membrane permeabilities of a particular cell type) to help focus particular experimental programs or to allow discarding specific explanations of an experimental observation. A computational model can also help researchers to differentiate between many possible hypotheses and identify new plausible hypotheses.

Modeling may also provide insight into fundamental questions in cancer biology and in the design of new experiments. As multiscale models which integrate intracellular processes with cell-level behaviors and tissue-level processes develop, insight may be gleaned on mechanisms for metastasis and resistance. As such, they may become effective tools in the development of new strategies for the identification of drug targets and the development of therapeutic strategies.

References

1. Downward J. The ins and outs of signalling. Nature. 2001;411(6839):759–62.
2. Hanahan D, Weinberg RA. The hallmarks of cancer. Cell. 2000;100(1):57–70.
3. Luo J, Solimini NL, Elledge SJ. Principles of cancer therapy: oncogene and non-oncogene addiction. Cell. 2009;136(5):823–37.
4. Anderson AR, Quaranta V. Integrative mathematical oncology. Nat Rev Cancer. 2008;8(3):227–34.
5. Hornberg JJ, Bruggeman FJ, Westerhoff HV, Lankelma J. Cancer: a systems biology disease. Biosystems. 2006;83(2–3):81–90.
6. Vogelstein B, Kinzler KW. Cancer genes and the pathways they control. Nat Med. 2004;10(8):789–99.
7. Rak J, Filmus J, Finkenzeller G, Grugel S, Marme D, Kerbel RS. Oncogenes as inducers of tumor angiogenesis. Cancer Metastasis Rev. 1995;14(4):263–77.
8. Hood L. Leroy Hood expounds the principles, practice and future of systems biology. Drug Discov Today. 2003;8(10):436–8.
9. Bialek W, Botstein D. Introductory science and mathematics education for 21st-century biologists. Science. 2004;303(5659):788–90.
10. Janes KA, Lauffenburger DA. A biological approach to computational models of proteomic networks. Curr Opin Chem Biol. 2006;10(1):73–80.
11. Kiran KL, Jayachandran D, Lakshminarayanan S. Mathematical modelling of avascular tumour growth based on diffusion of nutrients and its validation. Can J Chem Eng. 2009;87(5):732–40.
12. Ferreira SC, Martins ML, Vilela MJ. Reaction-diffusion model for the growth of avascular tumor. Phys Rev E. 2002;65(2):021907.

13. Levine HA, Smiley MW, Tucker AL, Nilsen-Hamilton M. A mathematical model for the onset of avascular tumor growth in response to the loss of p53 function. Cancer Inf. 2007;2:163–88.
14. Mac Gabhann F, Popel AS. Targeting neuropilin-1 to inhibit VEGF signaling in cancer: comparison of therapeutic approaches. PLoS Comput Biol. 2006;2(12):1649–62.
15. Peirce SM, Van Gieson EJ, Skalak TC. Multicellular simulation predicts microvascular patterning and in silico tissue assembly. FASEB J. 2004;18(6):731–3.
16. Alarcon T, Byrne HM, et al. A cellular automaton model for tumour growth in inhomogeneous environment. J Theor Biol. 2003;225(2):257–74.
17. Patel AA, Gawlinski ET, et al. A cellular automaton model of early tumor growth and invasion: the effects of native tissue vascularity and increased anaerobic tumor metabolism. J Theor Biol. 2001;213(3):315–31.
18. Giverso C, Scianna M, Preziosi L, Lo Buono N, Funaro A. Individual cell-based model for in-vitro mesothelial invasion of ovarian cancer. Math Model Nat Phenom. 2010;5(1):203–23.
19. Mansury Y, Deisboeck TS. Modeling tumors as complex biosystems: an agent-based approach; 2006. p. 573–602.
20. Szeto MD, Chakraborty G, Hadley J, Rockne R, Muzi M, Alvord EC, et al. Quantitative metrics of net proliferation and invasion link biological aggressiveness assessed by MRI with hypoxia assessed by FMISO-PET in newly diagnosed glioblastomas. Cancer Res. 2009;69(10):4502–9.
21. Chen LL, Zhang L, Yoon J, Deisboeck TS. Cancer cell motility: optimizing spatial search strategies. Biosystems. 2009;95(3):234–42.
22. Walker DC, Southgate J, et al. The epitheliome: agent-based modelling of the social behaviour of cells. Biosystems. 2004;76(1–3):89–100.
23. Knudson Jr AG. Mutation and cancer: statistical study of retinoblastoma. Proc Natl Acad Sci USA. 1971;68(4):820–3.
24. Lee WH, Bookstein R, Hong F, Young LJ, Shew JY, Lee EY. Human retinoblastoma susceptibility gene: cloning, identification, and sequence. Science. 1987;235(4794):1394–9.
25. Beerenwinkel N, Antal T, Dingli D, Traulsen A, Kinzler KW, Velculescu VE, et al. Genetic progression and the waiting time to cancer. PLoS Comput Biol. 2007;3(11):e225.
26. Ewens WJ. Mathematical population genetics. 2nd ed. New York: Springer; 2004.
27. Sjoblom T, Jones S, Wood LD, Parsons DW, Lin J, Barber TD, et al. The consensus coding sequences of human breast and colorectal cancers. Science. 2006;314(5797):268–74.
28. Robson M, Levin D, Federici M, Satagopan J, Bogolminy F, Heerdt A, et al. Breast conservation therapy for invasive breast cancer in Ashkenazi women with BRCA gene founder mutations. J Natl Cancer Inst. 1999;91(24):2112–7.
29. Rahko E, Blanco G, Bloigu R, Soini Y, Talvensaari-Mattila A, Jukkola A. Adverse outcome and resistance to adjuvant antiestrogen therapy in node-positive postmenopausal breast cancer patients – the role of p53. Breast. 2006;15(1):69–75.
30. Nagata Y, Lan KH, Zhou X, Tan M, Esteva FJ, Sahin AA, et al. PTEN activation contributes to tumor inhibition by trastuzumab, and loss of PTEN predicts trastuzumab resistance in patients. Cancer Cell. 2004;6(2):117–27.
31. Enderling H, Anderson ARA, Chaplain MAJ, Munro AJ, Vaidya JS. Mathematical modelling of radiotherapy strategies for early breast cancer. J Theor Biol. 2006;241(1):158–71.
32. Negrini S, Gorgoulis VG, Halazonetis TD. Genomic instability – an evolving hallmark of cancer [10.1038/nrm2858]. Nat Rev Mol Cell Biol. 2010;11(3):220–8.
33. Kinsella TJ. Coordination of DNA mismatch repair and base excision repair processing of chemotherapy and radiation damage for targeting resistant cancers. Clin Cancer Res. 2009;15(6):1853–9.
34. Martin LP, Hamilton TC, Schilder RJ. Platinum resistance: the role of DNA repair pathways. Clin Cancer Res. 2008;14(5):1291–5.
35. Seo Y, Yan T, Schupp JE, Colussi V, Taylor KL, Kinsella TJ. Differential radiosensitization in DNA mismatch repair-proficient and -deficient human colon cancer xenografts with 5-iodo-2-pyrimidinone-2′-deoxyribose. Clin Cancer Res. 2004;10(22):7520–8.
36. Gurkan E, Schupp JE, Aziz MA, Kinsella TJ, Loparo KA. Probabilistic modeling of DNA mismatch repair effects on cell cycle dynamics and iododeoxyuridine-DNA incorporation. Cancer Res. 2007;67(22):10993–1000.

37. Stites EC, Trampont PC, Ma Z, Ravichandran KS. Network analysis of oncogenic Ras activation in cancer. Science. 2007;318(5849):463–7.
38. Collins K, Jacks T, Pavletich NP. The cell cycle and cancer. Proc Natl Acad Sci USA. 1997;94(7):2776–8.
39. Tyson JJ, Csikasz-Nagy A, Novak B. The dynamics of cell cycle regulation. Bioessays. 2002;24(12):1095–109.
40. Qu Z, Weiss JN, MacLellan WR. Regulation of the mammalian cell cycle: a model of the G1-to-S transition. Am J Physiol Cell Physiol. 2003;284(2):C349–64.
41. Chassagnole C, Jackson RC, Hussain N, Bashir L, Derow C, Savin J, et al. Using a mammalian cell cycle simulation to interpret differential kinase inhibition in anti-tumour pharmaceutical development. Biosystems. 2006;83(2–3):91–7.
42. Rudin CM, Thompson CB. Apoptosis and disease: regulation and clinical relevance of programmed cell death. Annu Rev Med. 1997;48:267–81.
43. Albeck JG, Burke JM, Spencer SL, Lauffenburger DA, Sorger PK. Modeling a snap-action, variable-delay switch controlling extrinsic cell death. PLoS Biol. 2008;6(12):2831–52.
44. Janes KA, Albeck JG, Gaudet S, Sorger PK, Lauffenburger DA, Yaffe MB. A systems model of signaling identifies a molecular basis set for cytokine-induced apoptosis. Science. 2005;310(5754):1646–53.
45. Rehm M, Huber HJ, Dussmann H, Prehn JH. Systems analysis of effector caspase activation and its control by X-linked inhibitor of apoptosis protein. EMBO J. 2006;25(18):4338–49.
46. Albeck JG, Burke JM, Aldridge BB, Zhang M, Lauffenburger DA, Sorger PK. Quantitative analysis of pathways controlling extrinsic apoptosis in single cells. Mol Cell. 2008;30(1):11–25.
47. Campbell LL, Polyak K. Breast tumor heterogeneity: cancer stem cells or clonal evolution? Cell Cycle. 2007;6(19):2332–8.
48. Heppner GH, Miller BE. Tumor heterogeneity: biological implications and therapeutic consequences. Cancer Metastasis Rev. 1983;2(1):5–23.
49. Stein AM, Demuth T, Mobley D, Berens M, Sander LM. A mathematical model of glioblastoma tumor spheroid invasion in a three-dimensional in vitro experiment. Biophys J. 2007;92(1):356–65.
50. Bertuzzi A, Fasano A, Gandolfi A, Sinisgalli C. Necrotic core in EMT6/Ro tumour spheroids: Is it caused by an ATP deficit? J Theor Biol. 2010;262(1):142–50.
51. Sanga S, Sinek JP, Frieboes HB, Ferrari M, Fruehauf JP, Cristini V. Mathematical modeling of cancer progression and response to chemotherapy. Expert Rev Anticancer Ther. 2006;6(10):1361–76.
52. Rangarajan R, Zaman MH. Modeling cell migration in 3D: status and challenges. Cell Adh Migr. 2008;2(2):106–9.
53. Gatenby RA, Gawlinski ET. A reaction-diffusion model of cancer invasion. Cancer Res. 1996;56(24):5745–53.
54. Roose T, Chapman SJ, Maini PK. Mathematical models of avascular tumor growth. SIAM Rev. 2007;49(2):179–208.
55. Sander LM, Deisboeck TS. Growth patterns of microscopic brain tumors. Phys Rev E Stat Nonlin Soft Matter Phys. 2002;66(5 Pt 1):051901.
56. Bergers G, Benjamin LE. Tumorigenesis and the angiogenic switch. Nat Rev Cancer. 2003;3(6):401–10.
57. Lowengrub JS, Frieboes HB, Jin F, Chuang YL, Li X, Macklin P, et al. Nonlinear modelling of cancer: bridging the gap between cells and tumours. Nonlinearity. 2010;23(1):R1–91.
58. Peirce S. Computational and mathematical modeling of angiogenesis. Microcirculation. 2008;15(8):739–51.
59. Hogea CS, Murray BT, Sethian JA. Simulating complex tumor dynamics from avascular to vascular growth using a general level-set method. J Math Biol. 2006;53(1):86–134.
60. Miller-Kasprzak E, Jagodzinski PP. Endothelial progenitor cells as a new agent contributing to vascular repair. Arch Immunol Et Ther Exp. 2007;55(4):247–59.
61. Komarova NL, Mironov V. On the role of endothelial progenitor cells in tumor neovascularization. J Theor Biol. 2005;235(3):338–49.

62. Stamper IJ, Byrne HM, Owen MR, Maini PK. Modelling the role of angiogenesis and vasculogenesis in solid tumour growth. Bull Math Biol. 2007;69(8):2737–72.
63. An G, Mi Q, Dutta-Moscato J, Vodovotz Y. Agent-based models in translational systems biology. Wiley Interdiscip Rev Syst Biol Med. 2009;1(2):159–71.
64. Thorne BC, Bailey AM, Peirce SM. Combining experiments with multi-cell agent-based modeling to study biological tissue patterning. Brief Bioinform. 2007;8(4):245–57.
65. Athale C, Mansury Y, Deisboeck TS. Simulating the impact of a molecular "decision-process" on cellular phenotype and multicellular patterns in brain tumors. J Theor Biol. 2005;233(4):469–81.
66. Sanga S, Frieboes HB, Zheng X, Gatenby R, Bearer EL, Cristini V. Predictive oncology: a review of multidisciplinary, multiscale in silico modeling linking phenotype, morphology and growth. Neuroimage. 2007;37 Suppl 1:S120–34.
67. Zhang L, Athale CA, Deisboeck TS. Development of a three-dimensional multiscale agent-based tumor model: simulating gene-protein interaction profiles, cell phenotypes and multicellular patterns in brain cancer. J Theor Biol. 2007;244(1):96–107.
68. Peirce SM, Skalak TC, Papin JA. Multiscale biosystems integration: coupling intracellular network analysis with tissue-patterning simulations. IBM J Res Dev. 2006;50(6):601–15.
69. Jiang Y, Pjesivac-Grbovic J, Cantrell C, Freyer JP. A multiscale model for avascular tumor growth. Biophys J. 2005;89(6):3884–94.
70. Martins ML, Ferreira SC, Vilela MJ. Multiscale models for the growth of avascular tumors. Phys Life Rev. 2007;4(2):128–56.
71. Anderson AR, Weaver AM, Cummings PT, Quaranta V. Tumor morphology and phenotypic evolution driven by selective pressure from the microenvironment. Cell. 2006;127(5):905–15.
72. Auerbach W, Auerbach R. Angiogenesis inhibition: a review. Pharmacol Ther. 1994;63(3):265–311.
73. Zetter BR. Angiogenesis and tumor metastasis. Annu Rev Med. 1998;49:407–24.
74. Ebos JM, Lee CR, Cruz-Munoz W, Bjarnason GA, Christensen JG, Kerbel RS. Accelerated metastasis after short-term treatment with a potent inhibitor of tumor angiogenesis. Cancer Cell. 2009;15(3):232–9.
75. Loges S, Mazzone M, Hohensinner P, Carmeliet P. Silencing or fueling metastasis with VEGF inhibitors: antiangiogenesis revisited. Cancer Cell. 2009;15(3):167–70.
76. Jain RK, Duda DG, Willett CG, Sahani DV, Zhu AX, Loeffler JS, et al. Biomarkers of response and resistance to antiangiogenic therapy. Nat Rev Clin Oncol. 2009;6(6):327–38.
77. Zhu AX, Sahani DV, Duda DG, di Tomaso E, Ancukiewicz M, Catalano OA, et al. Efficacy, safety, and potential biomarkers of sunitinib monotherapy in advanced hepatocellular carcinoma: a phase II study. J Clin Oncol. 2009;27(18):3027–35.
78. Jain RK, Tong RT, Munn LL. Effect of vascular normalization by antiangiogenic therapy on interstitial hypertension, peritumor edema, and lymphatic metastasis: insights from a mathematical model. Cancer Res. 2007;67(6):2729–35.
79. Foo J, Michor F. Evolution of resistance to targeted anti-cancer therapies during continuous and pulsed administration strategies. PLoS Comput Biol. 2009;5(11):e1000557.
80. Sinek JP, Sanga S, Zheng XM, Frieboes HB, Ferrari M, Cristini V. Predicting drug pharmacokinetics and effect in vascularized tumors using computer simulation. J Math Biol. 2009;58(4–5):485–510.
81. Araujo RP, Petricoin EF, Liotta LA. A mathematical model of combination therapy using the EGFR signaling network. Biosystems. 2005;80(1):57–69.
82. Meads MB, Gatenby RA, Dalton WS. Environment-mediated drug resistance: a major contributor to minimal residual disease. Nat Rev Cancer. 2009;9(9):665–74.
83. Abbott LH, Michor F. Mathematical models of targeted cancer therapy. Br J Cancer. 2006;95(9):1136–41.
84. Jain HV, Nor JE, et al. Modeling the VEGF-Bcl-2-CXCL8 pathway in intratumoral angiogenesis. Bull Math Biol. 2008;70(1):89–117.

Chapter 7
Somatic Evolution of Acquired Drug Resistance in Cancer

John W. Pepper

Keywords Somatic evolution • Clonal selection • Systemic pathology • Cell motility • Public goods

Multilevel Selection and Cancer

Evolutionary processes operate on multiple levels in biology [1–3]. Selection among somatic cells occurs on the time scale of a human lifetime or less. Selection on organisms, over millennia, has led to adaptations that increase organismal fitness by constraining somatic evolution [4, 5]. Analysis of trade-offs in the conflicting levels of cellular and organismal selection helps to reveal not only our natural defenses against cancer but also the nature of remaining vulnerabilities to cancer [6–10]. Organismal selection has led to the evolution of general tumor-suppression mechanisms [11]. The role of organismal selection in shaping cancer biology was recently reviewed by Greaves [12]. Because of its central role in acquired drug resistance, this chapter will concentrate on selection and evolution within populations of cancer cells, rather than populations of individuals. Human cancer genetics differs from human population genetics in several ways: cancer cells tend to have high mutation rates due to their genetic instability [13], and they exhibit a wide diversity of genetic alterations. In addition to the point mutations typical of population genetics, other common somatic mutations in cancer include loss of heterozygosity, aneuploidy [14], and other copy number aberrations [15]. In addition to all these classes of genetic lesions, epigenetic lesions are also heritable across cell generations, impact cell phenotype, and are implicated in the somatic evolution of cancer [16, 17].

J.W. Pepper (✉)
Division of Cancer Prevention, National Cancer Institute, Bethesda, MD, USA
e-mail: pepperjw@mail.nih.gov

D. Gioeli (ed.), *Targeted Therapies: Mechanisms of Resistance*,
Molecular and Translational Medicine, DOI 10.1007/978-1-60761-478-4_7,
© Springer Science+Business Media, LLC 2011

Acquired Drug Resistance Arises Through Somatic Evolution

The molecular mechanisms of acquired drug resistance are many and diverse, but they all arise through the same processes of somatic evolution [18, 19]. They also all have similar clinical implications. Although each case is unique, most cancer drugs typically lose their effectiveness during therapy, and this fact accounts for much cancer mortality.

Somatic evolution is the evolution of a population of somatic cells within the body of a multicellular organism such as a human. Evolution by natural selection is both possible and inevitable in any population of reproducing entities that vary in heritable traits affecting their rate of reproduction. Somatic cells acquire heritable variation through somatic mutation, epigenetic changes, and sporadic somatic aneuploidy [14]. This variation is heritable through mitosis, and any variants that increase cell survival and replication thereby increase in frequency in somatic tissue, regardless of their ultimate effects on the health or fitness of the multicellular organism. Through this process, cancer therapies often select for acquired drug resistance, and this is the central problem in cancer therapy. For example, at relapse, mutant clones have been discovered in lung cancer, with point mutations in epidermal growth factor receptor (EGFR) that cause resistance to anilinoquinazoline EGFR inhibitors [20]. In chronic myeloid leukemia, an amino-acid change in BCR-ABL confers resistance to imatinib (Glivec) [21], and amplification of the thymidine synthase gene causes resistance to 5-fluorouracil in colorectal cancer [22]. This shows that therapies not only select for cancer stem cells [23], but specifically for cancer stem cells with resistance mutations [24]. The problem is especially acute for cytotoxins, because killing off drug-sensitive pathogen cells results in competitive release of any drug-resistant cells present, further increasing their fitness advantage and their proliferation [25, 26]. Thus, further development of new targeted cytotoxins is not a promising area of research [27].

Even targeted drugs remain subject to acquired drug resistance through somatic evolution. Because of their large numbers and high rates of somatic mutation, the cells in a human cancer typically harbor many drug-resistant mutations, even before treatment. Under the selective pressure of drugs that reduce fitness of drug-sensitive cells, this genetic diversity leads to rapid proliferation of drug-resistant cells, and thus to drug-resistant relapse after therapy. This was first observed in cytotoxic chemotherapies, and has proven equally true of the newer, more targeted compounds. As Chabner and Roberts [28] noted, "A vast array of resistance mechanisms … can defeat single agents, no matter how well designed and targeted."

This pitfall continues to dog even the most recent targeted therapies. One example is PLX4032. The only drug long approved by the United States Food and Drug Administration (FDA) for metastatic melanoma had only a 15% response rate. So when a trial for this new targeted molecular therapy reported a 70% response rate, it shocked the field, and was described as an astounding leap. Unfortunately, this trial also found that patients relapsed after about 9 months, and that a survival benefit was not demonstrated [29]. This illustrates that it is much easier to achieve an initial drug response than to save patient lives, due to the high frequency of resistant relapse.

Potential Solutions to the Problem

It would be a misleading oversimplification to say that acquired drug resistance is caused by somatic mutation, because this neglects the central role of somatic selection. Because of the large number of cancer cells present in a tumor, and their genetic instability, we must expect a cancer to produce mutations conferring resistance to virtually any agent it is exposed to. These mutant cells, however, only become a problem when they have a fitness advantage over neighboring cells, so that they proliferate into an expanding clonal cluster and eventually a completely drug-resistant tumor. This situation only arises when a therapeutic agent exerts a selective pressure by reducing the fitness of sensitive cells relative to resistant calls.

These facts might seem to present a hopeless dilemma. The only drugs that won't lose effectiveness are those that don't reduce the survival and proliferation of the specific cancer cells they act on. How could a drug possibly be useful if it didn't reduce the survival and proliferation of the cancer cells it acts on?

Cancer medicine often rests on the assumption that in order to reduce cancer mortality, we must use drugs that kill cancer cells, or at least directly impair their proliferation. If this assumption were correct, there would be no escaping the paradox that the most effective drugs will inevitably lose their effectiveness most rapidly [19]. Fortunately however, it is possible to escape both from this standard assumption, and from the dilemma it would lead to.

Agents That Help Patients Without Imposing Strong Somatic Selection Pressure

It is increasingly clear that many important pathological properties of cancer cells arise not solely from intrinsic properties of individual cells, but rather through the concerted action of populations of cells [30]. This insight suggests ways to disrupt cancer cell survival and proliferation without directly attacking the individual cells, and without thereby selecting for resistance mutations. Three specific avenues which will be discussed are: Preventing systemic pathology, preventing cell motility, and targeting cellular public goods.

The most direct causes of cancer mortality include systemic effects that could in principle be treated without killing cancer cells. For example, many cancer patients die wholly or in part from cachexia or wasting [31, 32], or from suppression of the immune system [33–36]. Both these pathologies are driven by tumor-derived factors, rather than directly by tumor cells themselves. These tumor-derived factors represent potentially important therapeutic targets. Therapies targeting tumor-derived factors would not necessarily reduce the fitness of the cancer cells producing them, and therefore should not select for therapeutic resistance.

The defining feature of a malignant cancer, as opposed to a benign neoplasm, is the destruction of normal tissue architecture caused by invasion of tumor cells into the surrounding tissue. Blocking this process would prevent progression to cancer, and in principle, would not require drugs with effects that would impose strong somatic selection for therapeutic resistance [50]. Investigations into the molecular mechanisms underlying tumor cell motility and invasion have identified some of the molecular pathways involved [37]. These molecular mechanisms represent potential therapeutic targets to prevent progression from benign growth to cancer. There may be some somatic selection favoring cell motility, which allows tumor cells to escape their depleted local environment and continue to proliferate. Such selection would also favor resistance to motility-blocking drugs. It seems likely though, that this selection would be much weaker than that imposed by drugs directly killing cancer cells or blocking their division. If so, motility-blocking drugs would be more robust against acquired resistance than would cyotoxic or cytostatic drugs.

Investigations of the molecular mechanisms underlying tumor cell motility and invasion have identified various molecular pathways involved in this cell behavior [37–39]. These molecular mechanisms represent potential therapeutic targets to prevent progression from benign growth to cancerous tumor. Indeed, specific molecules involved in cell motility have been suggested as targets for novel therapies; e.g., the human transmembrane protein podoplanin [40]. If reducing their motility does not directly and immediately reduce the fitness of tumor cells, then we can expect such therapies to reduce cancer mortality and morbidity, while also retaining effectiveness and avoiding the rapid onset of acquired drug resistance.

Cellular Public Goods as Drug Targets: Theory

As discussed above, the properties of cancer arise not solely through the properties of individual cancer cells, but also to a large extent through their interactions and the concerted actions of populations of cells. In particular, cancer cells cooperate by secreting external products (termed "public goods") into their microenvironments that are beneficial both to themselves and to other nearby cancer cells.

It has been proposed that drugs attacking such public goods would be less vulnerable to acquired resistance by pathogenic cells in general, including cancer cells [41]. Up to the present, most cancer therapy drugs have targeted molecules that are intrinsic to cancer cells, and that reduce the Darwinian fitness of the target cells by reducing their survival or replication. All such drugs inevitably act as strong selective agents by giving a large advantage to any mutant cells that are resistant to the therapeutic agent.

This proposed alternative approach exploits the fact that the survival and proliferation of cancer cells depends not only on their own intrinsic properties, but also on secreted metabolites that make their microenvironment more hospitable to all nearby cancer cells, including the producer. Such "public goods" provide a benefit to a larger group of cells than merely those producing them. Both theory and empirical observation of microbial evolution tells us that the selective pressure to maintain these traits in an effective form is much weaker than is the selection on intrinsic traits of cells. Mathematical theory quantifies the relative advantage to be expected

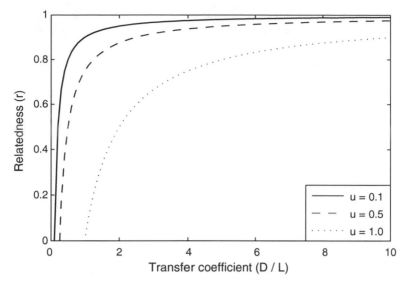

Fig. 7.1 The area above the curves represents the parameter space favoring the evolutionary maintenance of public goods production. D (diffusion coefficient), and L (diffusion length) from producers to neighboring cells. Relatedness quantifies the similarity among neighboring cells in whether or not they produce the public good. High transfer coefficients result in restrictive conditions for the evolutionary maintenance of public goods production. The three lines represent different values for the cellular uptake rate (u) of the public goods molecule. From Driscoll and Pepper [42]. Used with permission

from this approach in terms of the turnover rate of cells versus groups of cells, as well as the partitioning of genetic variance within versus between groups [41].

Further mathematical theory for the evolution of public goods traits has clarified why selection is stronger for the production and maintenance of private than public molecules [42]. Weaker selection for the maintenance of effective public goods will result in the slower somatic evolution of resistance to any therapeutic intervention that reduces it effectiveness. The evolutionary theory of public goods also shows there is in fact a continuum between public and private products excreted by cells. According to this body of theory, the tumor-produced and tumor-supporting extracellular products that are most "public," or widely shared, and thus against which resistance will evolve most slowly, are those characterized by high diffusion coefficients and short diffusion lengths among cells (Fig. 7.1).

Cellular Public Goods as Drug Targets: Examples

Many tumors cells secret angiogenesis factors that provide the benefit of increased blood and nutrient supply both to the specific cells secreting the factors, and to neighboring tumor cells. These factors are examples of public goods. Therapies designed to block tumor neoangiogenesis are the most prominent examples to date of therapies targeting public goods produced by cancer cells. As predicted by evolutionary theory, tumors do not typically develop rapid resistance to angiogenesis blockers, in contrast to the response to cytotoxic agents [43, 44].

In addition to the well-established example of angiogenesis blockers, many other opportunities exist for developing new therapies that will be robust against acquired resistance. Most tumors use anaerobic glycolytic metabolism as their energy source, and produce lactic acid that diffuses from the tumor into nearby normal tissue. This kills nearby normal cells and facilitates tumor invasion [45]. This acidification represents a tumor public good, and is a promising target for robust therapeutic intervention.

Various other public goods molecules secreted by cancer cells have been suggested as potential drug targets [41]. Among the most promising of these are secreted invasion factors (see also discussion above). Invasion factors in general have been suggested as therapeutic targets by other authors [46]. Indeed, specific targets and agents have been proposed, and tested successfully in animal models, such as Verapamil against matrix metalloproteinases [47]. What has not been tested yet is the theoretical prediction that such therapies, because they target cellular public goods, will be robust against somatic evolution of acquired resistance. Similarly, macrophage mobilization and infiltration into the tumor bed can facilitate tumor growth and invasion [48], and chemokines secreted by tumor cells that recruit macrophages represent another cancer public good. Neutralizing antibodies against monocyte chemoattractant protein I (CCL2) reduced tumor burden in an in vivo model of prostate cancer [49]. Again, the theoretical prediction remains to be tested that because such therapies are directed against cellular public goods, they will be robust against acquired therapeutic resistance.

Conclusions

Because of the large number of cells in the typical cancer, and their genetic instability and diversity, all targeted cytotoxins are expected to generate acquired resistance and consequent relapse. For such agents, initial drug response is not a strong predictor of reduced mortality. Other classes of agents are expected to be more robust against acquired resistance. These alternatives are more promising than cytotoxins as ways to reduce cancer mortality.

References

1. Lewontin RC. The units of selection. Annu Rev Ecol Syst. 1970;1:1–18.
2. Gould SJ. Gulliver's further travels: the necessity and difficulty of a hierarchical theory of selection. Philos Trans R Soc Lond B. 1998;353:307–14.
3. Keller LK. Levels of selection in evolution. Princeton: Princeton University Press; 1999.

4. Cairns J. Mutation selection and the natural history of cancer. Nature. 1975;255:197–200.
5. Leroi AM, Koufopanou V, Burt A. Cancer selection. Nat Rev Cancer. 2003;3:226–31.
6. Summers K, da Silva J, Farwell M. Intragenomic conflict and cancer. Med Hypotheses. 2002;59:170–9.
7. Weinstein BS, Ciszek D. The reserve-capacity hypothesis: evolutionary origins and modern implications of the trade-off between tumor-suppression and tissue-repair. Exp Gerontol. 2002;37:615–27.
8. Frank SA, Nowak MA. Problems of somatic mutation and cancer. Bioessays. 2004;26:291–9.
9. Campisi J. Aging, tumor suppression and cancer: high wire-act! Mech Ageing Dev. 2005;126:51–8.
10. Crespi B, Summers K. Evolutionary biology of cancer. Trends Ecol Evol. 2005;20:545–52.
11. Pepper JW, Sprouffske K, Maley CC. Animal cell differentiation patterns suppress somatic evolution. PLoS Comput Biol. 2007;3:2532–45.
12. Greaves M. Darwinian medicine: a case for cancer. Nat Rev Cancer. 2007;7:213–21.
13. Negrini S, Gorgoulis VG, Halazonetis TD. Genomic instability – an evolving hallmark of cancer. Nat Rev Mol Cell Biol. 2010;11:220–8.
14. Merlo LMF, Wang L, Pepper JW, Rabinovitch PS, Maley CC. Chapter 1: Polyploidy, aneuploidy and the evolution of cancer. In: Poon RYC, editor. Polyploidization and cancer. Austin: Landes Bioscience; 2010. p. 1–13.
15. Huang Q, Yu GP, McCormick SA, Mo J, Datta B, Mahimkar M, et al. Genetic differences detected by comparative genomic hybridization in head and neck squamous cell carcinomas from different tumor sites: construction of oncogenetic trees for tumor progression. Genes Chromosom Cancer. 2002;34:224–33.
16. Siegmund KD, Marjoram P, Woo YJ, Tavare S, Shibata D. Inferring clonal expansion and cancer stem cell dynamics from DNA methylation patterns in colorectal cancers. Proc Natl Acad Sci USA. 2009;106:4828–33.
17. Shackleton M, Quintana E, Fearon ER, Morrison SJ. Heterogeneity in cancer: cancer stem cells versus clonal evolution. Cell. 2009;138:822–9.
18. Merlo LMF, Pepper JW, Reid BJ, Maley CC. Cancer as an evolutionary and ecological process. Nat Rev Cancer. 2006;6:924–35.
19. Pepper JW, Findlay CS, Kassen R, Spencer SL, Maley CC. Cancer research meets evolutionary biology. Evol Appl. 2009;2(1):62–70.
20. Kobayashi S, Boggon TJ, Dayaram T, Janne PA, Kocher O, Meyerson M, et al. EGFR mutation and resistance of non-small-cell lung cancer to gefitinib. N Engl J Med. 2005;352:786–92.
21. Gorre ME, Mohammed M, Ellwood K, Hsu N, Paquette R, Rao PN, et al. Clinical resistance to STI-571 cancer therapy caused by BCR-ABL gene mutation or amplification. Science. 2001;293:876–80.
22. Wang TL et al. Digital karyotyping identifies thymidylate synthase amplification as a mechanism of resistance to 5-fluorouracil in metastatic colorectal cancer patients. Proc Natl Acad Sci USA. 2004;101:3089–94.
23. Donnenberg VS, Donnenberg AD. Multiple drug resistance in cancer revisited: the cancer stem cell hypothesis. J Clin Pharmacol. 2005;45:872–7.
24. Michor F, Hughes TP, Iwasa Y, Branford S, Shah NP, Sawyers CL, et al. Dynamics of chronic myeloid leukaemia. Nature. 2005;435:1267–70.
25. Williams PD. Darwinian interventions: taming pathogens through evolutionary ecology. Trends Parasitol. 2010;26:83–92.
26. Wargo AR, Huijben S, de Roode JC, Shepherd J, Read AF. Competitive release and facilitation of drug-resistant parasites after therapeutic chemotherapy in a rodent malaria model. Proc Natl Acad Sci USA. 2007;104:19914–9.
27. Gatenby RA. A change of strategy in the war on cancer. Nature. 2009;459:508–9.
28. Chabner BA, Roberts TG. Chemotherapy and the war on cancer. Nat Rev Cancer. 2005;5:65–72.

29. Garber K. Melanoma drug vindicates targeted approach. Science. 2009;326:1619.
30. Deisboeck TS, Couzin ID. Collective behavior in cancer cell populations. Bioessays. 2009;31:190–7.
31. Laviano A, Meguid MM, Inui A, Muscaritoli M, Rossi-Fanelli F. Therapy Insight: cancer anorexia-cachexia syndrome – when all you can eat is yourself. Nat Clin Pract Gastroenterol Hepatol. 2005;2:B158–65.
32. Muscaritoli M, Bossola M, Aversa Z, Bellantone R, Fanelli FR. Prevention and treatment of cancer cachexia: new insights into an old problem. Eur J Cancer. 2006;42:31–41.
33. Evans C, Dalgleish AG, Kumar D. Review article: immune suppression and colorectal cancer. Aliment Pharmacol Ther. 2006;24:1163–77.
34. Whiteside TL. Immune suppression in cancer: effects on immune cells, mechanisms and future therapeutic intervention. Semin Cancer Biol. 2006;16:3–15.
35. Herber DL, Nagaraj S, Djeu JY, Gabrilovich DI. Mechanism and therapeutic reversal of immune suppression in cancer. Cancer Res. 2007;67:5067–9.
36. Torres MP, Ponnusamy MP, Lakshmanan I, Batra SK. Immunopathogenesis of ovarian cancer. Minerva Medica. 2009;100:385–400.
37. Friedl P, Wolf K. Tumour-cell invasion and migration: diversity and escape mechanisms. Nat Rev Cancer. 2003;3:362–74.
38. Wang WG, Goswami S, Sahai E, Wyckoff JB, Segall JE, Condeelis JS. Tumor cells caught in the act of invading: their strategy for enhanced cell motility. Trends Cell Biol. 2005;15:138–45.
39. Mouneimne G, Brugge JS. Tensins: a new switch in cell migration. Dev Cell. 2007;13:317–9.
40. Wicki A, Christofori G. The potential role of podoplanin in tumour invasion. Br J Cancer. 2007;96:1–5.
41. Pepper JW. Defeating pathogen drug resistance: guidance from evolutionary theory. Evolution. 2008;62:3185–91.
42. Driscoll WW, Pepper JW. Theory for the evolution of diffusible external goods. Evolution. 2010;64:2682–7.
43. Kerbel RS. A cancer therapy resistant to resistance. Nature. 1997;390:335–6.
44. Boehm T, Folkman J, Browder T, O'Reilly MS. Antiangiogenic therapy of experimental cancer does not induce acquired drug resistance. Nature. 1997;390:404–7.
45. Gatenby RA, Gawlinski ET. The glycolytic phenotype in carcinogenesis and tumor invasion: insights through mathematical models. Cancer Res. 2003;63:3847–54.
46. Brunner N, Dano K. Invasion and metastasis factors in breast cancer. Breast Cancer Res Treat. 1993;24:173–4.
47. Farias EF, Ghiso JAA, Ladeda V, Joffe EBD. Verapamil inhibits tumor protease production, local invasion and metastasis development in murine carcinoma cells. Int J Cancer. 1998;78:727–34.
48. Loberg RD, Ying C, Craig M, Yan L, Snyder LA, Pienta KJ. CCL2 as an important mediator of prostate cancer growth in vivo through the regulation of macrophage infiltration. Neoplasia. 2007;9:556–62.
49. Loberg RD, Ying C, Craig M, Day LL, Sargent E, Neeley C, et al. Targeting CCL2 with systemic delivery of neutralizing antibodies induces prostate cancer tumor regression in vivo. Cancer Res. 2007;67:9417–24.
50. Aktipis CA, Maley CC, Pepper JW. Dispersal evolution in neoplasms: the role of disregulated metabolism in the evolution of cell motility. Cancer Prevention Res. 2011; in press.

Chapter 8
Interrogating Resistance to Targeted Therapy Using Genetically Engineered Mouse Models of Cancer

Edward Gunther

Keywords Targeted therapy • Mouse • Tumor escape • Drug resistance • Reversible

Reversible Cancer Models: Genetically Engineered Mouse Models of Targeted Anticancer Therapy

The latter part of the 1990s brought the first reports of clinical success using modern targeted anticancer agents [1]. Coincident with these therapeutic breakthroughs, novel transgenic mouse models of cancer were reported in which tumorigenesis was initiated by expression of an inducible oncogene [2–4]. Simulating "idealized" targeted therapy in these reversible cancer models (RCMs) by abrogating oncogene expression within established cancers typically triggered dramatic tumor regression, mirroring the wondrous responses sometimes achieved using targeted agents.

Tumor regression in RCMs was unquestionably a consequence of oncogene withdrawal, and not the confounding effect of a drug acting "off-target." Thus, RCMs provided a formal demonstration that initiating oncogenic lesions can remain essential for the maintenance of advanced tumors, thereby solidifying the concept of "oncogene addiction" [5]. More recently, a distinct class of RCMs was engineered to permit restoration of disrupted tumor suppressor gene function within established cancers [6–8]. Tumor regression seen in this context validates an inverse concept termed "tumor suppressor gene hypersensitivity" and supports anticancer strategies aimed at correcting signaling defects imposed by loss-of-function mutations [5, 9]. Thus far, oncogene withdrawal and tumor suppressor gene restoration appear to achieve a similar range of outcomes by activating an

E. Gunther (✉)
Department of Medicine, Pennsylvania State College of Medicine, Hershey, PA, USA
and
Jake Gittlen Cancer Research Foundation, Pennsylvania State College of Medicine,
Hershey, PA, USA
e-mail: eg12@psu.edu

D. Gioeli (ed.), *Targeted Therapies: Mechanisms of Resistance,*
Molecular and Translational Medicine, DOI 10.1007/978-1-60761-478-4_8,
© Springer Science+Business Media, LLC 2011

overlapping set of cellular programs. For simplicity, RCMs will be considered as a single group, and the term "oncogene withdrawal" will be used broadly to denote genetic simulation of targeted therapy via reversal of an oncogenic lesion.

Mirroring clinical experience, it soon became apparent that reversing an initiating oncogenic event in an RCM often fails to yield a cure. Sometimes, tumor regression is incomplete and short-lived [10–12]. Other times, regression leaves no trace of a clinically detectable tumor, but mice in remission remain at long-term risk for disease relapse [11–13]. Therefore, RCMs faithfully model the full range of clinical outcomes achieved with targeted therapy, where agents frequently encounter drug-resistant tumor cells de novo or select for their outgrowth over time. Accordingly, RCMs have emerged as important models for deciphering the molecular and cellular determinants of tumor regression and tumor escape [14, 15]. This chapter primarily explores clinically relevant insights derived from RCMs, and will not address the strategies employed to engineer reversible oncogenic lesions. These and related mouse modeling strategies have been reviewed elsewhere [16, 17].

Tumor Regression: Re-Engaging the Cellular Programs That Prevent Cancer

RCM studies reveal a striking overlap between the cellular mechanisms that curb tumorigenesis at its inception and those that mediate tumor regression due to oncogene withdrawal. Indeed, subsequent tumor escape likely involves selection for tumor cells that have acquired the means to bypass these familiar safeguards for a second time. Since the cellular mechanisms that initiate and maintain tumor regression represent barriers to disease relapse, they deserve close scrutiny. To date, numerous RCM studies have described short-term shifts in cell fate that immediately follow oncogene withdrawal and presumably initiate regression [18, 19]. A challenge for the future is to expand the use of RCMs to clarify which of these cell programs act long term to maintain regression.

Initiating Tumor Regression: The Short-Term Impact of Oncogene Withdrawal

Tumor regression in RCMs turns out to be quite complex. Presumably, this complexity reflects the fact that oncogenes network extensively with multiple signaling pathways. As such, oncogenic lesions do not correspond one-to-one with malignant traits [20]; rather, they act in a pleiotropic manner, simultaneously impacting diverse cell fate programs. This pleiotropy is supported by careful studies showing that inducible activation of Myc in keratinocytes is sufficient for synchronous and widespread tissue remodeling which rapidly yields a quasi-malignant microenvironment [4]. Similarly, in pancreatic islet cells, co-expressing Myc and just one additional oncogene (Bclxl, to counter Myc-induced apoptosis) yields angiogenic and invasive islet cell tumors [21].

Inversely, these early RCM studies indicated that oncogene withdrawal triggers complex "de-construction" of the malignant microenvironment, which includes a breakdown of tumor–host interactions. For example, regression of both Ras-driven melanomas and Myc-initiated islet cell tumors coincided with intratumoral collapse of host-derived vessels [2, 21]. These studies underscored cell nonautonomous functions of Ras and Myc that might easily elude detection in traditional cell culture studies. Similarly, liver cancers initiated by inducible p53 knockdown in the context of constitutive Ras pathway activation regressed when p53 expression was restored, and this regression required an innate immune response [8]. Immune cells appear to be critical for tumor regression in only a subset of RCMs, since several reports document efficient regression of RCM tumors propagated in immunodeficient host mice.

But what fates are imposed on actual tumor cells during oncogene withdrawal? Again, regression appears to be multifaceted. The tumor cell fates that predominate vary widely across RCMs, suggesting that the preferred cell fate programs depend, at least in part, upon which oncogenic pathway is perturbed and in what tumor type [19]. Oddly, even within a single malignancy, oncogene withdrawal drives tumor cells toward multiple cell fates. For example, reversal often triggers an increase in tumor cell death concurrent with a decrease in proliferation in RCM studies. So, at minimum, oncogene withdrawal routinely imposes cytocidal and cytostatic outcomes simultaneously. But when specific tumor cell fate programs are considered, the variety of outcomes is greater still. Early RCM studies typically documented cell death only by quantifying tumor cell apoptosis, leaving other cell death programs, including autophagy and necrosis, unexplored. Likewise, quantifying cell cycle arrest using traditional cell proliferation assays failed to discriminate between those cells that irreversibly exit the cell cycle (e.g., by following programs that culminate in senescence or terminal differentiation) versus those cells that enter quiescence and retain proliferative potential.

Irreversible Cell Cycle Arrest: Senescence and Terminal Differentiation

The cell senescence program, originally identified as a response to oncogene challenge in cell culture studies, is now known to serve an important tumor suppressor function in vivo [22]. Moreover, senescence has been implicated as a crucial mediator of tumor response to traditional cytotoxic chemotherapy [23]. With cell senescence markers and pathways coming into focus, investigators tested whether the senescence program contributes to tumor regression in RCMs. Remarkably, regression of a wide variety of RCM tumor types – including lymphomas, osteosarcomas [24], hepatocellular carcinomas [8], and medulloblastomas [25] – involved widespread tumor cell senescence. Intriguingly, in addition to its role in initiating regression, senescence appears to prevent delayed relapse of reversible lymphomas, presumably by enforcing sustained regression [26].

Triggering senescence, therefore, may involve a mechanism that senses high-magnitude swings in mitogenic signaling. Support for this notion comes from an RCM study employing mammary-directed expression of an inducible H-RAS^{G12V} allele. High, but not low, H-RAS^{G12V} expression triggered senescence, which arrested mammary ductal development. Low H-RAS^{G12V} expression triggered mammary epithelial cell proliferation and predisposed mice to mammary tumors over the long term [27]. But a jump in H-RAS^{G12V} expression seen in tumors suggested that progression-related events ultimately select for higher levels of Ras signaling. Studies employing a distinct RCM found that a similar threshold of oncogene expression levels dictated how diverse tissue compartments responded to inducer-dependent Myc expression [28]. These "oncogene-on" findings, coupled with findings from "oncogene-off" tumor regression studies suggest an interesting symmetry: the senescence program appears to be activated not only by abrupt *up*-regulation of oncogenic signaling (as seen in the context of untransformed cells), but also by abrupt *down*-regulation of oncogenic signaling (as seen in the context of malignancies). It follows that senescence may critically mediate the response to targeted therapy in some cases. This mechanistic insight offers an opportunity for potential clinical translation. Strategies aimed at reinforcing the senescence program may enhance tumor responses to targeted therapy, or may render these responses more durable.

Normal cells also can exit the cell cycle irreversibly upon terminal differentiation. Mutations that block differentiation programs clearly drive the pathogenesis of some cancers, such as childhood leukemias. Conversely, therapies that promote differentiation, such as retinoid therapy for promyelocytic leukemia, have established clinical roles. Thus, for some cell types, differentiation serves as an obstacle to transformation, and may, by extension, present a barrier to tumor escape. However, Myc-driven RCMs illustrate that the degree to which differentiation programs aid in maintaining tumor regression varies markedly across cell types. When MYC-initiated osteosarcomas were subjected to oncogene withdrawal, tumor cells differentiated into mature osteocytes. Remarkably, reactivating MYC expression in these differentiated tumor cells triggered widespread cell death, and tumors failed to recur [29]. By contrast, oncogene withdrawal in MYC-initiated hepatocellular cancers left traces of disease comprised of differentiated liver cells, but MYC re-expression in this context rapidly reconstituted cancers and reproduced the original tumor histopathology [30]. In this latter example, multilineage differentiation failed to provide a barrier against tumor escape.

Cell Fates Imposed by Oncogene Withdrawal: Surprising Intratumoral Diversity

The finding that, even within a single RCM tumor, oncogene withdrawal imposes varied cell fates poses a conundrum. Why does switching off a single oncogene within a clonal population of malignant cells lead to diverse outcomes? One possibility is that oncogene withdrawal forces cells to transit through several cell fate programs in succession (e.g., cell cycle arrest, followed by differentiation, then apoptosis). Alternatively, if multiple programs are engaged at the outset, the outcome for individual tumor cells might be strongly influenced by their interactions with neighboring cells and growth factors in the local microenvironment. In addition, diverse cell fate outcomes almost certainly reflect intrinsic tumor cell heterogeneity that awaits further characterization. Key questions remain regarding how such clinically distinct tumor cell subsets might arise. In particular, whether the differences that define these putative subsets are primarily genetically encoded (e.g., the consequence of clonal evolution) or epigenetically encoded (e.g., the remnant of a stem/progenitor cell hierarchy) remains an area of active inquiry. More detailed study of RCM tumors early in regression may bring rigorous data to bear on this question.

Ultimately, tumor regression is a dynamic process, and the relative contribution made by individual cytostatic and cytocidal programs will remain difficult to quantify so long as the assays only provide snapshot views. Emerging live cell imaging strategies may soon permit monitoring tumor cell fates during regression in real-time. It seems reasonable to surmise that both cell death and proliferation arrest contribute toward sustained disease remission. One possibility is that cytocidal programs figure prominently in tumor regression, whereas cytostatic programs subsequently become critical for maintaining regression in the surviving tumor cell fraction.

Maintaining Tumor Regression: Oncogene Withdrawal and Long-Term Tumor Dormancy

For the purpose of achieving cure, the cellular mechanisms that initiate regression and "de-bulk" the tumor may be less important than those that later maintain regression. Even the most potent targeted therapies appear incapable of eradicating all tumor cells. Imatinib can reduce CML cells to a nearly undetectable burden, yet relapses begin to accrue when the drug is stopped, showing that a malignant clone endures disease remission [31]. Similarly, persistence of so-called "minimal residual disease" (MRD) has long been recognized as the chief obstacle to cure of acute leukemias in adults treated with conventional chemotherapy. MRD also thwarts cure of solid tumors. In the case of breast cancer, disease remission is typically accomplished with surgery at the time of diagnosis, but MRD often persists and begets relapse years, even decades, later [32, 33].

A poorly understood phenomenon termed "tumor dormancy" has been proposed to account for prolonged periods of disease latency, during which subclinical cancer persists silently while retaining the capacity to seed relapse [34, 35]. A variety of mechanisms have been proposed to explain tumor dormancy with little in vivo evidence favoring one model over another. Some studies suggest that dormancy is enforced through complex interactions between tumor and host. For example, in some mouse models of sarcoma, disease latency can be maintained by a host immune response [36, 37]. Others have suggested that MRD remains dormant until a microscopic tumor focus can successfully recruit host vasculature by undergoing an "angiogenic switch" [38, 39]. If tumor–host interactions are important for maintaining dormancy, then modeling based exclusively on cancer cell lines propagated in culture may offer limited mechanistic insights.

By faithfully recapitulating clinical features of MRD, RCMs offer a unique opportunity to interrogate the biology of tumor dormancy. Thus far, dormancy appears to be a feature of most RCMs, as latent disease in the form of MRD typically persists after tumor regression (the Myc-initiated osteosarcoma model discussed above provides an important exception). The presence of dormant MRD can be documented readily by reactivating oncogenic signaling experimentally, which "awakens" sites of latent malignancy and typically yields rapidly growing tumors at previously affected sites. If oncogene withdrawal models "idealized" targeted therapy, then reactivation of oncogenic signaling is analogous to cessation of that therapy.

Reversible Cell Cycle Arrest: Is Dormant Malignancy Comprised of Dormant Tumor Cells?

An extended period of subclinical tumor dormancy is difficult to reconcile with the traditional concept that tumor cells proliferate in an unregulated manner [33]. One way to resolve this discrepancy is to posit that dormant disease lesions are maintained in a dynamic equilibrium wherein proliferating tumor cells fail to accumulate due to offsetting cell death. Alternatively, sites of dormant disease may be maintained by quiescent tumor cells, which exit the cell cycle indefinitely but retain their proliferative potential. Distinguishing between these models may be crucial to understanding treatment resistance. Most breast cancer patients receive adjuvant treatment with traditional cytotoxins following surgery with the goal of eradicating MRD. Determining whether malignant cells within MRD are actively cycling or quiescent may help in the rational design of improved adjuvant treatment strategies, since many anticancer agents act in a cell cycle phase-dependent manner.

Thus far, RCMs offer no direct in vivo evidence that oncogene withdrawal triggers tumor cell quiescence. Documenting quiescence poses a challenge since generally accepted cell markers are lacking. The value of quiescence markers in cancer research could rival that of senescence markers, leading several groups to pursue a molecular description of the quiescent cell [40, 41]. In the meanwhile, a functional demonstration of cell cycle re-entry is required to deem a cell population quiescent in the strict sense. Nonetheless, strong indirect evidence implies that oncogene withdrawal drives at least a subset of tumor cells into quiescence.

When dormant residual disease lesions that persisted after reversal of Wnt-initiated mammary tumors were implanted into the cleared mammary fat pads of host mice and maintained in the Wnt-off state, the resulting grafts regenerated normal-appearing, differentiation-competent ductal trees. When switched to the

Wnt-on state, these grafts rapidly and synchronously underwent morphologic transformation, begetting mammary tumors that were clonally related to the parental tumor [42]. Thus, cells residing in MRD that possess latent malignant potential participated in mammary gland reconstitution, a scenario most easily explained by invoking cellular quiescence within dormant disease lesions. Likewise, when mammary epithelial cells engineered to reversibly co-express Myc and Ras were propagated in 3D Matrigel culture, oncogene expression yielded solid, depolarized (i.e., tumor-like) cell clusters that regressed upon Myc/Ras withdrawal. The spherical monolayer of cells that survived de-induction appeared to be quiescent since they remained competent to expand in number during regeneration of a ductal tree in vivo [43].

Genetic Routes to Tumor Escape: Target Mutations, Rescue Mutations, and Off-Target Pathways

Excitement sparked by the spectacular success of targeted therapy against CML has been offset by concern that the most common and deadly solid tumors might present a far greater challenge [44]. CML is genetically homogeneous in that the BCR-ABL translocation serves as a driver mutation in nearly all cases, and relatively few additional genetic aberrations overlie this lesion. In the case of solid tumors, most mutations affecting individual driver genes are found at low prevalence, and those driver mutations that are prevalent across tumor sets are accompanied by numerous additional genetic aberrations [45]. Nonetheless, there are promising examples of targeted therapy triggering regression of complex solid tumors, and some important lessons learned from imatinib resistance apply to solid tumors as well.

Target Mutations: Validating and Overcoming Drug-Resistant Variants

Second-site mutations that modify the drug target are the best-studied mechanism of resistance to targeted agents. Sawyers and colleagues established this paradigm by showing that secondary mutations in the *BCR-ABL* fusion gene confer imatinib resistance [46]. They went on to render this observation clinically useful by identifying an agent, dasatinib, with potent activity against most imatinib-resistant BCR-ABL mutants [47]. With remarkable speed, dasatinib became established as a highly effective therapy for imatinib-resistant CML [1].

In 2004, several groups independently identified activating mutations in the epidermal growth factor receptor (EGFR) within a subset of lung adenocarcinomas that responded dramatically to EGFR antagonists [48–50]. Mirroring experience with imatinib, second-site EGFR mutations were soon identified as candidate drivers of drug-resistant disease relapse [51, 52]. Whereas second-line CML agents largely emerged from studies employing clinical specimens and cell lines, RCMs have assumed a central role in ongoing efforts to develop second-line treatments for EGFR-dependent lung cancers. Lung tumor-prone RCMs generated using mutant *EGFR* alleles have proven useful for both mechanistic studies and for preclinical testing of novel agents and drug combinations

RCMs engineered with lung-directed, Dox-inducible transgenes confirmed the central role played by mutant *EGFR* alleles in lung tumor maintenance. The two most common cancer-associated, activated EGFR alleles (*EGFR^{L858R}* and *EGFR^{delL747-S752}*) each were capable of initiating invasive lung tumors that regressed fully upon oncogene withdrawal [53, 54]. Notably, these models permitted idealized targeted therapy (simulated via abrogation of transgene expression) to be compared head-to-head with actual treatments using clinically important targeted agents. The mode and extent of tumor regression under each condition proved indistinguishable when assessed by serial magnetic resonance imaging (MRI) of live animals and by histopathology, indicating that oncogene withdrawal closely mimics the therapeutic effect of EGFR antagonists in vivo [53, 54].

After the recurring second-site *EGFR^{T790M}* mutation was identified in cases of acquired resistance to gefitinib or erlotinib, new RCMs were engineered incorporating the *EGFR^{T790M}* gatekeeper mutation. Whereas transgenic expression of a wild-type *EGFR* allele in mouse lungs failed to initiate tumors in preliminary experiments, expression of an *EGFR* allele harboring an isolated T790M mutation (*EGFR^{T790M}*) yielded lung tumors after an extended latency, supporting the notion that the T790M substitution by itself imparts modest EGFR activation [55]. Lung tumors initiated by the *EGFR^{T790M}* allele regressed upon abrogation of transgene expression, demonstrating their addiction to oncogenic EGFR signaling. However, these same tumors were resistant to treatment with erlotinib, validating the role of T790M mutations in conferring drug resistance. To model acquired second-site mutations, two separate groups engineered RCMs harboring double-mutant EGFR transgenes encoding the erlotinib-sensitizing L858R mutation in cis with the gatekeeper T790M mutation. These inducer-dependent *EGFR^{L858R+T790M}* alleles mirror those found in drug-resistant clinical specimens [55, 56]. Again, lung tumors arose that were transgene-dependent but erlotinib resistant, in keeping with clinical research findings.

RCMs initiated by the *EGFR^{L858R+T790M}* allele provide an important preclinical model for testing strategies aimed at overcoming T790M-mediated drug resistance. For example, in proof-of-principle experiments, the geldanamycin analogue 17-AAG showed modest activity against *EGFR^{L858R+T790M}*-dependent lung tumors and appeared to destabilize mutant EGFR protein [55]. These findings fit well with a model where 17-AAG inhibits the molecular chaperone hsp90, leading to enhanced degradation of mutant kinases [57]. In preclinical studies, irreversible inhibitors of the EGFR kinase domain showed promising antitumor activity in the *EGFR^{L858R+T790M}* model, especially when incorporated into combination therapy. One irreversible inhibitor, HKI-272, synergized strongly with rapamycin, revealing a role for mTOR signaling in T790M-mediated drug resistance [56]. Likewise, surprising synergy between BIBW-2992 and cetuximab indicated that the response to kinase inhibition may be enhanced by antibody-mediated depletion of the total EGFR pool [58]. Notably, neither rapamycin nor cetuximab synergized with the reversible EGFR inhibitor erlotinib, demonstrating that irreversible inhibitors offer a clear therapeutic advantage in the context of the T790M gatekeeper mutation.

More recently, RCMs harboring erlotinib-sensitizing *EGFR* alleles were used to examine mechanisms of acquired TKI resistance [59]. Lung tumors persisting after several rounds of intermittent erlotinib treatment were analyzed to identify escape mutations. Several tumors acquired the second-site T790M mutation, and one acquired *MET* amplification, consistent with RCM tumors traversing clinically relevant escape routes. Moreover, a majority of the tumors lacked target mutations, yet showed evidence of EGFR activation on immunohistochemistry. In-depth analysis of these tumors may yet reveal novel escape mechanisms responsible for acquired erlotinib resistance.

Rescue Mutations: Indirect Routes to Pathway Reactivation

Cancer genome resequencing studies performed on a variety of cancers reveal that a characteristic set of oncogenic pathways is dysregulated in each tumor type. But, even within narrowly defined cancer subtypes, tumor-to-tumor variability abounds. Though the same pathway may be disrupted repeatedly, individual tumors achieve this end by acquiring mutations in any one of multiple pathway components [45]. It follows that mutations affecting a variety of genes might suffice to reactivate oncogenic signaling and trigger tumor escape. One plausible alternative to target mutations that disrupts a drug–target interaction might be rescue mutations that restore oncogenic signaling indirectly by altering core signaling components elsewhere in the targeted pathway.

Have rescue mutations been identified that explain tumor escape encountered in the clinic? Amplification of *MET* may function as a rescue mutation in a subset of lung cancers that initially respond to EGFR antagonists [60]. However, some evidence suggest that *MET* amplification does not precisely substitute for EGFR loss of function, since a subset of relapsed tumors harbors *MET* amplification together with the drug-resistant T790M EGFR target mutation [61]. Thus, acquired MET-dependence may represent an example of "addiction-switching" where the activation of a second oncogenic pathway substitutes for targeted inhibition of the first [62].

RCM studies unambiguously demonstrate that rescue mutations can drive tumor escape. Interrogating escape mechanisms in a reversible Wnt1-initiated breast cancer model, most relapsed tumors were found to express Wnt pathway target genes, indicating reactivation of oncogenic Wnt signaling [63]. Half of these tumors reactivated *Wnt1* transgene expression, presumably via alterations in the tet regulatory module. However, the remaining relapses escaped without transgene reactivation, prompting a search for rescue mutations elsewhere in the Wnt pathway. Activating mutations in β(beta)-*catenin*, a key downstream component of the Wnt signaling cascade, were identified specifically in the subset of tumors that expressed Wnt target genes but lacked *Wnt1* transgene expression. Transgene re-expression and β-*catenin* mutations occurred in a mutually exclusive fashion, leaving little doubt that they represent alternative routes to restoring Wnt signaling. Thus, the β-*catenin* mutations identified in this model are *bona fide* rescue mutations [15].

In other RCMs, rescue mutations were identified that cause the reversible gene switch to malfunction. When Dox-dependent co-expression of *c-MYC* and *KRAS*[G12D] transgenes was used to drive mammary tumorigenesis, the relapses that arose after Dox withdrawal typically re-expressed both transgenes, pointing to corruption of the tet regulatory module [64]. Remarkably, point mutations in the reverse tetracycline transactivator (rtTA) were identified and shown capable of empowering rtTA to drive transgene expression in a Dox-independent manner. As in the case of β-catenin rescue mutations, these rtTA rescue mutations were identified exclusively in relapsed tumors and not in their antecedent primaries. Presumably, this reflects clonal selection for rare variants during tumor escape.

These studies document enormous selective pressure favoring the maintenance or reactivation of a targeted pathway during tumor escape. Important questions remain regarding when rescue mutations arise, and by what mechanism (see Fig. 8.1). In the case of CML, second-site BCR-ABL mutations capable of driving relapse exist prior to initiation of imatinib therapy. It seems likely that rescue mutations likewise precede oncogene withdrawal in RCMs. Because they act redundantly, superimposed on a previously activated oncogenic pathway, rescue mutations ought to be rare prior to oncogene withdrawal. They provide a tumor cell with little added fitness and a negligible impetus for clonal expansion. But, when potent targeted therapy is simulated, the selection pressure is suddenly and profoundly altered. That rare tumor cell harboring a rescue mutation enjoys a near-perfect remedy for oncogene withdrawal – one that precisely complements that which is lost.

Rescue mutations provide alternate routes to tumor escape, which may prove challenging to close off. Experience with CML has raised hope that combining drugs to suppress common second-site target mutations might prevent escape. However, as these drug cocktails approach "idealized" targeted therapy, selective pressure may

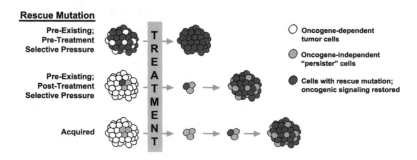

Fig. 8.1 Rescue mutations. When, where, and how do they arise?

build in favor of rescue mutations in downstream signaling components. In addition to the problems posed by an expanding number of available escape routes, identifying the genes that harbor rescue mutations may not be straightforward. The detailed molecular characterization of the Wnt signaling cascade in model systems provided a framework for zeroing in on β-catenin mutations as possible culprit lesions. Where signaling pathways are less well characterized, candidate gene approaches may not suffice. For example, the key downstream molecular transducers of HER2-dependent signaling in human breast cancer remain in doubt, so the candidate genes at greatest risk of sustaining rescue mutations in the context of anti-HER2 therapy are not clear. Identifying rescue mutations in RCM tumors and clinical specimens may require unbiased genome-wide DNA sequence comparisons between cancer samples obtained before and after tumor escape.

Off-Target Escape: A Key Role for p19^{ARF}-p53 Pathway Disruption and EMT

Pathway reactivation provides a clear mechanistic route to drug resistance, but some tumors mysteriously shed their dependence on a signaling pathway en route to relapse. For example, antihormonal treatment of advanced breast cancers with estrogen antagonists frequently triggers dramatic tumor regression, but drug-resistant relapse inevitably emerges. In a fraction of cases, relapsed disease responds to second-line estrogen antagonists, indicating that acquired resistance involved reactivation of estrogen-dependent signaling. But in other cases, relapsed disease proves to be resistant to all available antiestrogens, suggesting that lesions in an off-target pathway render estrogen-dependent signaling dispensable. A key question in clinical oncology centers on whether each tumor achieves off-target resistance by a unique molecular route, or whether off-target escape involves recurring lesions affecting a limited number of key pathways.

Since p19^{Arf}-p53 pathway function serves as an important determinant of tumor response following treatment with conventional cytotoxic agents, several groups have explored how disrupting this pathway impacts tumor regression and relapse in RCMs. p53 itself was found to be dispensable for regression triggered by oncogene withdrawal in several studies spanning different oncogenes and different tissue compartments. Regression of K-Ras^{G12D}-dependent lung tumors and Wnt1-dependent mammary tumors occurred even in mice that inherited two null p53 alleles [3, 11]. Similarly, p53-independent regression occurred in cases where tumors were rendered functionally p53-null by an acquired somatic mutation [11, 65]. In mice inheriting a single p53-null allele (*p53$^{(+/-)}$*), most Wnt1-initiated mammary tumors and c-Myc-initiated lymphomas remained reversible, including tumors whose wild-type *p53* allele was deleted by a loss-of-heterozygosity event. But, in both RCMs, p53-deficiency correlated with increased residual disease burden. For example, 40% of the Wnt1-initiated mammary tumors that arose in *p53$^{(+/-)}$* mice regressed incompletely upon oncogene withdrawal, whereas complete regression occurred in nearly all mice carrying two wild-type *p53* alleles. The palpable tumor remnants that persist in *p53*[(+/−)] mice soon regrew in an oncogene-independent manner.

Even when Wnt-initiated mammary tumors arising on *p53*[(+/−)] mice regressed to become clinically undetectable, p53-deficiency strongly promoted tumor escape over an extended monitoring period. Remarkably, relapsed tumors arising in *p53*[(+/−)] mice nearly always showed histological and molecular features characteristic of an epithelial-to-mesenchymal transition (EMT), whereas only a minority of relapsed tumors from *p53* wild-type mice bore EMT hallmarks [11, 63]. Analysis of Wnt pathway transcriptional targets showed that EMT-type relapses reactivate Wnt signaling only rarely, implying that EMT compensates for the loss of Wnt signaling by a mechanism that is indirect, and as yet undefined. Subsequent work showed that p19[Arf] operates upstream of p53 to suppress oncogene-independent tumor escape, since *p19*[Arf]-deficiency phenocopied *p53*-deficiency by promoting EMT-associated relapse [63].

The EMT mode of oncogene-independent tumor escape is not restricted to Wnt1-initiated tumors. Relapses in an RCM of Neu-initiated mammary tumorigenesis frequently involved EMT, even in *p53* wild-type mice [13]. Notably, this work showed that EMT can play a causal role in tumor escape. Neu-dependent tumor cells transduced with retrovirus encoding the transcription factor *Snail*, a master regulator of EMT, regressed upon oncogene withdrawal but rapidly regrew in a Neu-independent manner. Since EMT appears to enable relapse following withdrawal of a variety of oncogenes, EMT may be a general mode of escape that broadly predisposes mammary tumors to treatment failure. Supporting this notion, recent preclinical and clinical studies implicate EMT in treatment-resistant breast cancer [66, 67].

Tumor Cell Nonautonomous Effects of p19[ARF]-p53 Pathway Disruption

Unexpectedly, disruption of the p19[Arf]-p53 pathway can promote tumor escape by altering tumor–host interactions. For instance, *p19*[Arf] loss altered Bcr-Abl-dependence in a mouse model of acute lymphoblastic leukemia by acting in a cell-nonautonomous manner [68, 69]. Retroviral transduction of *Bcr-Abl* into wild-type bone marrow cells initiated imatinib-sensitive lympholeukemias, whereas the more aggressive leukemias that arose upon transducing *p19*[Arf]-deficient marrow were imatinib-refractory. Remarkably, imatinib sensitivity was restored when *p19*[Arf]-deficient leukemias were propagated in vitro, pointing to a cell-extrinsic mechanism underlying drug resistance in mice. This resistance appeared to involve cytokine signaling in the leukemic microenvironment, since transducing Bcr-Abl into *p19*[Arf]-deficient marrow that is additionally deficient in the cytokine receptor common γ(gamma)-chain yielded imatinib-sensitive disease. Therefore, drugs that disrupt cytokine-mediated signaling may enhance imatinib activity against acute lymphoblastic leukemias, which are often rendered $p19^{ARF}$-deficient due to *CDKN2A* locus deletions [70].

In a similar vein, RCM mice studies showed that full regression of Myc-driven lymphomas requires reversal of an angiogenic switch downstream of p53 [65]. As mentioned earlier, when Myc-initiated lymphomas lacked p53 expression, they left behind a greater burden of residual tumor following oncogene withdrawal and relapsed more quickly than their p53-intact counterparts. Lymphomas that lacked p53 expression likewise lacked expression of Tsp-1, a key p53-regulated antagonist of angiogenesis. Restoring either p53 or Tsp1 expression in Myc-dependent lymphoma cell lines abrogated Myc-independent angiogenesis, enabling complete and sustained regression of cell line-derived lymphomas upon Myc withdrawal. Together, these findings underscore once again how studies based solely on in vitro propagation of tumor cell lines may overlook important mechanisms of tumor escape.

Epigenetic Routes to Tumor Escape: The Stem-Persister Phenotype and Epithelial-Mesenchymal Transition

Somatic mutations are unlikely to be the only clinically important source of tumor cell heterogeneity. Returning to the CML paradigm, imatinib treatment of chronic phase disease reduces tumor burden by several orders of magnitude, but does not eradicate the malignant clone [31]. Latent disease appears to be maintained by a small population of imatinib-refractory malignant stem cells. Disease remission is maintained so long as these aberrant stem cells primarily yield differentiated progeny that remain imatinib-sensitive. Thus, a vestige of the stem cell hierarchy operative during normal hematopoiesis yields clinically important tumor cell heterogeneity. Whether stem cell hierarchies serve as a clinically important source of tumor cell heterogeneity in solid cancers remains controversial. Some evidence from RCMs offer indirect support for a cancer stem cell model operating in cancers of the breast and liver [30, 42].

Recent findings from disparate models offer an intriguing link between the stem-progenitor cell phenotype and epithelial-mesenchymal transition (EMT) [66, 71]. Furthermore, p53 pathway disruption not only enables EMT in RCMs but also enables reacquisition of stem cell properties during transcription factor-mediated reprogramming of somatic cells [72]. Whether EMT in cancer models is triggered by genetic or epigenetic events remains unclear, but an epigenetic route seems more likely if EMT changes are indeed reversible and highly context-dependent, as has been proposed [73]. A definitive role for EMT in the progression of human cancers remains to be firmly established. Unlike RCM tumors, human breast cancers at relapse do not ordinarily bear hallmarks of a full-blown EMT. Here, RCMs may fall short as faithful models of human cancers, with discrepancies possibly reflecting important mouse-human species differences that stem from the greater plasticity of mouse cell lineages.

Forward Genetic Screens for Mediators of Tumor Escape

A substantial fraction of solid tumors that become resistant to targeted therapy do so without acquiring second-site mutations in the drug target. The design of second-line drugs for such tumors is made problematic by the need to counter escape mechanisms that remain poorly defined. Unfortunately, this problem is as old as the practice of medical oncology. Traditional cytotoxic agents yield dramatic tumor remissions when used in combination against a number of advanced malignancies (e.g., acute myelogenous leukemia, small cell lung cancer), but most patients subsequently develop treatment-refractory disease relapse. Though several important mechanisms underlying resistance to individual cytotoxins have been identified, translating these findings into improved treatment regimens remains challenging.

Several groups have turned to mouse models to identify genes that drive tumor escape. Toward this end, a genetic complementation assay was devised which allows candidate genes to be tested for their ability to rescue tumor maintenance in the face of oncogene withdrawal [74]. This strategy used avian retroviral vectors that enabled repeated infection of cells from mice transgenic for the avian retroviral receptor, TVA. To establish proof of principle, p53-deficient mouse embryo fibroblasts were engineered such that retroviral infection imparted Dox-dependent expression of a $K-Ras^{G12D}$ transgene. Infected cells gave rise to Dox-dependent tumors when implanted on the flanks of nude mice, as expected. Notably, superinfection of these tumor cells with a virus harboring a constitutively expressed $K-Ras^{G12D}$ allele rendered tumors resistant to Dox withdrawal, whereas tumors superinfected with control retrovirus remained Dox-dependent. This flexible model might be adapted to assay complementation for a variety of oncogenes across a spectrum of tissues.

Others have employed quasi-random insertional mutagenesis strategies to screen genome-wide for genes that confer drug resistance. For example, retroviral infection was used to introduce Bcr-Abl into transplanted bone marrow, creating a mouse model of CML. Imatinib therapy triggered disease remission, but ultimately mice relapsed with imatinib-resistant leukemia. Intriguingly, imatinib was shown to select for clones of leukemic cells harboring retroviral integration near the *Runx3* promoter [75], suggesting that retroviral activation of *Runx3* expression may contribute to imatinib resistance. Indeed, Runx3 expression was shown to protect Bcr-Abl-positive cell lines from imatinib-induced apoptosis. Taking a similar tack, retroviral transduction of mouse bone marrow was used to accelerate the onset of leukemias in an Nf1-deficient model [76]. A subset of these leukemias underwent transient remission upon treatment with an MEK inhibitor, and the retroviral integrations sites mapped in relapsed disease implicated several genes and pathways in drug-resistant tumor progression.

As yet, forward screens for tumor escape genes have employed drugs, but it is easy to envision adapting RCMs for this purpose in cases where potent targeted therapies remain under development. Cooperating genetic events might be superimposed on existing RCMs using retroviral infections as above. Alternatively, RCMs might be modified such that Sleeping Beauty-mediated transposition cooperates in tumorigenesis and relapse [77]. Using these and other tools, unbiased genome-wide screens for tumor escape genes are likely to be taken to saturation over the next decade. It will be interesting to see whether each initiating oncogenic pathway and tissue type yields a unique set of escape routes, or whether a limited set of escape routes provides well-worn paths to disease relapse.

The Big Question: Which Sources of Tumor Cell Diversity Are Clinically Important?

In the end, RCMs will be most useful if they aid in deciphering and combating mechanisms of tumor escape that actually thwart targeted therapy in the clinic. The discovery of second-site and rescue mutations highlights the role of tumor cell genetic diversity in tumor escape. Since multiple sources of genetic diversity have been described, there is a compelling need to clarify which sources most commonly drive relapse (Fig. 8.2). Second-site gatekeeper mutations account for only a fraction of kinase inhibitor-resistant relapses, so other mechanisms of escape await discovery. Along these lines, an elegant study recently showed that introducing chromosomal instability into RCM lung tumors via transient overexpression of Mad2 hastened subsequent relapse [78]. These findings have ominous implications, since the chromosomal instability modeled here likely arises early in tumorigenesis. Conversely, treatment-induced mutations may be a key, late-arising source of tumor cell diversity which clinicians can hope to modify. Most clinically important cytotoxins are potent mutagens and carcinogens in their own right. The concept that treatment-associated mutations drive tumor escape, though attractive, remains unproved.

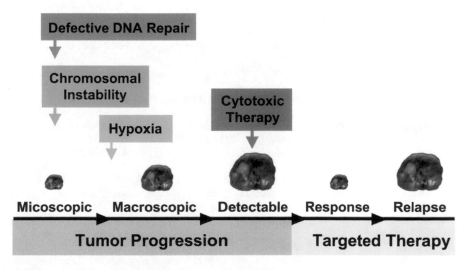

Fig. 8.2 Potential sources of tumor cell genetic heterogeneity

Validating the concept with well-characterized RCMs would have profound implications for optimizing the sequential administration of cytotoxins and targeted agents. Finally, with continued refinement, RCMs ought to emerge as key research tools for delving into potential epigenetic sources of tumor cell diversity and exploring their clinical relevance.

References

1. Sawyers CL. Shifting paradigms: the seeds of oncogene addiction. Nat Med. 2009;15:1158–61.
2. Chin L et al. Essential role for oncogenic Ras in tumour maintenance. Nature. 1999;400: 468–72.
3. Fisher GH et al. Induction and apoptotic regression of lung adenocarcinomas by regulation of a K-Ras transgene in the presence and absence of tumor suppressor genes. Genes Dev. 2001;15:3249–62.
4. Pelengaris S, Littlewood T, Khan M, Elia G, Evan G. Reversible activation of c-Myc in skin: induction of a complex neoplastic phenotype by a single oncogenic lesion. Mol Cell. 1999;3:565–77.
5. Weinstein IB. Cancer. Addiction to oncogenes – the Achilles heal of cancer. Science. 2002;297:63–4.
6. Martins CP, Brown-Swigart L, Evan GI. Modeling the therapeutic efficacy of p53 restoration in tumors. Cell. 2006;127:1323–34.
7. Ventura A et al. Restoration of p53 function leads to tumour regression in vivo. Nature. 2007;445:661–5.
8. Xue W et al. Senescence and tumour clearance is triggered by p53 restoration in murine liver carcinomas. Nature. 2007;445:656–60.
9. Kastan MB. Wild-type p53: tumors can't stand it. Cell. 2007;128:837–40.
10. Pelengaris S et al. Brief inactivation of c-Myc is not sufficient for sustained regression of c-Myc-induced tumours of pancreatic islets and skin epidermis. BMC Biol. 2004;2:26.
11. Gunther EJ et al. Impact of p53 loss on reversal and recurrence of conditional Wnt-induced tumorigenesis. Genes Dev. 2003;17:488–501.
12. Boxer RB, Jang JW, Sintasath L, Chodosh LA. Lack of sustained regression of c-MYC-induced mammary adenocarcinomas following brief or prolonged MYC inactivation. Cancer Cell. 2004;6:577–86.
13. Moody SE et al. The transcriptional repressor Snail promotes mammary tumor recurrence. Cancer Cell. 2005;8:197–209.
14. Chin L, DePinho RA. Flipping the oncogene switch: illumination of tumor maintenance and regression. Trends Genet. 2000;16:147–50.
15. van Amerongen R, Berns A. Targeted anticancer therapies: mouse models help uncover the mechanisms of tumor escape. Cancer Cell. 2008;13:5–7.
16. Vargo-Gogola T, Rosen JM. Modelling breast cancer: one size does not fit all. Nat Rev Cancer. 2007;7:659–72.
17. Frese KK, Tuveson DA. Maximizing mouse cancer models. Nat Rev Cancer. 2007;7:645–58.
18. Felsher DW. Cancer revoked: oncogenes as therapeutic targets. Nat Rev Cancer. 2003;3:375–80.
19. Shachaf CM, Felsher DW. Rehabilitation of cancer through oncogene inactivation. Trends Mol Med. 2005;11:316–21.
20. Hanahan D, Weinberg RA. The hallmarks of cancer. Cell. 2000;100:57–70.
21. Pelengaris S, Khan M, Evan GI. Suppression of Myc-induced apoptosis in beta cells exposes multiple oncogenic properties of Myc and triggers carcinogenic progression. Cell. 2002;109:321–34.

22. Evan GI, d'Adda di Fagagna F. Cellular senescence: hot or what? Curr Opin Genet Dev. 2009;19:25–31.
23. Schmitt CA et al. A senescence program controlled by p53 and p16INK4a contributes to the outcome of cancer therapy. Cell. 2002;109:335–46.
24. Wu CH et al. Cellular senescence is an important mechanism of tumor regression upon c-Myc inactivation. Proc Natl Acad Sci USA. 2007;104:13028–33.
25. Swartling FJ et al. Pleiotropic role for MYCN in medulloblastoma. Genes Dev. 2010;24: 1059–72.
26. van Riggelen J et al. The interaction between Myc and Miz1 is required to antagonize TGFbeta-dependent autocrine signaling during lymphoma formation and maintenance. Genes Dev. 2010;24:1281–94.
27. Sarkisian CJ et al. Dose-dependent oncogene-induced senescence in vivo and its evasion during mammary tumorigenesis. Nat Cell Biol. 2007;9:493–505.
28. Murphy DJ et al. Distinct thresholds govern Myc's biological output in vivo. Cancer Cell. 2008;14:447–57.
29. Jain M et al. Sustained loss of a neoplastic phenotype by brief inactivation of MYC. Science. 2002;297:102–4.
30. Shachaf CM et al. MYC inactivation uncovers pluripotent differentiation and tumour dormancy in hepatocellular cancer. Nature. 2004;431:1112–7.
31. Michor F et al. Dynamics of chronic myeloid leukaemia. Nature. 2005;435:1267–70.
32. Demicheli R, Biganzoli E, Boracchi P, Greco M, Retsky MW. Recurrence dynamics does not depend on the recurrence site. Breast Cancer Res. 2008;10:R83.
33. Demicheli R. Tumour dormancy: findings and hypotheses from clinical research on breast cancer. Semin Cancer Biol. 2001;11:297–306.
34. Uhr JW, Scheuermann RH, Street NE, Vitetta ES. Cancer dormancy: opportunities for new therapeutic approaches. Nat Med. 1997;3:505–9.
35. Aguirre-Ghiso JA. Models, mechanisms and clinical evidence for cancer dormancy. Nat Rev Cancer. 2007;7:834–46.
36. Koebel CM et al. Adaptive immunity maintains occult cancer in an equilibrium state. Nature. 2007;450:903–7.
37. Teng MW, Swann JB, Koebel CM, Schreiber RD, Smyth MJ. Immune-mediated dormancy: an equilibrium with cancer. J Leukoc Biol. 2008;84:988–93.
38. Udagawa T, Fernandez A, Achilles EG, Folkman J, D'Amato RJ. Persistence of microscopic human cancers in mice: alterations in the angiogenic balance accompanies loss of tumor dormancy. FASEB J. 2002;16:1361–70.
39. Watnick RS, Cheng YN, Rangarajan A, Ince TA, Weinberg RA. Ras modulates Myc activity to repress thrombospondin-1 expression and increase tumor angiogenesis. Cancer Cell. 2003;3:219–31.
40. Coller HA, Sang L, Roberts JM. A new description of cellular quiescence. PLoS Biol. 2006;4:e83.
41. Harmes DC, DiRenzo J. Cellular quiescence in mammary stem cells and breast tumor stem cells: got testable hypotheses? J Mammary Gland Biol Neoplasia. 2009;14:19–27.
42. Gestl SA, Leonard TL, Biddle JL, Debies MT, Gunther EJ. Dormant Wnt-initiated mammary cancer can participate in reconstituting functional mammary glands. Mol Cell Biol. 2007;27:195–207.
43. Jechlinger M, Podsypanina K, Varmus H. Regulation of transgenes in three-dimensional cultures of primary mouse mammary cells demonstrates oncogene dependence and identifies cells that survive deinduction. Genes Dev. 2009;23:1677–88.
44. Kaelin Jr WG. Gleevec: prototype or outlier? Sci STKE. 2004;2004:12.
45. Stratton MR, Campbell PJ, Futreal PA. The cancer genome. Nature. 2009;458:719–24.
46. Gorre ME et al. Clinical resistance to STI-571 cancer therapy caused by BCR-ABL gene mutation or amplification. Science. 2001;293:876–80.
47. Shah NP et al. Overriding imatinib resistance with a novel ABL kinase inhibitor. Science. 2004;305:399–401.

48. Lynch TJ et al. Activating mutations in the epidermal growth factor receptor underlying responsiveness of non-small-cell lung cancer to gefitinib. N Engl J Med. 2004;350:2129–39.
49. Paez JG et al. EGFR mutations in lung cancer: correlation with clinical response to gefitinib therapy. Science. 2004;304:1497–500.
50. Pao W et al. EGF receptor gene mutations are common in lung cancers from "never smokers" and are associated with sensitivity of tumors to gefitinib and erlotinib. Proc Natl Acad Sci USA. 2004;101:13306–11.
51. Kobayashi S et al. EGFR mutation and resistance of non-small-cell lung cancer to gefitinib. N Engl J Med. 2005;352:786–92.
52. Pao W et al. Acquired resistance of lung adenocarcinomas to gefitinib or erlotinib is associated with a second mutation in the EGFR kinase domain. PLoS Med. 2005;2:e73.
53. Ji H et al. The impact of human EGFR kinase domain mutations on lung tumorigenesis and in vivo sensitivity to EGFR-targeted therapies. Cancer Cell. 2006;9:485–95.
54. Politi K et al. Lung adenocarcinomas induced in mice by mutant EGF receptors found in human lung cancers respond to a tyrosine kinase inhibitor or to down-regulation of the receptors. Genes Dev. 2006;20:1496–510.
55. Regales L et al. Development of new mouse lung tumor models expressing EGFR T790M mutants associated with clinical resistance to kinase inhibitors. PLoS One. 2007;2:e810.
56. Li D et al. Bronchial and peripheral murine lung carcinomas induced by T790M-L858R mutant EGFR respond to HKI-272 and rapamycin combination therapy. Cancer Cell. 2007;12:81–93.
57. Sawai A et al. Inhibition of Hsp90 down-regulates mutant epidermal growth factor receptor (EGFR) expression and sensitizes EGFR mutant tumors to paclitaxel. Cancer Res. 2008;68:589–96.
58. Regales L et al. Dual targeting of EGFR can overcome a major drug resistance mutation in mouse models of EGFR mutant lung cancer. J Clin Invest. 2009;119:3000–10.
59. Politi K, Fan PD, Shen R, Zakowski M, Varmus H. Erlotinib resistance in mouse models of epidermal growth factor receptor-induced lung adenocarcinoma. Dis Model Mech. 2010;3:111–9.
60. Engelman JA et al. MET amplification leads to gefitinib resistance in lung cancer by activating ERBB3 signaling. Science. 2007;316:1039–43.
61. Bean J et al. MET amplification occurs with or without T790M mutations in EGFR mutant lung tumors with acquired resistance to gefitinib or erlotinib. Proc Natl Acad Sci USA. 2007;104:20932–7.
62. Sharma SV, Settleman J. Oncogene addiction: setting the stage for molecularly targeted cancer therapy. Genes Dev. 2007;21:3214–31.
63. Debies MT et al. Tumor escape in a Wnt1-dependent mouse breast cancer model is enabled by p19Arf/p53 pathway lesions but not p16 Ink4a loss. J Clin Invest. 2008;118:51–63.
64. Podsypanina K, Politi K, Beverly LJ, Varmus HE. Oncogene cooperation in tumor maintenance and tumor recurrence in mouse mammary tumors induced by Myc and mutant Kras. Proc Natl Acad Sci USA. 2008;105:5242–7.
65. Giuriato S et al. Sustained regression of tumors upon MYC inactivation requires p53 or thrombospondin-1 to reverse the angiogenic switch. Proc Natl Acad Sci USA. 2006;103:16266–71.
66. Mani SA et al. The epithelial-mesenchymal transition generates cells with properties of stem cells. Cell. 2008;133:704–15.
67. Creighton CJ et al. Residual breast cancers after conventional therapy display mesenchymal as well as tumor-initiating features. Proc Natl Acad Sci USA. 2009;106:13820–5.
68. Williams RT, Roussel MF, Sherr CJ. Arf gene loss enhances oncogenicity and limits imatinib response in mouse models of Bcr-Abl-induced acute lymphoblastic leukemia. Proc Natl Acad Sci USA. 2006;103:6688–93.
69. Williams RT, den Besten W, Sherr CJ. Cytokine-dependent imatinib resistance in mouse BCR-ABL+, Arf-null lymphoblastic leukemia. Genes Dev. 2007;21:2283–7.
70. Dorshkind K, Witte ON. Linking the hematopoietic microenvironment to imatinib-resistant Ph+ B-ALL. Genes Dev. 2007;21:2249–52.

71. Sharma SV et al. A chromatin-mediated reversible drug-tolerant state in cancer cell subpopulations. Cell. 2010;141:69–80.
72. Krizhanovsky V, Lowe SW. Stem cells: the promises and perils of p53. Nature. 2009;460: 1085–6.
73. Polyak K, Weinberg RA. Transitions between epithelial and mesenchymal states: acquisition of malignant and stem cell traits. Nat Rev Cancer. 2009;9:265–73.
74. Pao W, Klimstra DS, Fisher GH, Varmus HE. Use of avian retroviral vectors to introduce transcriptional regulators into mammalian cells for analyses of tumor maintenance. Proc Natl Acad Sci USA. 2003;100:8764–9.
75. Miething C et al. Retroviral insertional mutagenesis identifies RUNX genes involved in chronic myeloid leukemia disease persistence under imatinib treatment. Proc Natl Acad Sci USA. 2007;104:4594–9.
76. Lauchle JO et al. Response and resistance to MEK inhibition in leukaemias initiated by hyperactive Ras. Nature. 2009;461:411–4.
77. Largaespada DA. Transposon-mediated mutagenesis of somatic cells in the mouse for cancer gene identification. Methods. 2009;49:282–6.
78. Sotillo R, Schvartzman JM, Socci ND, Benezra R. Mad2-induced chromosome instability leads to lung tumour relapse after oncogene withdrawal. Nature. 2010;464:436–40.

Chapter 9
microRNA: A Potential Therapy Able to Target Multiple Cancer Pathways

Benjamin Kefas and Benjamin W. Purow

Keywords Cancer • microRNA • Apoptosis • Therapy • Oncogenes • Tumor suppressors • Glioma • Notch • EGFR

Targeted Cancer Therapy

Cancer is a complex disease in which cells display uncontrolled growth and invade adjacent tissues, sometimes spreading to other locations in the body. Data over the years have indicated that the transformation of cells from normal to cancer cells is a multistep process where the malignant cell accumulates genetic and epigenetic lesions in oncogenes (genes that promote cancer) and tumor suppressors (genes that prevent cancer) [1]. At the end of their transformation process, the cancer cells lose their cellular identity and acquire growth independence and resistance to apoptosis (programmed cell death).

Because of the invasive nature of most cancer cells and their heterogeneous composition, they often are very difficult to treat using conventional means such as radiation and chemotherapy [1]. Recent studies have been focused on the inhibition of specific genes or pathways that are altered in given tumors, an approach broadly termed targeted cancer therapy [2]. The pathways and molecules altered in tumors include, among others, growth factors, anti-apoptotic, cell adhesion molecules, cell fate determination factors, and metabolic pathways.

Unlike normal cells, tumor cells do not depend on exogenous growth stimulation. They instead produce their own growth factors, which make them less dependent on their microenvironment. Such factors depend on the type of tumors. For instance, platelet-derived growth factor (PDGF) and tumor growth factor alpha (TGFα[alpha]) are produced by glioblastoma and sarcomas respectively [1].

B.W. Purow (✉)
Department of Neurology, University of Virginia, Charlottesville, VA, USA
e-mail: bwp5G@virginia.edu

D. Gioeli (ed.), *Targeted Therapies: Mechanisms of Resistance*,
Molecular and Translational Medicine, DOI 10.1007/978-1-60761-478-4_9,
© Springer Science+Business Media, LLC 2011

Cell surface receptors that transduce the signals from growth factors in the cells are also altered and deregulated during the process of tumorigenesis. The deregulation and overexpression of these receptors make tumor cells very sensitive and hyperresponsive to ambient amounts of growth factors that do not typically trigger proliferation of normal cells. This condition favors tumor cell proliferation [1]. The most prominent growth factor receptors deregulated in tumors are those containing tyrosine kinase components.

The deregulation of growth factor receptors could either be growth factor dependent or independent. In the case of growth factor-dependent tumors, both ligands and their respective receptors are overexpressed [2]. In the case of growth factor-independent tumors, their growth is driven by ligand-independent receptors that have been converted to oncogenic, constitutively active kinases [1, 2].

Both growth factor-dependent and independent tumors display activation of downstream pathways such as the phosphoinositide kinase (PI3K)/AKT and Ras pathways. These pathways have been specifically targeted in tumors. However, the results have been disappointing. Several theories have been proposed, ranging from compensatory pathways to the fact that most of these drugs work on the kinase activity of the targeted protein and leave other functions of this protein intact [2]. It may be possible to overcome these obstacles with a therapeutic approach that can target multiple pathways at once, and that can block expression of the targeted proteins. Exogenous delivery of microRNAs, small noncoding RNAs recently discovered to regulate much of the genome, has the potential to do both.

microRNA Discovery, Biogenesis and Function

The first microRNA (miRNA), lin-4, was discovered as a small noncoding RNA molecule that regulates the development of *Caenorhabditis elegans* (*C. elegans*) [3, 4]. At that time, they were considered to be peculiar to nematodes, until the subsequent discovery of their homologs in humans and other animals [4, 5].

miRNAs range from 17 to 25 nucleotides and are growing in numbers, function, and diversity. Computational modeling has predicted that there exist over 1,000 miRNAs [6, 7]. There are, however, around 533 microRNAs that have been documented [8].

In humans, miRNAs are distributed all over the genome and are encoded in both introns and intergenic regions [9]. For instance, the mature microRNA-7 is encoded in three different loci: mir-7-1 in the intron of heterogeneous nuclear ribonucleoprotein K (hnRNP-K) [10], mir-7-3 in the intron of pituitary gland-specific factor 1a (PGSF1) [11], and mir-7-2 in the intron of a long non-protein coding transcript on chromosome 15 [9]. The expression of miRNAs in the introns of genes suggests a parallel transcription of host genes and miRNAs takes place, and thus similar expression patterns for host gene and miRNAs may often be observed. This has been observed for several miRNAs and their host genes [9], such as miR-326 and its host gene beta-arrestin in glioblastomas [12].

Most miRNAs are transcribed as long primary transcripts, primary RNA (pri-miRNAs), by RNA polymerase II in the cell nucleus [13].They have a 5′ 7-methylguanosine cap and a 3′ polyadenylated tail folded into a long stem-like structure with a hairpin [13, 14] (Fig. 9.1). After transcription of pri-miRNAs, excision of part of the stem is performed in the nucleus by an enzymatic microprocessor complex that includes Drosha (RNase III enzyme) and DGCR8, leaving 65–85 nucleotide intermediate pre-miRNAs [15] (Fig. 9.1). The pre-miRNAs, which are short RNA hairpins bearing a 2–3 nucleotide overhang, are bound and transported out of the nucleus to the cytoplasm by a nuclear exporting protein Exportin 5 [16]. In the cytoplasm, the enzyme Dicer removes the hairpin loop and generates a 19–22 base pair double stranded RNA, mature miRNA [17–19]. One of the mature miRNA strands is incorporated into the large RNA-induced silencing complex (RISC). The mature miRNA in the RISC guides the complex to the target messenger RNAs (mRNAs) to repress the expression of targeted genes [20, 21]. The repression of mRNA is achieved in two different ways, depending on the complementarity

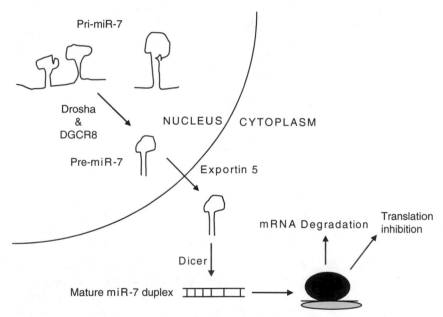

Fig. 9.1 Overview of microRNA biogenesis and function. The transcription of miRNA gene is facilitated by RNA polymerase II in the nucleus. The resulting transcript (primary miRNA >1 kb) is then cleaved by Drosha and DGCR8 to a pre-miRNA (70 nt). The pre-miRNA is exported out of the nucleus to the cytoplasm by exportin 5. The pre-miRNA undergoes processing, which involves the removal of the hairpin loop by dicer yielding a mature miRNA duplex. One of the mature miRNA strands is incorporated into the risc complex and guides it to the target miRNA. A partial complementarity leads to translational inhibition, while a near-perfect one leads to mRNA degradation

between the so-called "seed" region (bases 2–8 or 1–7) of the miRNA and the target [22]. In the cases where the miRNA seed region binds with near-perfect complementarity to the 3'-UTR of its target gene, the mRNA is cut and degraded. In the usual situation, there is imperfect complementarity between the miRNA and the 3'-UTR of its target, resulting in translational inhibition [23]. Also, recent studies have uncovered five general features of site context on the 3'UTR of genes that influence site efficacy: AU-rich nucleotide composition near the site, proximity to sites for coexpressed miRNAs (which leads to cooperative action), proximity to residues pairing to miRNA nucleotides 13–16, positioning within the 3'-UTR at least 15 nucleotides from the stop codon, and positioning away from the center of long UTRs [24].

microRNAs and Cancer

The first direct evidence for the involvement of miRNAs in cancer came from the observation that the chromosome region 13q14 is deleted in a majority of chronic lymphocytic leukemia (CLL). This deletion suggested the presence of a tumor suppressor in the locus, but a relevant tumor suppressor gene could not be found in this region. It was recently uncovered that this region encodes miR-15 and miR-16 in its intron, and it was discovered that 68% of patients with CLL have reduced abundance of these miRNAs [25]. Further studies confirm miR-15 and miR-16 as tumor suppressors in CLL targeting the oncogenic BCL2 [26].

Several other miRNAs have been either mapped to chromosomal regions involved in or found to be downregulated in cancers, such as let-7 in lung, ovarian, and liver tumors [27–30]. Furthermore, the levels of let-7 have been correlated to cancer prognosis [30–33]. The reason for this correlation has been linked to the targeting of the oncogenes RAS and myc by let-7 miRNA family [28, 34] (Table 9.1) [12, 25, 26, 28, 34–53]. RAS genes encode protein kinases that bind guanine nucleotides and they are important signal transducers in cells. It is mutated in about 20–30% of all human tumors [54]. Myc genes encode transcription factors with a basic Helix-Loop-Helix Leucine Zipper (bHLH/LZ) domain. Through their bHLH domain, they can bind to DNA, while the leucine zipper domain allows the dimerization with its partner Max, another bHLH transcription factor. They are important in cellular proliferation, apoptosis, and metabolism [55–57]. More importantly, they are deregulated in a broad range of human cancers and are often associated with poor prognosis [55, 56]. Another important target of let-7 is the high mobility group A2 (HMGA2) protein, known to be overexpressed in gastric, lung, and ovarian cancers [30, 58, 59] (Table 9.1). The relevance of let-7 as a tumor suppressor targeting HMGA2 came from studies that forcibly expressed let-7 in cancer cells. Also, one of the studies identified seven let-7 sites on the 3'-UTR of HMGA2. Transfection of tumor cells with let-7 led to decreased levels of HMGA2 and cancer cell proliferation, and the disruption of the regulation of HMGA2 by let-7 led to tumor formation in mice [35–37].

Table 9.1 Selected microRNAs dysregulated in cancer. A selection from the literature of microRNAS dysregulated in cancers. Oncogenic microRNAS upregulated in multiple cancers with their targets are shown at the top of the chart. At the bottom are microRNAs with potential tumor suppressive function with their targets

Oncogenic microRNA	Example of target genes	Selected tumors	References
miR-21	PTEN, PDCD4, TPM1, and TGFβ	Breast, lung, glioblastoma, colon, prostate, and cervical	[49, 78, 80–83]
miR-17-92 cluster	BIM	Lymphoma, lung, and colon	[53–55]
miR-221/222	P27^{Kip1}	Breast	[46]
miR-155	SOCS1 and APC	Breast	[40]
Tumor suppressor microRNA			
miR-15/16	Bcl-2, CDK-1, and CDK-2	Chronic lymphocytic leukemia	[25, 26]
Let-7	RAS, Myc, and HMGA2	Lung, ovarian, and liver	[28, 34–37]
miR-34a	c-met, Notch-1, Notch-2, and SIRT1	Glioblastoma, pancreatic, and prostate	[38, 45, 53]
miR-7	EGFR, IRS-1, IRS-2	Glioblastoma and breast	[12, 47]
miR-326	Notch-1, Notch-2, and MRP-1	Glioblastoma and breast	[41, 47]
miR-128	Bmi-1	Glioblastoma	[39]
miR-10b	BDNF and SHC1	Breast	[40]
miR-125b	YES, AKT3, and FGFR2	Breast	[40]
miR-145	Cyclin D2, MYCN, FOS, and FLI1	Breast	[40]

Tumors tend to downregulate genes that have the ability to prevent their growth or survival. It is therefore to be expected that miRNAs that have tumor suppressive abilities will be downregulated in tumors, as observed above with let-7. In other examples, the levels of miR-7, miR-34a, miR-128, and miR-326 were found to be downregulated in the most aggressive form of brain tumors, glioblastoma [12, 38, 39, 60–62], and miR-10b, miR-125b and miR-145 levels are decreased in breast cancer [40]. It is conceivable that these miRNAs are downregulated in tumors because they target putative oncogenic pathways. This seems to be the case for numerous downregulated miRNAs in glioblastoma, as they target pro-survival and pro-proliferative pathways such as AKT, EGFR signaling, Bmi-1, E2f-3a, and Notch [12, 38, 39, 41, 60, 61, 63, 64] (Table 9.1). For breast cancer, the putative oncogenic targets for downregulated miRNAs include FLT1 and the v-crk homolog, growth factor BDNF and SHC1 for miR-10b; YES, AKT3, and FGFR2 for miR-125b; and MYCN, FOS, cyclin D2, and FLI1 for miR-145 [40] (Table 9.1).

As mentioned earlier, the mechanism(s) behind miRNAs downregulation is rarely understood in tumors, but a few studies have indicated possible explanations. For instance, transcription of the host gene beta-arrestin of miR-326 is downregulated in brain tumors, accounting for miR-326 downregulation. For the let-7 family, an inhibitor of their processing, lin-28, is upregulated in tumors [34, 62].

Chromosomal regions that bear oncogenic proteins are often amplified in tumors. miR-17-92 is a cluster of seven miRNAs, generated from the polycistronic transcript of C13orf25 in the 13q31.3 chromosomal region. This region is frequently amplified in several tumors, including B-cell lymphomas [42, 43]; lymphoma cells and patient samples carrying amplification in this region had high levels of miR-17-92 transcript [42–44]. To test its oncogenic potential, these authors investigated a mouse model of B-cell lymphoma generated by overexpression of the oncogenic c-myc protein. Coexpression of the miR-17-92 cluster and c-myc accelerated lymphomagenesis in this mouse model [42].

microRNA Dysregulation Contributes to Cancer Treatment Resistance

While important advances have been made in the war on cancer in recent decades, treatment resistance frequently limits treatment effectiveness. We mentioned earlier some of the reasons why tumors are resistant to present available therapies, and recent studies have also implicated the dysregulation of miRNAs in the resistance to anticancer drugs.

Like other tumors, the prostate cancer line PC3 is resistant to treatment with chemotherapeutic agents such as camptothecin. The overexpression of silent mating type information regulation 2 homolog 1 (*SIRT1*) has been suggested to be involved in the resistance of prostate cancer cells to camptothecin [65]. Coincidentally, *SIRT1* is one of the predicted targets of miR-34a (Table 9.1), and not surprisingly miR-34a levels are downregulated in this tumor. Exogenous reexpression of miR-34a decreased *SIRT1* mRNA and protein levels and attenuated the resistance of PC3 to camptothecin-induced apoptosis [45].

The fight against breast cancer has continued to expand around the world, as breast cancer accounts for 31% of all cancers in women and is ultimately resistant to chemotherapy. The addition of tamoxifen to chemotherapy has been found to be effective against breast cancers positive for estrogen receptor [46]. However, recent studies have uncovered resistance to treatment even with the addition of tamoxifen in some estrogen receptor-positive breast cancer patients. As mentioned earlier, some miRNAs are down or upregulated in breast cancer, as in other cancers. Using miRNA microarray and quantitative polymerase chain reaction (qPCR), eight miRNAs were found to be upregulated and seven downregulated in breast cancer cells that are resistant to tamoxifen treatment [46]. Among the downregulated was the oncogenic miR-21, and among the upregulated was miR-221/222. The resistance to tamoxifen was attributed to the downregulation of the cell cycle regulator protein p27[Kip1] (Table 9.2) [45, 46, 65–68] caused by the induction of miR-221/222 during treatment. The resistance of the tumor cells to tamoxifen treatment was abrogated by reexpression of p27[Kip1] [46]. Another study looked at the relationship between the multidrug-resistant gene (MDR1) and miRNA expression and found miR-27a and miR-451 to be induced in multidrug-resistant

Table 9.2 Chart of microRNAs and their targets that are dysregulated in cancer and are associated with anticancer drug resistance

Cancer type	miRNAs	Targets	References
Prostate	miR-34a	SIRT1	[45, 46, 65]
	miR-221/222	p27^{Kip1}	
Gastric	miR-15b, miR-16	Bcl-2	[67]
Ovarian	miR-130a	M-CSF	[68]
Breast	miR-326	MRP-1	[66]

cancer cells when compared to their parental cells [69]. The induction or exogenous reexpression of miR-27a and miR-451 caused the upregulation of multidrug-resistant genes, MDR1 and p-glycoprotein. This suggests that the targets of miR-27a and miR-451 are endogenous inhibitors of MDR1 and p-glycoprotein. Treatment of these cells with antagomirs of miR-27a or miR-451 decreased the levels of MDR1 and p-glycoprotein and sensitized them to chemotherapy-induced cell death [69].

Advanced estrogen receptor-negative breast cancer cells are frequently resistant to currently available chemotherapeutic agents, such as VP-16 and doxorubicin [47]. The resistance of these cells has been associated with the increased expression of multidrug resistance (MDR)-associated protein (MRP-1) [47, 66]. MRP-1 confers resistance to chemotherapeutic drugs by acting as an efflux pump, pumping drugs out of cancer cells [47]. The level of MRP-1 was found to be higher in advanced breast cancer cells resistant to VP-16 and doxorubicin as compared to their parent nonresistant cells. MRP-1 is a predicted target of the tumor suppressive miRNA, miR-326. The quantification of miRNAs in these cells revealed the tumor-suppressive miR-326 to be downregulated in the resistant cells, consistent with the high expression of MRP-1 [66]. The transfection of miR-326 into the advanced breast cancers cells sensitized them to VP-16 and doxorubicin-induced cell death [66].

The involvement of miRNAs in MDR was also observed in gastric cancer. In this study, the authors also examined the expression of different miRNAs in MDR gastric cancer cells and found miR-16 and miR-15b to be downregulated. The anti-apoptotic gene Bcl2 is a target of miR-16 and miR15b (Table 9.2). It is logical to postulate that the levels of Bcl2 would be increased in gastric cancer cells and contribute to their resistance to chemotherapy [67]. This was indeed demonstrated in gastric cancer cells resistant to chemotherapy [70].

Ovarian cancer is the leading cause of gynecological cancer deaths. The preferred form of treatment of this tumor is chemotherapeutic drugs such as cisplatin. However, a successful complete response is impeded by resistance [67]. Several miRNAs were found to be dysregulated in cisplatin-resistant tumor cells, including miR-130a. The downregulation of miR-130a was linked to the upregulation of a known ovarian cancer chemo-resistance gene, M-CSF [68] (Table 9.2).

Figure 9.2 describes a potential strategy for sensitizing chemo-resistant cancers to drug treatment.

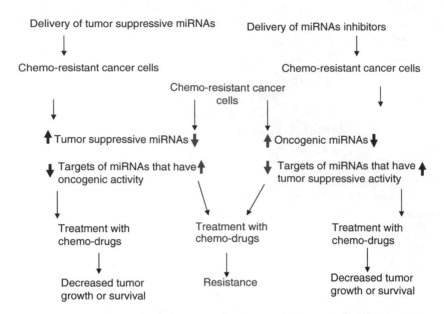

Fig. 9.2 Schematic of treatment of chemo-resistant cancer cells using microRNA delivery or inhibition as a strategy. Resistance to chemotherapy markedly worsens prognosis in cancer patients. microRNAs are dysregulated in chemo-resistant cancer cells. Basic strategies for utilizing microRNAs as a therapy for chemo-resistant cells include the following: (1) for chemo-resistant cells that overexpress oncogenic miRNAs and thus have decreased tumor suppressors, the strategy will be to deliver microRNA inhibitors. The delivery of microRNA inhibitors will increase the expression of the targets (tumor suppressors) of miRNAs that are being inhibited, and thus make the cells susceptible to chemo-drugs. (2) For tumors that underexpress tumor suppressive microRNAs, the treatment strategy will be to deliver synthetic tumor-suppressive microRNAs. This will induce or up-regulate pro-apoptotic genes leading to the cells becoming sensitive to chemotherapy

microRNA as a Targeted Therapeutic Tool for Cancer Treatment

Several studies have suggested small interfering RNAs (siRNAs) that target specific endogenous mRNAs as possible therapeutic tools for treating tumors [71]. Recent studies have suggested that using or targeting miRNAs may have advantages. Unlike siRNA, one miRNA can target several genes at once, and miRNAs do not elicit an interferon response [72, 73]. Thus one miRNA can be used to target several oncogenes instead of delivering several siRNAs. This is especially relevant given recent work indicating that simultaneous inhibition of multiple oncogenic pathways may be necessary to treat cancer [74]. Additionally, since microRNAs are dysregulated in cancer, normalizing their levels or activity represents a potentially nontoxic approach to therapy.

Use of Inhibitors of miRNAS

Perhaps the most commonly used inhibitors of miRNAs are the modified anti-miRNA antisense oligonucleotides (AMOs) known as the antagomirs. These are a class of chemically engineered small synthetic RNAs that are perfectly complementary to the specific miRNA targets with either mispairing at the cleavage site of Argonaute 2 (Ago2) or some sort of base modification to inhibit Ago2 cleavage. Also, the antagomirs have other modifications that make them more resistant to degradation and allow effective delivery in vivo [75–77]. Modifications that increase resistance to nuclease degradation include the removal of the 2-OH residue on the ribose, the addition of 2'-O-methyl (2'-Ome), 2'-O-methoxyethyl (2'-MOE), and locked nucleic acid (LNA), as well as phosphorothioate backbone modification [78, 79]. Another modification is the addition of a cholesteryl group at the 3' end of the antagomir, to enhance cellular uptake and stability in the presence of serum [80, 81]. It is unclear how exactly antagomirs inhibit miRNA activity, but they are believed to inhibit by irreversibly binding miRNAs. Multiple steps in the processing, generation, and function of the miRNA pathway could be targeted with AMOs, depending on whichever yields the best result [82].

Several investigators have used various AMOs to target miRNAs in both animal models and cell lines. Even though there are not yet many in vivo studies using AMOs, a recent promising report showed that intravenous delivery of cholesterol-conjugated AMOs successfully inhibited miR-122 expression and activity in several tissues, excluding the central nervous system [76]. The lack of effect in the central nervous system has been linked to lack of accessibility due to the blood–brain barrier [76]. Local delivery to brain tumors appears to overcome this problem, however, as shown by recent studies with a miR-21 inhibitor [83]. As of now, most of the studies using AMOs to target miRNAs in tumors have been done in cancer cell lines.

Endogenously expressed miRNAs have been thought to have either pro- or anti-proliferative/apoptotic effects in human cells and tumors. In an effort to understand and clarify which effects are elicited by which miRNAs, an early study used a panel of microRNA inhibitors to screen for miRNAs that might be important for the growth and survival of Hela cells [48]. In this study, over 200 mammalian miRNAs were found to be expressed in Hela cells, but only a few had physiological relevance for growth and survival [48]. Of the over 200 miRNAs found, the inhibition of 19 caused a decrease in cellular growth, the inhibition of miR-24 increased the growth, and the inhibition of seven other miRNAs decreased the apoptosis of Hela cells. In lung carcinoma line A549, the inhibition of eight miRNAs profoundly downregulated growth and the inhibition of nine others increased growth [48].

Gene profiling of neuroblastoma, glioblastoma, colorectal, lung, breast, and pancreatic cancer found miR-21 to be overexpressed in these tumors. Further studies identified miR-21 to be oncogenic, as its inhibition with miR-21 oligonucleotide alone or in combination with neural precursor cells bearing a soluble form of tumor necrosis factor-related apoptosis inducing ligand (TRAIL) resulted in increased apoptosis in glioblastoma cells [49, 84]. Also, inhibition of miR-21 in breast cancer cells increased their apoptosis and slowed their growth [84]. Studies in cancer cells using a miR-21 inhibitor to elucidate its oncogenic mechanisms identified the tumor suppressors tropomysin 1 and PTEN as potential targets [50, 51]. One of the functions of TPM1 protein is to stabilize microfilaments of the cellular cytoskeleton and control growth. Tumors downregulate TPM1, thus destabilizing the cytoskeleton and leading to uncontrolled growth. The inhibition of miR-21 resulted in increased PTEN and TPM1 levels and decreased tumor growth. The increase in PTEN levels observed with miR-21 inhibition led to a decrease in tumor cell migration and invasiveness [50]. PTEN protein is deleted in several tumors, including glioblastoma, and it is thought to be involved in tumorigenesis [52]. This suggests that downregulation of tumor suppressors tropomysin 1 (TPM1) and PTEN in cancer cells by miR-21 could be responsible for its oncogenicity [50, 51, 84]. In addition, miR-21 inhibition led to an increase in programmed cell death 4 (PDCD4) protein and a subsequent decrease in tumor cell invasion [85]. This observation fits with the known role of PDCD4 as a tumor suppressor that is overexpressed during apoptosis [86, 87]. Furthermore, miR-21 was found to be highly expressed and PDCD4 expression low in colorectal cancer, confirming that PDCD4 is an important target of miR-21 [85] and that miR-21 functions as an oncogene in tumors.

Taken together, the above data suggest that the inhibition of miRNAs could be a viable therapeutic goal in tumors. The next hurdle will be effective delivery of these miRNA inhibitors into tumors, either systemically or locally, to inhibit their growth or cause their death.

One final but nonspecific strategy for the inhibition of miRNAs is to downregulate a component of the miRNA processing machinery using either siRNA or small molecules. This can be done by targeting Drosha, Dicer, or other key proteins in miRNA processing that might be responsible for the generation of sets of miRNAs considered as oncogenic in a given tumor.

Delivery of Synthetic Pre-miRNA and Mature miRNA and Induction of Endogenous miRNAs

As discussed above, the expression levels of some miRNAs quantified by northern blotting or qPCR are altered in tumors, including some considered as tumor suppressors or oncogenes [12, 38, 41, 88]. We have discussed the use of inhibitors to block microRNAs that are highly expressed in tissues or tumors. One therapeutic alternative takes the opposite approach, the delivery of miRNAs downregulated in tumors and functioning as tumor suppressors. One strategy involves the delivery of the miRNAs themselves, either using vectors expressing a specific miRNA or by transient transfection of hairpin pre-miR or double-stranded mature miRNA. A second strategy is the induction of endogenous miRNAs in cells or tissues. Several microRNAs have been shown to have tumor-suppressive activity. Let-7 miRNAs have been found to be downregulated almost universally in cancer cells, and their delivery is cytotoxic [12, 38, 41, 53, 89]. The miR-34 family of miRNAs was recently identified as targets of p53, the so-called "guardian of the genome." p53 is activated in response to cellular stress and DNA damage, and it is involved in the regulation of cellular apoptosis and proliferation [90]. miR-34a is upregulated by p53 in response to DNA damage and promotes apoptosis. Also, the delivery of miR-34 reduced the growth of tumor cells [38, 42, 90].

In brain tumor cell lines and surgical samples, several microRNAs have been found to be downregulated and to act as possible tumor suppressors, including miR-7, miR-326, and miR-34a [12, 38, 62]. Computational prediction and transient transfection of these miRNAs in glioma cells identified the Notch, EGFR, AKT, and MET pathways as possible targets of these miRNAs [12, 38, 41]. These pathways, as mentioned earlier, are dysregulated in brain tumors and act in an oncogenic fashion. Supporting the idea that these miRNAs are tumor suppressors, transient transfection of glioma cells with miRs-7, -326, and -34a significantly induced their death and reduced their growth in vitro, and in some cases in vivo in mouse models [12, 38, 41]. This suggests that these miRNAs are potential tumor suppressors, and their delivery may have utility as tools for the treatment of glioblastoma.

The next step researchers are taking is the delivery of these miRNAs in vivo into tumors. A recent work studied the effects of systemic delivery of synthetic miR-16 in a xenograft mouse model. miR-16 targets the pro-survival gene Bcl2 as well as cell cycle regulators cyclin-dependent kinase-1/2 (CDK-1 and CDK-2) in metastatic prostate tumor [91]. The tail vein injection of miR-16 with atelocollagen significantly inhibited the growth of prostate cancer metastatic to bone in mice [91]. Also, the delivery of let-7 into lung cancer cells has been shown to reduce tumor growth in xenograft lung cancer mouse models [92, 93].

In the second strategy, it may be possible to induce expression of miRNAs by deleting or inhibiting proteins that suppress their expression. This type of strategy is exemplified in a recent study on the regulation of miR-326 by Notch [62].

Notch is an oncogenic pathway in glioblastomas and other cancers, and its inhibition slows growth and causes apoptosis in these settings. Notch inhibition increases levels of miR-326, and this miR-326 elevation can partially mediate the cytotoxic effects of Notch inhibition in glioma cells [62, 63].

Conclusion

Although miRNAs were discovered not long ago, their importance in cancer pathogenesis, diagnosis, and resistance to chemotherapy is becoming obvious. Recent studies by several investigators have shown that miRNAs are dysregulated in tumors, and the comparison of miRNA levels in tumors and normal tissues may correlate with their functions as oncogenes or tumor suppressors. miRNA levels may also shed light on the sensitivity of tumors to chemotherapy, depending on their targets. This suggests that miRNA profiling of tumors will allow us to choose better drug combinations for tumors that are normally resistant to chemotherapy. In addition, the modulation of miRNA levels in tumors, either by inhibition or exogenous delivery, may become an important new therapy targeting multiple pathways in treatment-resistant cancers.

References

1. Hanahan D, Weinberg RA. The hallmarks of cancer. Cell. 2000;100(1):57–70.
2. Hynes NE, Lane HA. ERBB receptors and cancer: the complexity of targeted inhibitors. Nat Rev Cancer. 2005;5(5):341–54.
3. Lee RC, Feinbaum RL. The *C. elegans* heterochronic gene lin-4 encodes small RNAs with antisense complementarity to lin-14. Cell. 1993;75(5):843–54.
4. Reinhart BJ, Slack FJ, Basson M, et al. The 21-nucleotide let-7 RNA regulates developmental timing in *Caenorhabditis elegans*. Nature. 2000;403(6772):901–6.
5. Pasquinelli AE, Reinhart BJ, Slack F, et al. Conservation of the sequence and temporal expression of let-7 heterochronic regulatory RNA. Nature. 2000;408(6808):86–9.
6. Berezikov E, van Tetering G, Verheul M, et al. Many novel mammalian microRNA candidates identified by extensive cloning and RAKE analysis. Genome Res. 2006;16(10):1289–98.
7. Berezikov E, Cuppen E, Plasterk RH. Approaches to microRNA discovery. Nat Genet. 2006;38(Suppl):S2–7.
8. Bentwich I, Avniel A, Karov Y, et al. Identification of hundreds of conserved and nonconserved human microRNAs. Nat Genet. 2005;37(7):766–70.
9. Rodriguez A, Griffiths-Jones S, Ashurst JL, Bradley A. Identification of mammalian microRNA host genes and transcription units. Genome Res. 2004;14(10A):1902–10.
10. Aravin AA, Lagos-Quintana M, Yalcin A, et al. The small RNA profile during *Drosophila melanogaster* development. Dev Cell. 2003;5(2):337–50.
11. Farh KK, Grimson A, Jan C, et al. The widespread impact of mammalian microRNAs on mRNA repression and evolution. Science. 2005;310(5755):1817–21.
12. Kefas B, Godlewski J, Comeau L, et al. microRNA-7 inhibits the epidermal growth factor receptor and the Akt pathway and is down-regulated in glioblastoma. Cancer Res. 2008;68(10):3566–72.
13. Bartel DP. MicroRNAs: genomics, biogenesis, mechanism, and function. Cell. 2004;116(2):281–97.
14. Lee Y, Kim M, Han J, et al. MicroRNA genes are transcribed by RNA polymerase II. EMBO J. 2004;23(20):4051–60.
15. Gregory RI, Yan KP, Amuthan G, et al. The Microprocessor complex mediates the genesis of microRNAs. Nature. 2004;432(7014):235–40.
16. Yi R, Qin Y, Macara IG, Cullen BR. Exportin-5 mediates the nuclear export of pre-microRNAs and short hairpin RNAs. Genes Dev. 2003;17(24):3011–6.
17. Hutvagner G, Zamore PD. A microRNA in a multiple-turnover RNAi enzyme complex. Science. 2002;297(5589):2056–60.
18. Ketting RF, Fischer SE, Bernstein E, Sijen T, Hannon GJ, Plasterk RH. Dicer functions in RNA interference and in synthesis of small RNA involved in developmental timing in *C. elegans*. Genes Dev. 2001;15(20):2654–9.
19. Hammond SM. Dicing and slicing: the core machinery of the RNA interference pathway. FEBS Lett. 2005;579(26):5822–9.
20. Martinez J, Tuschl T. RISC is a 5′ phosphomonoester-producing RNA endonuclease. Genes Dev. 2004;18(9):975–80.
21. Hammond SM, Bernstein E, Beach D, Hannon GJ. An RNA-directed nuclease mediates post-transcriptional gene silencing in *Drosophila* cells. Nature. 2000;404(6775):293–6.

22. Lai EC, Tam B, Rubin GM. Pervasive regulation of *Drosophila* Notch target genes by GY-box-, Brd-box-, and K-box-class microRNAs. Genes Dev. 2005;19(9):1067–80.
23. Yekta S, Shih IH, Bartel DP. MicroRNA-directed cleavage of HOXB8 mRNA. Science. 2004;304(5670):594–6.
24. Grimson A, Farh KK, Johnston WK, Garrett-Engele P, Lim LP, Bartel DP. MicroRNA targeting specificity in mammals: determinants beyond seed pairing. Mol Cell. 2007;27(1):91–105.
25. Calin GA, Ferracin M, Cimmino A, et al. A MicroRNA signature associated with prognosis and progression in chronic lymphocytic leukemia. N Engl J Med. 2005;353(17): 1793–801.
26. Cimmino A, Calin GA, Fabbri M, et al. miR-15 and miR-16 induce apoptosis by targeting BCL2. Proc Natl Acad Sci USA. 2005;102(39):13944–9.
27. Jiang J, Lee EJ, Gusev Y, Schmittgen TD. Real-time expression profiling of microRNA precursors in human cancer cell lines. Nucleic Acids Res. 2005;33(17):5394–403.
28. Johnson SM, Grosshans H, Shingara J, et al. RAS is regulated by the let-7 microRNA family. Cell. 2005;120(5):635–47.
29. Shah YM, Morimura K, Yang Q, Tanabe T, Takagi M, Gonzalez FJ. Peroxisome proliferator-activated receptor alpha regulates a microRNA-mediated signaling cascade responsible for hepatocellular proliferation. Mol Cell Biol. 2007;27(12):4238–47.
30. Shell S, Park SM, Radjabi AR, et al. Let-7 expression defines two differentiation stages of cancer. Proc Natl Acad Sci USA. 2007;104(27):11400–5.
31. Yanaihara N, Caplen N, Bowman E, et al. Unique microRNA molecular profiles in lung cancer diagnosis and prognosis. Cancer Cell. 2006;9(3):189–98.
32. Takamizawa J, Konishi H, Yanagisawa K, et al. Reduced expression of the let-7 microRNAs in human lung cancers in association with shortened postoperative survival. Cancer Res. 2004;64(11):3753–6.
33. Yu SL, Chen HY, Chang GC, et al. MicroRNA signature predicts survival and relapse in lung cancer. Cancer Cell. 2008;13(1):48–57.
34. Sampson VB, Rong NH, Han J, et al. MicroRNA let-7a down-regulates MYC and reverts MYC-induced growth in Burkitt lymphoma cells. Cancer Res. 2007;67(20):9762–70.
35. Mayr C, Hemann MT, Bartel DP. Disrupting the pairing between let-7 and Hmga2 enhances oncogenic transformation. Science. 2007;315(5818):1576–9.
36. Peng Y, Laser J, Shi G, et al. Antiproliferative effects by Let-7 repression of high-mobility group A2 in uterine leiomyoma. Mol Cancer Res. 2008;6(4):663–73.
37. Lee YS, Dutta A. The tumor suppressor microRNA let-7 represses the HMGA2 oncogene. Genes Dev. 2007;21(9):1025–30.
38. Li Y, Guessous F, Zhang Y, et al. MicroRNA-34a inhibits glioblastoma growth by targeting multiple oncogenes. Cancer Res. 2009;69(19):7569–76.
39. Godlewski J, Nowicki MO, Bronisz A, et al. Targeting of the Bmi-1 oncogene/stem cell renewal factor by microRNA-128 inhibits glioma proliferation and self-renewal. Cancer Res. 2008;68(22):9125–30.
40. Iorio MV, Ferracin M, Liu CG, et al. MicroRNA gene expression deregulation in human breast cancer. Cancer Res. 2005;65(16):7065–70.
41. Kefas B, Comeau L, Floyd DH, Seleverstov O, Godlewski J, Schmittgen T, et al. The neuronal microRNA miR-326 acts in a feedback loop with notch and has therapeutic potential against brain tumors. J Neurosci. 2009;29:15161–18.
42. He L, Thomson JM, Hemann MT, et al. A microRNA polycistron as a potential human oncogene. Nature. 2005;435(7043):828–33.
43. Ota A, Tagawa H, Karnan S, et al. Identification and characterization of a novel gene, C13orf25, as a target for 13q31-q32 amplification in malignant lymphoma. Cancer Res. 2004;64(9):3087–95.
44. Inomata M, Tagawa H, Guo YM, Kameoka Y, Takahashi N, Sawada K. MicroRNA-17-92 down-regulates expression of distinct targets in different B-cell lymphoma subtypes. Blood. 2009;113(2):396–402.

45. Fujita Y, Kojima K, Hamada N, et al. Effects of miR-34a on cell growth and chemoresistance in prostate cancer PC3 cells. Biochem Biophys Res Commun. 2008;377(1):114–9.
46. Miller TE, Ghoshal K, Ramaswamy B, et al. MicroRNA-221/222 confers tamoxifen resistance in breast cancer by targeting p27Kip1. J Biol Chem. 2008;283(44):29897–903.
47. Szakacs G, Paterson JK, Ludwig JA, Booth-Genthe C, Gottesman MM. Targeting multidrug resistance in cancer. Nat Rev Drug Discov. 2006;5(3):219–34.
48. Cheng AM, Byrom MW, Shelton J, Ford LP. Antisense inhibition of human miRNAs and indications for an involvement of miRNA in cell growth and apoptosis. Nucleic Acids Res. 2005;33(4):1290–7.
49. Chan JA, Krichevsky AM, Kosik KS. MicroRNA-21 is an antiapoptotic factor in human glioblastoma cells. Cancer Res. 2005;65(14):6029–33.
50. Meng F, Henson R, Wehbe-Janek H, Ghoshal K, Jacob ST, Patel T. MicroRNA-21 regulates expression of the PTEN tumor suppressor gene in human hepatocellular cancer. Gastroenterology. 2007;133(2):647–58.
51. Zhu S, Si ML, Wu H, Mo YY. MicroRNA-21 targets the tumor suppressor gene tropomyosin 1 (TPM1). J Biol Chem. 2007;282(19):14328–36.
52. Maehama T. PTEN: its deregulation and tumorigenesis. Biol Pharm Bull. 2007;30(9): 1624–7.
53. Gaur A, Jewell DA, Liang Y, et al. Characterization of microRNA expression levels and their biological correlates in human cancer cell lines. Cancer Res. 2007;67(6):2456–68.
54. Malumbres M, Barbacid M. RAS oncogenes: the first 30 years. Nat Rev Cancer. 2003;3(6):459–65.
55. Pelengaris S, Khan M, Evan G. c-MYC: more than just a matter of life and death. Nat Rev Cancer. 2002;2(10):764–76.
56. Schmidt EV. The role of c-myc in cellular growth control. Oncogene. 1999;18(19):2988–96.
57. Van de Casteele M, Kefas BA, Cai Y, et al. Prolonged culture in low glucose induces apoptosis of rat pancreatic beta-cells through induction of c-myc. Biochem Biophys Res Commun. 2003;312(4):937–44.
58. Motoyama K, Inoue H, Nakamura Y, Uetake H, Sugihara K, Mori M. Clinical significance of high mobility group A2 in human gastric cancer and its relationship to let-7 microRNA family. Clin Cancer Res. 2008;14(8):2334–40.
59. Sarhadi VK, Wikman H, Salmenkivi K, et al. Increased expression of high mobility group A proteins in lung cancer. J Pathol. 2006;209(2):206–12.
60. Cui JG, Zhao Y, Sethi P, et al. Micro-RNA-128 (miRNA-128) down-regulation in glioblastoma targets ARP5 (ANGPTL6), Bmi-1 and E2F-3a, key regulators of brain cell proliferation. J Neurooncol. 2009;98:297–304.
61. Zhang Y, Chao T, Li R, et al. MicroRNA-128 inhibits glioma cells proliferation by targeting transcription factor E2F3a. J Mol Med. 2009;87(1):43–51.
62. Kefas B, Comeau L, Floyd DH, et al. The neuronal microRNA miR-326 acts in a feedback loop with notch and has therapeutic potential against brain tumors. J Neurosci. 2009;29(48):15161–8.
63. Purow BW, Haque RM, Noel MW, et al. Expression of Notch-1 and its ligands, Delta-like-1 and Jagged-1, is critical for glioma cell survival and proliferation. Cancer Res. 2005;65(6):2353–63.
64. Dancey JE, Freidlin B. Targeting epidermal growth factor receptor – are we missing the mark? Lancet. 2003;362(9377):62–4.
65. Kojima K, Ohhashi R, Fujita Y, et al. A role for SIRT1 in cell growth and chemoresistance in prostate cancer PC3 and DU145 cells. Biochem Biophys Res Commun. 2008;373(3): 423–8.
66. Liang Z, Wu H, Xia J, et al. Involvement of miR-326 in chemotherapy resistance of breast cancer through modulating expression of multidrug resistance-associated protein 1. Biochem Pharmacol. 2010;79(6):817–24.
67. Xia L, Zhang D, Du R, et al. miR-15b and miR-16 modulate multidrug resistance by targeting BCL2 in human gastric cancer cells. Int J Cancer. 2008;123(2):372–9.

68. Sorrentino A, Liu CG, Addario A, Peschle C, Scambia G, Ferlini C. Role of microRNAs in drug-resistant ovarian cancer cells. Gynecol Oncol. 2008;111(3):478–86.
69. Zhu H, Wu H, Liu X, et al. Role of MicroRNA miR-27a and miR-451 in the regulation of MDR1/P-glycoprotein expression in human cancer cells. Biochem Pharmacol. 2008;76(5): 582–8.
70. Legge F, Ferrandina G, Salutari V, Scambia G. Biological characterization of ovarian cancer: prognostic and therapeutic implications. Ann Oncol. 2005;16 Suppl 4:iv95–101.
71. Mocellin S, Costa R, Nitti D. RNA interference: ready to silence cancer? J Mol Med. 2006;84(1):4–15.
72. Jackson AL, Burchard J, Schelter J, et al. Widespread siRNA "off-target" transcript silencing mediated by seed region sequence complementarity. RNA. 2006;12(7):1179–87.
73. Grimm D, Streetz KL, Jopling CL, et al. Fatality in mice due to oversaturation of cellular microRNA/short hairpin RNA pathways. Nature. 2006;441(7092):537–41.
74. Pelicano H, Martin DS, Xu RH, Huang P. Glycolysis inhibition for anticancer treatment. Oncogene. 2006;25(34):4633–46.
75. Boutla A, Delidakis C, Tabler M. Developmental defects by antisense-mediated inactivation of micro-RNAs 2 and 13 in *Drosophila* and the identification of putative target genes. Nucleic Acids Res. 2003;31(17):4973–80.
76. Krutzfeldt J, Rajewsky N, Braich R, et al. Silencing of microRNAs in vivo with 'antagomirs'. Nature. 2005;438(7068):685–9.
77. Czech MP. MicroRNAs as therapeutic targets. N Engl J Med. 2006;354(11):1194–5.
78. Davis S, Lollo B, Freier S, Esau C. Improved targeting of miRNA with antisense oligonucleotides. Nucleic Acids Res. 2006;34(8):2294–304.
79. Hutvagner G, Simard MJ, Mello CC, Zamore PD. Sequence-specific inhibition of small RNA function. PLoS Biol. 2004;2(4):E98.
80. Yang M, Mattes J. Discovery, biology and therapeutic potential of RNA interference, microRNA and antagomirs. Pharmacol Ther. 2008;117(1):94–104.
81. Bijsterbosch MK, Rump ET, De Vrueh RL, et al. Modulation of plasma protein binding and in vivo liver cell uptake of phosphorothioate oligodeoxynucleotides by cholesterol conjugation. Nucleic Acids Res. 2000;28(14):2717–25.
82. Wu H, Lima WF, Zhang H, Fan A, Sun H, Crooke ST. Determination of the role of the human RNase H1 in the pharmacology of DNA-like antisense drugs. J Biol Chem. 2004;279(17):17181–9.
83. Corsten MF, Miranda R, Kasmieh R, Krichevsky AM, Weissleder R, Shah K. MicroRNA-21 knockdown disrupts glioma growth in vivo and displays synergistic cytotoxicity with neural precursor cell delivered S-TRAIL in human gliomas. Cancer Res. 2007;67(19): 8994–9000.
84. Si ML, Zhu S, Wu H, Lu Z, Wu F, Mo YY. miR-21-mediated tumor growth. Oncogene. 2007;26(19):2799–803.
85. Asangani IA, Rasheed SA, Nikolova DA, et al. MicroRNA-21 (miR-21) post-transcriptionally downregulates tumor suppressor Pdcd4 and stimulates invasion, intravasation and metastasis in colorectal cancer. Oncogene. 2008;27(15):2128–36.
86. Lankat-Buttgereit B, Goke R. Programmed cell death protein 4 (pdcd4): a novel target for antineoplastic therapy? Biol Cell. 2003;95(8):515–9.
87. Mudduluru G, Medved F, Grobholz R, et al. Loss of programmed cell death 4 expression marks adenoma-carcinoma transition, correlates inversely with phosphorylated protein kinase B, and is an independent prognostic factor in resected colorectal cancer. Cancer. 2007;110(8):1697–707.
88. Lu J, Getz G, Miska EA, et al. MicroRNA expression profiles classify human cancers. Nature. 2005;435(7043):834–8.
89. Medina PP, Slack FJ. microRNAs and cancer: an overview. Cell Cycle. 2008;7(16): 2485–92.
90. Chang TC, Wentzel EA, Kent OA, et al. Transactivation of miR-34a by p53 broadly influences gene expression and promotes apoptosis. Mol Cell. 2007;26(5):745–52.

91. Takeshita F, Patrawala L, Osaki M, et al. Systemic delivery of synthetic microRNA-16 inhibits the growth of metastatic prostate tumors via downregulation of multiple cell-cycle genes. Mol Ther. 2009;18:181–7.
92. Esquela-Kerscher A, Trang P, Wiggins JF, et al. The let-7 microRNA reduces tumor growth in mouse models of lung cancer. Cell Cycle. 2008;7(6):759–64.
93. Kumar MS, Erkeland SJ, Pester RE, et al. Suppression of non-small cell lung tumor development by the let-7 microRNA family. Proc Natl Acad Sci USA. 2008;105(10):3903–8.

Chapter 10
Rational Combination of Targeted Agents to Overcome Cancer Cell Resistance

Yun Dai and Steven Grant

Keywords Leukemia • Targeted agents • Drug resistance • Signal transduction • Combination therapy

Introduction

Targeted therapies refer to chemotherapeutic strategies directed specifically at the dysregulated pathways or oncogenic proteins responsible for the transformation process. The development of imatinib mesylate (Gleevec) for the treatment of chronic myelogenous leukemia (CML) [1] is often viewed as the prototype for this approach, but in reality targeted therapy was initiated long before this approach was developed. For example, it has long been recognized that supraphysiologic concentrations of all-trans retinoic acid (ATRA) could overcome the block to differentiation conferred by the promyelocytic leukemia (PML) protein in leukemia cells exhibiting the 15:17 translocation, and the success of ATRA in patients with acute PML is well established [2]. These successes have led to the hope that similar strategies could be applied to a wide variety of, and potentially all, malignancies, if only the underlying dysregulated proteins and pathways could be identified. A major theoretical advantage of such approaches over standard, cytotoxic chemotherapy therapy is that, in contrast to the latter, which disrupt critical cellular processes required by both normal and neoplastic cells, targeted approaches can be specifically directed against the dysregulated pathways responsible for transformation. Consequently, they may display the highly desirable characteristic of therapeutic selectivity.

However, while excitement about the prospect of targeted therapy persists, enthusiasm has been tempered by the realization that the success of imatinib

S. Grant(✉)
Department of Internal Medicine, Hematology/Oncology, Virginia
Commonwealth University, Richmond, VA, USA
e-mail: stgrant@vcu.edu

D. Gioeli (ed.), *Targeted Therapies: Mechanisms of Resistance*,
Molecular and Translational Medicine, DOI 10.1007/978-1-60761-478-4_10,
© Springer Science+Business Media, LLC 2011

mesylate in CML may be difficult to duplicate in other malignancies. Moreover, even those patients who initially respond to imatinib mesylate generally develop resistance to this agent, often due to the acquisition (or preexistence) of point mutations in the Bcr/Abl protein which prevent imatinib mesylate binding [3]. While such cells may respond to second-generation Bcr/Abl kinase inhibitors, other mutations (e.g., gatekeeper mutations such as T315I) may confer resistance to these second-generation agents [4]. Even more problematic is the fact that the oncogenic Bcr/Abl tyrosine kinase in CML is unusual in that it occupies an apical position in the transformation process, and CML cells have become addicted to it for survival. The nature and origin of this addiction phenomenon is intimately related to the question of resistance (see below). Furthermore, it is likely that in the large majority of malignancies, multiple oncogenes cooperate to trigger transformation, reducing the dependence of transformed cells upon a single pathway. For example, while Ras mutations commonly occur in diverse malignancies [5], agents that target this pathway such as farnesyltransferase inhibitors have shown relatively little activity in this setting [6], in striking contrast to the case of imatinib mesylate in CML or ATRA in PML.

The basis for resistance to targeted agents can be divided into two broad categories: intrinsic vs. acquired, and target-dependent vs. target-independent. Of the two classification systems, the latter two categories are closely linked to oncogene addiction, a phenomenon in which tumor cells become dependent for their survival upon the dysregulation of a particular oncogenic protein or pathway [7]. In target-dependent forms of resistance, cells escape the lethal effects of agents through perturbations that prevent the agent of interest from inhibiting a critical survival pathway. Examples include the development of mutations that prevent binding of an inhibitor to its target [8], upregulation of the oncogene in question, or pharmacokinetic mechanisms preventing achievement of adequate inhibitor concentrations [9]. However, the tumor cell remains dependent upon the oncogenic pathway for survival. In contrast, target-independent resistance mechanisms involve release of the tumor cell from its dependence upon the critical survival pathway e.g., by a compensatory mechanism, often involving activation of a complementary pathway capable of transmitting survival signals sufficient to overcome the lethal consequences of interruption of the primary pathway. An example of the latter is the ability of hyperactivation of the PTEN/AKT pathway (e.g., by PTEN mutations) to overcome the otherwise lethal consequences of blockade of the Ras/RAF/MEK1/2/ERK1/2 pathway in transformed cells [10]. Alternatively, upregulation of anti-apoptotic members of the Bcl-2 family e.g., Bcl-2, Bcl-xL, XIAP, Mcl-1, etc., can abrogate the lethal effects of interruption of a critical oncogenic pathway. The significance of such a phenomenon is that this form of resistance represents a fundamental change in the nature of the neoplastic cell inasmuch as it is no longer dependent for survival upon the signals that originally contributed to its transformation. An important corollary of this notion is that conventional strategies designed to overcome resistance e.g., increasing the degree or duration of target inhibition by pharmacokinetic means or developing more potent inhibitors, are doomed to failure under these conditions. Instead, just as the cell has developed evasive mechanisms to overcome its dependence on a particular oncogene, fundamentally different approaches, most likely involving the identification of alternative targets, will be required to reestablish the cell death program in this setting.

The notion of resistance to targeted agents is intimately connected with the concept of oncogene addiction [11], which is in turn linked to our understanding of the hallmarks of cancer, initially described by Weinberg in 2000 [12] and subsequently updated and expanded by Elledge [13]. Although the mechanism by which oncogene addiction occurs has not been elucidated with certainty, one theory holds that the genes responsible for transformation have certain lethal functions that must be overridden in order for transformed cells to survive [14]. An example would be the well-described oncogene c-Myc, which promotes cell proliferation but which exerts pro-apoptotic actions in certain settings. Under these conditions, overexpression of the anti-apoptotic gene Bcl-2 may cooperate with dysregulated c-Myc to allow survival of c-Myc-driven transformed cells [15]. Thus, such cells are addicted to Bcl-2, and may be susceptible to strategies that inhibit the function of this protein. In addition, transformed cells may operate under increased stresses (e.g., oxidative, replicative, etc.) which must be overcome in order to preserve their proliferative and survival advantages over their normal counterparts [13]. An alternative, but potentially compatible view holds that the phenomenon of oncogene addiction stems from the disparate kinetics of the disappearance of pro- vs. anti-apoptotic proteins following interruption of a critical transforming pathway [16]. For example, if a particular oncogene signals to both pro- and anti-apoptotic downstream targets, and if the half-lives of the former are longer than those of the latter, interruption of the pathway at a proximal site may shift the balance away from cell survival to cell death.

Despite the uncertainty about the nature of resistance and the basis for oncogene addiction, several concepts are emerging in ongoing efforts to circumvent loss of sensitivity to targeted agents by transformed cells. For example, it is clear that strategies will have to be tailored specifically to the mechanism(s) responsible for resistance. For example, improving drug pharmacokinetics through the use of alternative drug schedules or doses [17], or developing analogs capable of inhibiting mutant kinases resistant to first generation kinase inhibitors may be effective in target-dependent tumors but not in the setting of target-independent ones. An alternative strategy is to attack critical survival-related targets downstream of the mutant oncoprotein to circumvent the primary resistance mechanism. However, accumulating evidence suggests that for both target-dependent and target-independent forms of resistance, inhibition of dual signaling/survival pathways may represent the most promising strategy. For example, in the case of target-dependent resistance, such a combinatorial approach might involve inhibition of additional survival or cell cycle regulatory pathways which can lower the threshold for cell death triggered by the initial targeted agent. Similar strategies may also be effective in the setting of target-independent resistance. For example, dual inhibition of two complementary survival pathways (e.g., Ras/Raf/MEK1/2/ERK1/2 and PI3K/AKT/mTOR) may be effective when inhibition of a single pathway is no longer capable of triggering cell death [18]. A key question to be resolved in such approaches is the relative benefits of dual inhibition of two nodes within a linear survival pathway ("linear inhibition") vs. inhibition of two complementary pathways ("parallel inhibition"). A variation on this theme is the concept of inhibiting "orthogonal" pathways that each contribute, in a fundamentally different way, to the transformed state [13]. A prototype of this strategy might entail simultaneous inhibition of an oncoprotein in conjunction with disruption of a second target responsible for overcoming oncogene-related stress characteristic of transformed cells. Disrupting the cooperation that occurs between such oncogenic proteins might account for or contribute to the antitumor synergism that occurs between inhibitors of survival and cell cycle regulatory signaling [19].

This chapter is not intended to represent a comprehensive summary of resistance to targeted agents or strategies to circumvent this phenomenon; reviews dealing with this subject have recently appeared [20]. Instead, its goal is to outline mechanisms by which transformed cells escape the lethal effects of such agents, and how rational and individualized strategies can be designed to overcome this problem. A particular emphasis will be placed on the evolving concept of inhibiting dual signaling/cell cycle regulatory pathways as a means to circumvention of resistance to targeted agents. Mechanisms of resistance to targeted agents and proposed strategies to circumvent them are summarized in Fig. 10.1.

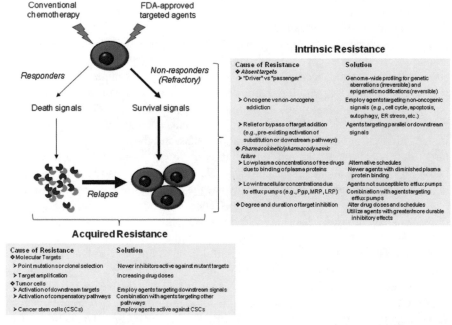

Fig. 10.1 Mechanisms of resistance to targeted agents and proposed strategies designed to circumvent them

Intrinsic vs. Acquired Resistance

As in the case of more conventional chemotherapeutic agents, resistance to targeted agents may be either intrinsic or acquired. In the case of the latter, resistance may stem from the development of point mutations in oncogenic proteins that prevent drug binding to the active site of the protein. The classic example is the development of point mutations in the Bcr/Abl tyrosine kinase ATP binding domain, which confer resistance to imatinib mesylate [21]. However, the distinction between acquired vs. intrinsic resistance may be blurred in view of evidence that cells bearing such mutations may preexist, and be selected for during the course of tyrosine kinase therapy [22]. Both intrinsic or acquired resistance may be related to increased expression of an oncogenic protein, as reported in the case of Bcr/Abl-related malignancies [23]. Strategies effective against these mechanisms, whether intrinsic or acquired, include increasing drug doses, developing kinase inhibitors active against mutant oncoproteins [24], or combining drugs with inhibitors of other signaling (e.g., farnesyltransferase inhibitors) [25] or cell cycle regulatory pathways (e.g., CDK inhibitors such as flavopiridol) [26]. Finally, another potentially promising strategy directed against either intrinsic or acquired mechanisms of resistance involves the inhibition of critical pathways downstream of the original target. For example, recent studies suggest that Polo-like kinase 1 (PLK-1) operates downstream of Bcr/Abl, and that PLK-1 inhibitors induce apoptosis in imatinib mesylate-resistant cells exhibiting various forms of resistance, including those resulting from the T315I gatekeeper mutation [27]. The advantage of such a strategy is that inhibiting such a downstream target eliminates the need to circumvent the initial resistance mechanism, irrespective of its origin.

Pharmacokinetic/Pharmacodynamic Mechanisms of Resistance to Targeted Agents

Since inhibition of an oncoprotein by a targeted agent is generally a dose-dependent phenomenon, such targeted agents will only be effective if: (a) sufficiently high plasma concentrations (of free drug) can be achieved and (b) if the agent of interest can be transported intracellularly. For example, in the case of the multi-kinase inhibitor UCN-01, which inhibits PKC, CDKs, PDK1, and Chk1, among other targets [28], extensive binding of the drug to plasma proteins (e.g., α_1-acidic glycoprotein) results in a very prolonged plasma half-life (e.g., 4–6 weeks) and diminished efficacy at least in the case of prolonged administration schedules [29]. Alternative schedules may circumvent this problem [30]. Similar issues have been identified in the case of the CDK inhibitor flavopiridol, which also binds extensively to plasma proteins, and which has been shown to be minimally effective with prolonged infusion schedules [31]. However, recent results suggest that administration of a loading dose followed by a relatively brief (4 h) infusion may overcome problems associated with prolonged infusions, and initial results of significantly improved efficacy of flavopiridol have been reported in the case of chronic lymphocytic leukemia (CLL) [32]. An alternative approach is to select agents that are less susceptible to inactivation through plasma protein binding. For example, a large number of Chk1 inhibitors have now been developed that do not exhibit the pharmacokinetic problems encountered with UCN-01 [33].

The intracellular disposition of many targeted agents e.g., tyrosine kinase inhibitors (TKIs) such as imatinib mesylate are regulated by natural product efflux pumps e.g., those related to Pgp, MRP, LRP, etc. [34]. Approaches to this problem include the selection of agents that are not susceptible to such efflux pumps, or combination with agents that interfere with efflux.

Degree and Duration of Target Inhibition

For targeted agents, the degree and duration of target inhibition may play a critical role in determining whether cells live or die in the face of inhibition of a critical signaling pathway. For example, in the case of FLT3 mutant acute myeloid leukemia (AML), the failure of FLT3 inhibitors to achieve responses in patients has been attributed to the failure to achieve sufficiently high drug concentrations for an adequate interval, and to recapitulate the drug duration and levels capable of inducing apoptosis in leukemia cells in vitro [35]. Thus, in this setting, FLT3 mutant cells may not be intrinsically resistant to a FLT3 inhibitor, but only to the agent when administered at pharmacologically achievable concentrations and for a limited duration. One approach to circumventing this form of resistance would be to alter drug doses and schedules; another would be to employ alternative inhibitors whose pharmacokinetics permit either greater target inhibition, more durable target inhibition, or both. Interestingly, the question of the relative importance of the degree vs. the duration of target inhibition has been investigated directly in the case of CML. Notably, it was found that in the case of certain Bcr/Abl kinase inhibitors, a relatively brief exposure to a high inhibitor concentration which triggered virtually complete target blockade was as effective, if not more so, than a considerably longer exposure to a lower drug concentration [17]. Consequently, in this instance, a threshold for cell death appeared to exist which depended upon the degree of target inhibition but was relatively independent of duration. Based upon these disparate results, it is clear that the relative importance of drug concentration vs. duration of target inhibition will very likely vary with the inhibitor as well as the malignant cell type in question.

Target-Specific Mechanisms of Resistance

Much attention has been focused on attempts to understand mechanisms of resistance to receptor tyrosine kinases such as HER2 in breast cancer and EGFR in lung cancer [36]. Interventions generally take two forms: small molecule inhibitors and monoclonal antibody approaches. A complicating factor stems from the fact that both common and disparate resistance mechanisms may exist for these agents. For example, in the case of monoclonal antibodies e.g., the HER2 MoAb trastuzumab, resistance can stem from alterations in the receptor (e.g., the presence of mutant forms that do not bind to the MoAb, competition with endogenous ligands, activation of parallel or downstream pathways, or other immunological mechanisms) [20]. Similarly, in the case of TKIs (e.g., gefitinib in the case of EGFR), resistance can stem from amplification or mutation of the kinase, activation of downstream targets, compensatory activation of parallel pathways (e.g., Ras/Raf/MEK/ERK) or PTEN/PI3K/AKT, or a combination of these factors.

Several recent clinical observations have shed light on the reciprocal nature of resistance and sensitivity to targeted agents in various settings. For example, colon cancer patients with *K-Ras* mutations are unlikely to respond to TKIs directed against EGFR [37]. A likely explanation for this phenomenon is that activation of the Ras/Raf/MEK/ERK pathway, which lies downstream to EGFR, may relieve transformed cells of their addiction to EGFR activation. Preclinical studies suggest that similar considerations may apply to the case of the PTEN/PI3K/AKT/mTOR pathway, which is also activated downstream of EGFR [10]. The development or preexistence of PTEN mutations may, as in the case of mutant Ras, relieve cells of their addiction to EGFR signaling. At the preclinical level, interventions capable of interrupting the PTEN/PI3K/AKT pathway (e.g., administration of PI3K inhibitors) have been shown to be effective in this setting [38]. Efforts to test such a strategy in the clinic are currently ongoing.

Another intriguing finding stems from the observation that patients with lung cancer expressing certain activating EGFR mutations are much more likely to respond to EGFR inhibitors than patients whose cells do not exhibit these mutations e.g., from ~10 to 70–80% [36]. Thus, such tumors appear to be particularly addicted to EGFR signaling for survival. The mechanisms underlying this phenomenon, which are currently the subject of intense investigation, remain to be fully elucidated. One speculative possibility is that for reasons not yet understood, such activating mutations do not require or induce activation of "orthogonal" protective pathways, as may occur in tumors developing without such mutations. Consequently, the absence of such activated compensatory parallel or downstream signaling pathways may render interruption of the mutant tyrosine kinase particularly lethal. It should be kept in mind that while TKIs display significant activity in patients with EGFR mutants, these agents are not curative, and patients ultimately die of their disease. This raises the possibility that even in the case of susceptible EGFR mutant disease, interrupting complementary survival signaling pathways in conjunction with TKI administration may improve results further.

While certain mutations predict for activity of EGFR inhibitors, others, such as the T790M mutation, confer resistance through interference with drug binding [39]. Approaches to circumvention of such forms of resistance include identification of TKIs that inhibit mutant tyrosine kinase activity, or the use of agents that inhibit either parallel or downstream pathways that cooperate with the kinase in promoting transformed cells survival.

Dysregulation of the Apoptotic Machinery in Targeted Agent Resistance

The Bcl-2 family of pro- and anti-apoptotic proteins are ultimately responsible for determining cell fate. Anti-apoptotic proteins such as Bcl-2, Bcl-xL, Mcl-1, and A1 are multidomain proteins that promote cell survival either directly by preserving mitochondrial integrity, or indirectly, by binding to and/or blocking the activity of pro-apoptotic proteins [40]. The pro-apoptotic proteins include multidomain proteins such as Bak and Bax, and BH3-only proteins such as Puma, Noxa, Hrk, Bid, Bik, Bad, and Bim [41]. Pro-apoptotic proteins may be further subcategorized as direct activator proteins (Bid, Puma, Bim), which may directly induce mitochondrial injury, or sensitizer proteins (e.g., Bad), which antagonize the survival functions of multidomain anti-apoptotic proteins [42]. The pro-apoptotic actions of targeted agents that disrupt growth factor-related or other survival signaling pathways are believed to be integrated at the level of pro- and anti-apoptotic proteins. For example, the intracellular disposition of Bad and Bim is regulated by phosphorylation via multiple signaling pathways, particularly Ras/Raf/MEK/ERK and PI3K/AKT/mTOR [10]. It has been shown that increased lethality in neoplastic cells resulting from simultaneous interruption of these pathways may stem from enhanced accumulation of Bad and Bim [10, 18]. Approaches to circumvention of resistance to targeted agents due to increased expression of anti-apoptotic proteins have included coadministration of small molecule BH3 mimetics such as ABT-737, obatoclax, or AT-101 [43]. An alternative strategy is to bypass blockade of the intrinsic, mitochondrial apoptotic pathway by triggering the extrinsic apoptotic cascade e.g., by administration of agents (e.g., histone deacetylase inhibitors) that upregulate and activate death receptors [44].

Autophagy-Related Cell Death Mechanisms

Autophagy, a term literally meaning "self-eating," represents a process in which various cellular stresses trigger a program in which cellular constituents are catabolized in lysosomal vesicles, providing a source of energy to maintain critical cellular functions [45]. Autophagy can therefore serve to protect cells from diverse environmental insults [46]. On the other hand, autophagy can also contribute to the cell death under other circumstances. One possible explanation for these disparate roles is that initially, autophagy represents a defensive response to damage which is extensive, or when cellular energy sources (e.g., ATP) are depleted; autophagy becomes toxic and contributes to the cell's demise. Under conditions in which autophagy protects cells from the lethal effects of targeted agents, administration of autophagy antagonists may dramatically increase cell death. For example, inhibitors such as chloroquine or 3-MA have been shown to enhance the lethality of histone deacetylase inhibitors by blocking autophagy in human leukemia cells [47].

Linear vs. Parallel Pathway Inhibition

Inhibition of multiple targets can take at least two forms. Linear inhibition refers to blockade of components of a single pathway at two separate sites. Examples include simultaneous inhibition of PI3K and AKT or mTOR [48]; inhibition of Bcr/Abl and a downstream target (e.g., PLK-1) [27]; or EGFR and MEK1/2 inhibitors [10]. This approach may be particularly appropriate when inhibition of a single component of a survival pathway is incomplete and insufficient to trigger cell death. Under these conditions, interruption of the pathway at a second, downstream site may reduce survival signals below threshold necessary to support survival. On the other hand, interruption of such a pathway at both upstream and downstream sites may be redundant, and could, at least theoretically, be counterproductive. For example, the lethal consequences of interruption of an upstream node such as PI3K may depend upon signaling imbalances stemming from persistent, if only transient, activation of downstream targets such as AKT or mTOR. Interruption of such conflicting signals (e.g., by addition of AKT or mTOR inhibitors) could potentially attenuate the lethal consequences of PI3K interruption.

An alternative approach, designated parallel inhibition, involves the simultaneous interruption of complementary parallel pathways which cooperate to maintain transformed cell survival. As noted previously, a classic example of such cooperativity involves the Ras/Raf/MEK/ERK and PI3K/AKT/mTOR pathways, which may prevent cell death by promoting phosphorylation (and subsequent degradation) of pro-death proteins (e.g., Bad and Bim) at separate sites. Several recent studies have demonstrated that regimens consisting of PI3K or AKT inhibitors and MEK1/2 inhibitors potently induce cell death in both solid tumor and hematologic malignancies [38, 49].

Dual Pathway Inhibition by Targeted Agents

Since the large majority of targeted agents have multiple targets, attempts to understand the basis of interactions between them have been hindered by their complexity. Nevertheless, due to a variety of factors, including the development of resistance or the presence or emergence of compensatory survival pathways, the need to interrupt two or more such pathways to achieve meaningful clinical results is now generally acknowledged. What follows below is not intended to be a complete overview of all such efforts, but rather prototypical examples of some of the more rationally based approaches. Representative examples of dual pathway inhibition by targeted agents are briefly summarized in Table 10.1 [10, 18, 19, 26, 38, 44, 49–90].

Table 10.1 Dual pathway inhibition by targeted agents

Rationales	Examples	Mechanisms	References
Survival signals and cell cycle regulatory pathways	Imatinib mesylate/IM + flavopiridol (CML)	Downregulation of p21^{CIP1}	[26]
DNA damage checkpoints	Cisplatin or gemcitabine + Chk1 inhibitors	Abrogation of G2/M or S phase checkpoints	[50]
Checkpoint and Ras/Raf/ MEK/ERK pathway inhibition	Chk1 inhibitors + MEK inhibitors or FTIs	Prevention of Bim phosphorylation and degradation Promotion of DNA damage	[19, 51–54]
HDAC inhibitor-based combination regimens	HDACIs + TRAIL	Upregulation of DR4 and DR5	[44, 55]
	HDACIs + topoisomerase poisons	Relaxation of chromatin	[56]
	HDACIs + TKIs	Disruption of chaperone function	[57–61]
	HDACIs + aurora kinase inhibitors	Potentiation of aurora kinase inhibition	[62, 63]
	HDACIs + flavopiridol	Downregulation of Mcl-1, p21^{CIP1} by inhibition of RNA Pol II	[64–66]
	HDACIs + IKK inhibitors	Prevention of NF-κB activation by blocking RelA acetylation	[67]
	HDACIs + Bcl-2 antagonists	Upregulation and reactivation of Bim	[69]
Proteasome inhibitor-based combination regimens	Proteasome inhibitors + HDACIs	Inhibition of NF-κB activation	[68, 72, 73]
		Aggresome disruption	[70]
		Induction of ER stress	[71]
		Bim upregulation	[68]
	Proteasome inhibitors + flavopiridol	Activation of SAPK/JNK	[74]
		Potentiation of NF-κB inhibition	[75–77]
	Proteasome inhibitors + Bcl-2 antagonists	Downregulation of Mcl-1	[78–81]
		Activation of SAPK/JNK	
		ROS induction	
Bcl-2 antagonist combinations	Bcl-2 antagonists + MEK inhibitors	Downregulation of Mcl-1	[82]
	Bcl-2 antagonists + CDK inhibitors	Downregulation of Mcl-1 by inhibition of RNA Pol II	[83, 84]
	Bcl-2 inhibitors + sorafenib	Downregulation of Mcl-1	[84]
		Upregulation of Bim	[85]
MEK inhibitor-based combinations	MEK inhibitors + IM	Potentiated inhibition of Bcr/Abl downstream signals	[86]
	MEK inhibitors + mTOR inhibitors	Prevention of ERK activation	[18, 38]
	MEK inhibitors + perifosine	Upregulation of Bim	[49, 87]
	MEK inhibitors + sorafenib	Prevention of ERK activation	[88]
PI3K/Akt inhibitor-based combinations	PI3K/Akt inhibitors + TKIs	Prevention of Bad degradation	[10]
	PI3K/Akt inhibitors + HDACIs	Interruption of MEK/ERK signal	[89]
	PI3K/Akt inhibitors + Bcl-2 antagonists	Disability of Bcl-xL	[90]

Interruption of Cell Signaling and Cell Cycle Regulatory Pathways

Numerous links exist between the cell cycle and survival signaling regulatory apparatus. For example, the Ras/Raf/MEK/ERK pathway has been implicated in regulating G_2M progression and in governing the disposition of cyclin D1, which is critically involved in progression into the cell cycle from G_0G_1 [91]. Consequently, simultaneous disruption of the survival signaling pathways in conjunction with interference with the cell cycle machinery is an attractive concept. In this context, it has been shown that the CDK inhibitor flavopiridol induces a pronounced increase in the lethality of imatinib mesylate in Bcr/Abl+ leukemia cells in association with downregulation of the endogenous CDK inhibitor p21^{CIP1} [26]. Clinical trials designed to evaluate the efficacy of this strategy in patients with CML have been initiated.

Another strategy targeting cell cycle and survival signaling pathways involves inhibition of cell cycle checkpoints, most notably Chk1. Chk1 is an important component of the DNA damage response (DDR) and is responsible for triggering cell cycle arrest in cells subjected to genotoxic insults, allowing repair to occur if the damage is limited, or apoptosis if it is severe. Chk1 has been a major target for therapeutic intervention because it is involved in essentially all DNA damage checkpoints, and may also contribute to cell survival in a more direct manner [33]. To date, most strategies involving Chk1 inhibitors involve combination with various DNA damaging agents such as topoisomerase inhibitors, cisplatin, or gemcitabine [50]. However, it has been shown that in malignant hematopoietic and epithelial tumor cells, Chk1 inhibition elicits a compensatory activation of the Ras/Raf/MEK/ERK pathway [51]. Significantly, abrogation of this pathway at downstream sites (e.g., by MEK1/2 inhibitors) or at more upstream sites (e.g., by farnesyltransferase inhibitors) dramatically increases Chk1 inhibitor lethality [19, 52]. Recently, this phenomenon has been specifically linked to potentiation of Chk1 inhibitor-mediated DNA damage, manifested by a striking increase in expression of γH2A.X [53], a marker for double-stranded DNA damage, as well as upregulation of the pro-apoptotic protein Bim [54]. Such findings raise the possibility that in transformed cells, disruption of cell cycle checkpoints, which are often dysregulated in neoplasia, triggers a compensatory activation of the Ras/Raf/MEK/ERK pathway allowing them to survive. Consequently, disabling this pathway (e.g., by farnesyltransferase or MEK1/2 inhibitors) lowers the threshold for DNA damage-induced cell death.

Histone Deacetylase Inhibitor-Based Combination Regimens

Histone deacetylase inhibitors (HDACIs) are truly pleiotropic agents in that they induce neoplastic cell death through multiple pathways. These include, among others, induction of death receptors, generation of reactive oxygen species, inhibition of DNA repair via acetylation of DNA repair proteins (e.g., Ku70), acetylation of chaperone proteins (e.g., Hsp90) and downregulation of survival-related proteins (e.g., Raf, AKT), disruption of cell cycle checkpoints, and induction of pro-apoptotic proteins (e.g., Bim) [92]. It is therefore not surprising that HDACIs have been shown to interact synergistically with multiple other targeted agents as well as more conventional agents. A summary of representative interactions follows below.

HDACIs and Death Receptor Agonists

The ability of HDACIs to upregulate death receptors (e.g., DR4 and DR5) in malignant cells has been exploited by attempts to combine them with activators of the extrinsic apoptotic pathway e.g., TRAIL. For example, synergistic interactions between TRAIL and HDACIs have been observed in human leukemia cells; moreover, this process selectively spared normal hematopoietic cells [44, 93]. Synergism between TRAIL and HDACIs has also been attributed to simultaneous activation of the intrinsic and extrinsic apoptotic pathways [55].

HDACIs and Topoisomerase Inhibitors

Synergistic interactions have been reported between HDACIs and topoisomerase poisons in various malignant cell types, particularly when HDACI exposure precedes administration of DNA damaging agents. This phenomenon has been attributed to HDACI-mediated relaxation of chromatin, and the resulting enhanced susceptibility of DNA to genotoxic agents [56].

HDACIs and TKIs

Numerous studies have demonstrated that HDACIs, particularly pan-HDACIs or inhibitors of HDAC6, potentiate the effects of TKIs in malignant hematopoietic cells. This action may reflect the capacity of pan-HDACIs and HDAC6 inhibitors to acetylate Hsp90, disrupt its chaperone function, and induce downregulation of mutant oncoproteins, which are particularly dependent upon normal chaperone function for their survival [57]. For example, HDACIs have been shown to interact synergistically with Bcr/Abl kinase inhibitors such as imatinib and dasatinib in CML cells [58, 59], and with FLT3 inhibitors in human leukemia cells expressing mutant FLT3 [60]. Potentiation of the activity of EGFR inhibitors has also been observed in the case of epithelial malignancies [61].

HDACIs and Aurora Kinase Inhibitors

The ability of HDACIs to induce mitotic slippage [94] and to interfere with cell cycle checkpoints provides a theoretical basis for interactions between these agents and inhibitors of aurora kinase, a protein that plays a key role in chromosome segregation and the mitotic process in general. In addition, HDACIs have been shown to induce downregulation of aurora kinases in malignant cells [62]. Indeed, synergistic interactions between HDACIs and aurora kinase inhibitors have been observed in malignant hematopoietic cells, including Bcr/Abl+ leukemias [63]. This interaction has been attributed to multiple factors, including potentiation of Bcr/Abl kinase inhibition, enhanced interference with aurora kinase function, manifested by diminished phosphorylation of histone H3, upregulation of Bim, and potentiation of cell death in endoreduplicated cells.

HDACIs and CDK Inhibitors

Synergistic interactions have been described between HDACIs and cyclin-dependent kinase inhibitors such as flavopiridol, particularly CDK inhibitors that disrupt the P-TEFb (CDK9/cyclin T) transcriptional regulatory apparatus by inhibiting the phosphorylation of the carboxy-terminal domain (CTD) of RNA Pol II [64]. Such agents, by inhibiting transcription, downregulate several short-lived proteins such as Mcl-1 and p21^{CIP1} which may be induced by HDACIs [65]. By preventing induction of these proteins, CDK inhibitors lower the threshold for HDACI-induced cell death. Several clinical trials combining flavopiridol with HDACIs such as vorinostat are in progress in patients with acute leukemia or solid tumors to test the in vivo relevance of these findings [66].

HDACIs and Inhibitors of the NF-κB Pathway

HDACIs acetylate, and thereby in addition to HDACs, multiple proteins involved in cell survival decisions, might be more accurately characterized as protein acetylases [95]. One such protein is RelA/p65, the most abundant member of the NF-κB family. Acetylation of RelA has been invoked to explain the sustained activation of NF-κB that occurs in cells exposed to HDACIs, in contrast to the early termination of NF-κB activation observed in the case of TNFα [96]. This stems from enhanced binding of acetylated RelA to DNA and diminished affinity for IκBα [97]. Notably, IKK inhibitors, which are currently being developed as anti-inflammatory and anticancer agents, by blocking IκBα phosphorylation and degradation, interfere with RelA acetylation and nuclear translocation, resulting in downregulation of NF-κB-dependent proteins, such as SOD2, XIAP, and Bcl-xL [67]. This leads to a marked increase in HDACI lethality, raising the possibility that such agents may enhance the antitumor activity of HDACIs. An alternative strategy to block IκBα degradation would be to prevent its proteasomal degradation i.e., by proteasome inhibitors. Indeed, proteasome inhibitors such as bortezomib have been shown to prevent HDACI-mediated NF-κB activation in malignant hematopoietic cells (e.g., CLL cells) [68]. However, it is likely that additional mechanisms are involved in the synergism that occurs with combined HDAC and proteasome inhibition (see below).

HDACIs and Bcl-2 Antagonists

Among their numerous actions, HDACIs modulate the expression of pro- and anti-apoptotic proteins, and in so doing, may enhance the lethality of other targeted agents. For example, HDACIs have been shown to upregulate Bim in transformed cells through an E2F1-dependent mechanism [98]. In this context, HDACIs have been shown to potentiate the lethality of TKIs in transformed cells through a Bim-dependent mechanism [99]. In addition, synergistic interactions between HDACIs and the BH3-mimetic and Bcl-2/Bcl-xL antagonist ABT-737 have recently been attributed to upregulation of Bim in human leukemia and myeloma cells [69].

Proteasome Inhibitor-Based Combinations

Proteasome inhibitors, exemplified by the boronic anhydride bortezomib (Velcade) disrupt protein disposition by the 26S proteasome, and kill transformed cells by multiple mechanisms. Bortezomib has recently been approved for the treatment of refractory multiple myeloma and mantle cell lymphoma [100]. Notably, proteasome inhibitors have been shown to exhibit selective lethality toward transformed cells compared to their normal counterparts [101]. Proteasome inhibitors kill transformed cells through diverse mechanisms, including inhibition of NF-κB, induction of oxidative injury, disruption of DNA repair, and induction of endoplasmic reticulum (ER) stress, among others [100]. The pleiotropic actions of proteasome inhibitors make them particularly suitable candidates for combination strategies.

Proteasome Inhibitors and HDAC Inhibitors

Synergistic interactions have been described between proteasome inhibitors and HDACIs in both solid tumor and hematologic malignancies. Three major mechanisms have been proposed to account for such interactions. First, proteasome inhibitors, by blocking IκBα degradation, can prevent HDACI-mediated NF-κB induction, and in so doing abrogate cytoprotective responses. Second, HDACIs which inhibit HDAC6, can disrupt aggresome function, and amplify the lethal consequences of interference with protein disposition [70]. Lastly, combined proteasome and HDAC inhibition can promote ER stress [71]. In this context, synergistic interactions between proteasome inhibitors and HDACIs have been described in multiple myeloma cells [72], and the results of a recent trial in which bortezomib was combined with the HDACI vorinostat in patients with refractory multiple myeloma appeared promising [73]. In addition, highly synergistic interactions between bortezomib and the HDACI romidepsin in primary CLL cells [68], and trials combining these agents in multiple myeloma and CLL are underway. Recently, highly synergistic interactions between the second-generation, irreversible proteasome inhibitor carfilzomib (PR-171) and HDACIs including vorinostat and SNDX-275 have been described in diffuse large B-cell lymphoma (DLBCL) cells, including those resistant to bortezomib [74]. A clinical trial combining carfilzomib and vorinostat in patients with refractory non-Hodgkin's lymphoma is currently underway. Finally, synergistic interactions between proteasome inhibitors and HDACIs have been observed in myeloid leukemia cells [102, 103], suggesting that this strategy may warrant attention in myeloid malignancies.

Proteasome and CDK Inhibitors

Preclinical studies have demonstrated highly synergistic interactions between the proteasome inhibitor bortezomib and the pan-CDK inhibitor flavopiridol in malignant hematopoietic cells [75]. This interaction was associated with a marked increase in activation of the stress-related JNK pathway. Notably, combination of bortezomib with flavopiridol, which also acts as an IKK inhibitor [76], markedly diminished NF-κB activation in malignant cells [75]. This raises the possibility that diminishing NF-κB activation below a level sufficient for cell survival may underlie or contribute to the lethality of this regimen. Early clinical trials of bortezomib and flavopiridol in patients with refractory multiple myeloma, mantle cell lymphoma, or indolent non-Hodgkin's lymphoma have yielded encouraging results [77].

Proteasome Inhibitors and Bcl-2 Antagonists

A variety of BH3-mimetic inhibitors of anti-apoptotic members of the Bcl-2 family (e.g., Bcl-2, Bcl-xL, A1, Mcl-1) have been developed which lower the threshold for apoptosis induced by both conventional cytotoxic agents as well as targeted therapies. These include ABT-737, AT-101, and GX15-070 (obatoclax), among others [78, 104]. In multiple myeloma cells, bortezomib was shown to interact synergistically with the BH3-mimetic HA14-1 in association with induction of oxidative injury and activation of JNK [79]. Similar interactions have been described between ABT-737 and the epoxyketone proteasome inhibitor carfilzomib in non-Hodgkin's lymphoma and mantle cell lymphoma cells [80]. The latter study demonstrated in vivo activity for this strategy with acceptable toxicity. Synergism between bortezomib and obatoclax has also been described in multiple myeloma cells [81].

Bcl-2 Antagonist Combinations

As noted above, BH3 mimetics variably disable anti-apoptotic members of the Bcl-2 family. Certain of these agents e.g., ABT-737 or its clinically relevant analog, ABT-263, potently inhibit Bcl-2 and Bcl-xL, but have little affinity for Mcl-1 [104]. Consequently, the activity of these agents is inversely related to expression of Mcl-1 in tumor cells [105]. A corollary of this notion is that agents or interventions capable of downregulating Mcl-1 should increase the activity of ABT-737 or analogous agents. Indeed, multiple studies have demonstrated synergistic interactions between such agents and ABT-737 in various tumor cell types.

Bcl-2 Antagonists and MEK1/2 Inhibitors

Phosphorylation of Mcl-1 via the MEK1/2/ERK1/2 pathway may, under some circumstances, spare Mcl-1 from proteasomal degradation; conversely, inhibition of Mcl-1 phosphorylation may lead to diminished Mcl-1 expression. Consistent with this notion, pharmacologic MEK1/2 inhibitors have been shown to downregulate Mcl-1 levels in human leukemia cells, leading to a marked increase in apoptosis for the combination [82].

Bcl-2 Antagonists and CDK Inhibitors

As discussed previously, several CDK inhibitors, particularly those that inhibit CDK9 and by extension, block phosphorylation of the CTD of RNA Pol II by inhibiting the CDK9/cyclin T P-TEFb complex. As a consequence, they act as transcriptional repressors, and induce downregulation of proteins with short half-lives, such as Mcl-1. Synergistic interactions between such CDK inhibitors and ABT-737 have been described. For example, the CDK inhibitor roscovitine, or seliciclib, the R-enantiomer of roscovitine, have been shown to downregulate Mcl-1 expression in human multiple myeloma, leukemia cells, and other neoplastic cells, resulting in a high degree of synergism with ABT-737 [83, 84]. The possibility also arises that downregulation of other short-lived anti-apoptotic proteins such as XIAP may contribute to interactions between these agents.

Bcl-2 Antagonists and Sorafenib

As noted previously, although sorafenib was originally developed as a B-Raf inhibitor, its other mechanisms of action have been identified, including inhibition of angiogenesis and induction of ER stress [106]. In fact, the ability of sorafenib to induce ER stress, accompanied by inhibition of translation and Mcl-1 downregulation, have been shown to be the primary mechanisms of lethality toward malignant human hematopoietic cells, rather than interruption of the Raf/MEK1/2/ERK1/2 pathway [107]. Therefore, sorafenib represents a logical agent to employ in combination with Bcl-2 antagonists whose actions may be limited by Mcl-1 expression in tumor cells. Indeed, synergistic interactions between sorafenib and ABT-737 have been described in human lung cancer and leukemia cells [84, 85]. The ability of sorafenib to inhibit FLT3 provides an additional rationale for combining sorafenib with Bcl-2 antagonists such s ABT-737 in human leukemia, particularly in patients whose cells exhibit mutant FLT3.

MEK1/2 Inhibitor-Based Combinations

The Raf/MEK1/2/ERK1/2 pathway signals downstream to regulate multiple survival and pro-proliferative proteins, including Bim, Bad, cyclin D1, caspase-9, and RSK, among others [108]. Consequently, it is not surprising that synergistic interactions between MEK1/2 inhibitors and other targeted agents have been reported in multiple transformed cell types, in addition to those described above in the case of Chk1 inhibitors and Bcl-2 antagonists. For example, MEK1/2 inhibitors have been shown to potentiate the lethality of TKIs such as imatinib mesylate in Bcr/Abl+ human leukemia cells [86]. In addition, cooperation between MEK1/2 inhibitors and inhibitors of the PI3K/AKT/mTOR pathway has been described in both hematologic and nonhematologic malignancies. For example, exposure to mTOR inhibitors can trigger a cytoprotective ERK1/2 response via growth factor receptors, which limits lethality. In the case of prostate and breast cancer cells, coadministration of mTOR and MEK1/2 inhibitors resulted in a marked increase in lethality [18, 38]. Analogously, in human leukemia cells, administration of an AKT inhibitor (perifosine) resulted in a marked increase in ERK1/2 activation; prevention of the latter event e.g., by MEK1/2 inhibitors synergistically enhanced apoptosis [49]. Similar interactions between perifosine and MEK1/2 inhibitors have been observed in multiple myeloma cells [87].

Interestingly, similar interactions may occur between MEK1/2 inhibitors and inhibitors of upstream components of the Ras/Raf/MEK1/2/ERK1/2 pathway. For example, recent studies indicate that in melanoma and other transformed cells bearing the V600E B-Raf mutation, B-Raf inhibitors inhibit cell growth and trigger apoptosis. However, in cells without this mutation and/or with mutated Ras, B-Raf inhibitors paradoxically activate ERK1/2 through a C-Raf-dependent mechanism [109]. It is tempting to speculate that under these circumstances, coadministration of a MEK1/2 inhibitor might lead to a marked increase in lethality. In this context, the B-Raf inhibitor sorafenib has recently been shown to induce activation, rather than inactivation, of ERK1/2 in human DLBCL cells [88]. In accord with the latter hypothesis, coadministration of MEK1/2 inhibitors blocked sorafenib-mediated ERK1/2 activation, and resulted in a dramatic increase in lethality [88]. Therefore, coadministration of sorafenib with MEK1/2 inhibitors may not represent a linear blockade of a signaling pathway; instead, it may reflect inhibition of parallel cytoprotective pathways.

PI3K/AKT Inhibitor-Based Combinations

Activation of the PI3K/AKT pathway (e.g., in cells exhibiting mutant PTEN) may allow transformed cells to survive interruption of other survival signaling pathways such as the Ras/Raf/MEK1/2/ERK1/2 pathway. As described previously, activation of the PI3K/AKT pathway can protect cells from the lethal effects of inhibitors of growth factor receptors e.g., EGFR inhibitors, possibly by promoting degradation of the pro-apoptotic protein Bad [10]. In such settings, inhibition of PI3K can restore sensitivity of cells to TKIs.

Inhibitors of PI3K have also been shown to promote the lethality of HDACIs in both epithelial as well as malignant hematopoietic cells [89]. Interestingly, the latter effect was found to be more closely related to inhibition of the MEK1/2/ERK1/2 than the PI3K/AKT pathway.

PI3K/AKT inhibitors have also been reported to potentate the activity of Bcl-2 antagonists (e.g., ABT-737) in malignant cells via a Bcl-xL-related mechanism [90].

Summary and Future Directions

Results to date suggest that with rare exceptions (e.g., Bcr/Abl inhibitors in CML), interruption of a single survival pathway will be insufficient to achieve meaningful clinical responses in most tumor types. As in the case of cytotoxic chemotherapy, where combinations of agents have been required for cures of diseases such as testicular cancer, DLBCL, Hodgkin's disease, and acute myeloid and lymphoid leukemias, it seems quite likely that analogous approaches will be necessary in the case of targeted agents. Although it seems logical that targeted agents may have the capacity to enhance the activity of conventional cytotoxic agents or regimens, results with this strategy have not yet realized their potential. On the other hand, the rational combination of targeted agents, particularly those capable of blocking complementary survival signaling or cell cycle regulatory pathways, represents a very appealing alternative approach. Aside from the intrinsic logic of this mechanism-based strategy, the tools are currently available to perform correlative laboratory studies capable of determining the basis for the success or failure of individual regimens. In addition, the notion of targeting pathways specifically implicated in transformation offers the prospect of both individualized therapy as well as the potential for therapeutic selectivity.

Optimization of this strategy will require addressing a number of unanswered questions. A key question is whether a targeted agent must display single agent activity in a particular disease in order to be of benefit in a combination regimen. In the case of conventional targeted agents, it has long been assumed, although never formally proven, that individual agents must have activity in a particular disease in order to enhance the activity of a combination regimen. While it is possible that this may be the case for targeted agents, it is nevertheless conceivable that agents inactive alone may potentiate the activity of another targeted agent if they disable an important compensatory pathway, even if interruption of this pathway is not by itself lethal. For example, while HDACIs have not yet shown single agent activity in multiple myeloma, preliminary evidence raises the possibility that they might enhance the efficacy of bortezomib in this setting [73].

Another key question is the role of agents that disrupt so-called "orthogonal," cancer-related stress pathways should play in such strategies. The latter ameliorate the otherwise lethal effects of oxidative, proteotoxic, DNA damage-related and other forms of stress that accompany activation of oncogenes such as Ras and c-Myc [13]. Although inhibitors of such pathways are not as specific as those disabling oncoproteins directly responsible for transformation (e.g., mutant FLT3 in the case of AML or Bcr/Abl in the case of CML), they may still play a critical role in maintaining the transformed phenotype. Consequently, interruption of such pathways could play an important adjunctive role in combination with inhibitors of transforming oncoproteins.

The bulk of attention in this area has thus far focused on the simultaneous interruption of two complementary survival signaling pathways to achieve enhanced transformed cell killing. However, many of the successes of combination chemotherapy involving conventional cytotoxic agents have involved more than two agents e.g., the CHOP regimen in the case of DLBCL [110]. Furthermore, emerging evidence suggests that analogous to this model, simultaneous interruption of more than two signaling pathways may be required for optimal cell killing of transformed cells [111]. To put this in the context of the hallmarks of cancer, which currently number at least 12 [13], maintenance of the transformed state may require multiple aberrations in signaling pathways. Consequently, eradication of such cells may require simultaneous blockade of three or more such pathways. A future paradigm for such approaches may involve combining inhibitor of oncoproteins directly implicated in development of a malignancy (e.g., FLT3 or Bcr/Abl inhibitors in the case of AML or CML respectively), with an inhibitor of potential compensatory survival pathway (e.g., a MEK1/2 inhibitors) in conjunction with an inhibitor of an orthogonal proteotoxic or DNA damage-related stress pathway (e.g., an HDAC or Chk1 inhibitor).

Finally, successful curative approaches to neoplastic diseases may ultimately depend upon the eradication of cancer stem cells, which have been well characterized in the case of hematopoietic malignancies (e.g., AML) [112], but which are being actively investigated in the case of epithelial malignancies [113]. Interestingly, stem cell survival and maintenance may depend upon unique pathways not shared by the population of tumor cells as a whole. For example, in the case of leukemia, stem cells may require activation of certain developmental pathways for their survival (e.g., members of the Wnt family) [114]. Indeed, recent preclinical studies suggest that combining antagonists of such pathways with inhibitors of oncoproteins directly implicated in pathogenesis of the disease (e.g., Bcr/Abl inhibitors) may yield results superior to those obtained with either agent alone or may overcome imatinib resistance [114, 115]. A logical extension of this approach would be to incorporate inhibitors of stem cell-dependent pathways into the multiagent regimens described above. Given the large number of agents capable of inhibiting existing and new targets currently available, the number of such regimens is obviously very large. Nevertheless, this approach may offer the best chance of achieving long-lasting remissions or even cures in a group of diseases otherwise considered fatal. Future progress in this effort is awaited with considerable anticipation.

Acknowledgments This work was supported by awards CA63753, CA93738, CA100866, and P50CA130805 from the National Institutes of Health; award R6059-06 from the Leukemia and Lymphoma Society of America; Lymphoma SPORE award P50CA130805; and an award from the V Foundation.

References

1. Kantarjian H, Sawyers C, Hochhaus A, et al. Hematologic and cytogenetic responses to imatinib mesylate in chronic myelogenous leukemia. N Engl J Med. 2002;346(9):645–52.
2. Tallman MS. Current management and new approaches in the treatment of APL. Clin Adv Hematol Oncol. 2003;1(10):580–1.
3. Gorre ME, Mohammed M, Ellwood K, et al. Clinical resistance to STI-571 cancer therapy caused by BCR-ABL gene mutation or amplification. Science. 2001;293(5531):876–80.
4. Young MA, Shah NP, Chao LH, et al. Structure of the kinase domain of an imatinib-resistant Abl mutant in complex with the Aurora kinase inhibitor VX-680. Cancer Res. 2006;66(2):1007–14.
5. Giehl K. Oncogenic Ras in tumour progression and metastasis. Biol Chem. 2005;386(3): 193–205.
6. Sebti SM, Hamilton AD. Farnesyltransferase and geranylgeranyltransferase I inhibitors and cancer therapy: lessons from mechanism and bench-to-bedside translational studies. Oncogene. 2000;19(56):6584–93.
7. Weinstein IB, Joe AK. Mechanisms of disease: oncogene addiction – a rationale for molecular targeting in cancer therapy. Nat Clin Pract Oncol. 2006;3(8):448–57.
8. Gorre ME, Ellwood-Yen K, Chiosis G, Rosen N, Sawyers CL. BCR-ABL point mutants isolated from patients with imatinib mesylate-resistant chronic myeloid leukemia remain sensitive to inhibitors of the BCR-ABL chaperone heat shock protein 90. Blood. 2002;100(8):3041–4.
9. Sausville EA. Dragons round the fleece again: STI571 versus alpha1 acid glycoprotein. J Natl Cancer Inst. 2000;92(20):1626–7.
10. She QB, Solit DB, Ye Q, O'Reilly KE, Lobo J, Rosen N. The BAD protein integrates survival signaling by EGFR/MAPK and PI3K/Akt kinase pathways in PTEN-deficient tumor cells. Cancer Cell. 2005;8(4):287–97.
11. Sharma SV, Settleman J. Oncogene addiction: setting the stage for molecularly targeted cancer therapy. Genes Dev. 2007;21(24):3214–31.
12. Hanahan D, Weinberg RA. The hallmarks of cancer. Cell. 2000;100(1):57–70.
13. Luo J, Solimini NL, Elledge SJ. Principles of cancer therapy: oncogene and non-oncogene addiction. Cell. 2009;136(5):823–37.
14. Sharma SV, Settleman J. Oncogenic shock: turning an activated kinase against the tumor cell. Cell Cycle. 2006;5(24):2878–80.
15. Vaux DL, Cory S, Adams JM. Bcl-2 gene promotes haemopoietic cell survival and cooperates with c-myc to immortalize pre-B cells. Nature. 1988;335(6189):440–2.
16. Sharma SV, Fischbach MA, Haber DA, Settleman J. "Oncogenic shock": explaining oncogene addiction through differential signal attenuation. Clin Cancer Res. 2006;12(14 Pt 2):4392s–5.
17. Shah NP, Kasap C, Weier C, et al. Transient potent BCR-ABL inhibition is sufficient to commit chronic myeloid leukemia cells irreversibly to apoptosis. Cancer Cell. 2008;14(6):485–93.
18. Carracedo A, Ma L, Teruya-Feldstein J, et al. Inhibition of mTORC1 leads to MAPK pathway activation through a PI3K-dependent feedback loop in human cancer. J Clin Invest. 2008;118(9):3065–74.
19. Dai Y, Landowski TH, Rosen ST, Dent P, Grant S. Combined treatment with the checkpoint abrogator UCN-01 and MEK1/2 inhibitors potently induces apoptosis in drug-sensitive and -resistant myeloma cells through an IL-6-independent mechanism. Blood. 2002;100(9):3333–43.
20. Ellis LM, Hicklin DJ. Resistance to targeted therapies: refining anticancer therapy in the era of molecular oncology. Clin Cancer Res. 2009;15(24):7471–8.
21. Shah NP. Advanced CML: therapeutic options for patients in accelerated and blast phases. J Natl Compr Canc Netw. 2008;6 Suppl 2:S31–6.
22. Roche-Lestienne C, Preudhomme C. Mutations in the ABL kinase domain pre-exist the onset of imatinib treatment. Semin Hematol. 2003;40(2 Suppl 2):80–2.

23. Quintas-Cardama A, Kantarjian H, Cortes J. Imatinib and beyond – exploring the full potential of targeted therapy for CML. Nat Rev Clin Oncol. 2009;6(9):535–43.
24. O'Hare T, Shakespeare WC, Zhu X, et al. AP24534, a pan-BCR-ABL inhibitor for chronic myeloid leukemia, potently inhibits the T315I mutant and overcomes mutation-based resistance. Cancer Cell. 2009;16(5):401–12.
25. Daley GQ. Towards combination target-directed chemotherapy for chronic myeloid leukemia: role of farnesyl transferase inhibitors. Semin Hematol. 2003;40(2 Suppl 2):11–4.
26. Yu C, Krystal G, Dent P, Grant S. Flavopiridol potentiates STI571-induced mitochondrial damage and apoptosis in BCR-ABL-positive human leukemia cells. Clin Cancer Res. 2002;8(9):2976–84.
27. Gleixner KV, Ferenc V, Peter B, et al. Polo-like kinase 1 (Plk1) as a novel drug target in chronic myeloid leukemia: overriding imatinib resistance with the Plk1 inhibitor BI 2536. Cancer Res. 2010;70(4):1513–23.
28. Sato S, Fujita N, Tsuruo T. Interference with PDK1-Akt survival signaling pathway by UCN-01 (7-hydroxystaurosporine). Oncogene. 2002;21(11):1727–38.
29. Fuse E, Tanii H, Takai K, et al. Altered pharmacokinetics of a novel anticancer drug, UCN-01, caused by specific high affinity binding to alpha1-acid glycoprotein in humans. Cancer Res. 1999;59(5):1054–60.
30. Kummar S, Gutierrez ME, Gardner ER, et al. A phase I trial of UCN-01 and prednisone in patients with refractory solid tumors and lymphomas. Cancer Chemother Pharmacol. 2010;65(2):383–9.
31. Senderowicz AM. Flavopiridol: the first cyclin-dependent kinase inhibitor in human clinical trials. Invest New Drugs. 1999;17(3):313–20.
32. Byrd JC, Lin TS, Dalton JT, et al. Flavopiridol administered using a pharmacologically derived schedule is associated with marked clinical efficacy in refractory, genetically high-risk chronic lymphocytic leukemia. Blood. 2007;109(2):399–404.
33. Dai Y, Grant S. New insights into Chk kinase 1 in the DNA damage repair (DDR) signaling network: rationale for employing Chk1 inhibitors in cancer chemotherapy. Clin Cancer Res. 2010;16(2):376–83.
34. Mahon FX, Belloc F, Lagarde V, et al. MDR1 gene overexpression confers resistance to imatinib mesylate in leukemia cell line models. Blood. 2003;101(6):2368–73.
35. Pratz KW, Cortes J, Roboz GJ, et al. A pharmacodynamic study of the FLT3 inhibitor KW-2449 yields insight into the basis for clinical response. Blood. 2009;113(17):3938–46.
36. Sharma SV, Bell DW, Settleman J, Haber DA. Epidermal growth factor receptor mutations in lung cancer. Nat Rev Cancer. 2007;7(3):169–81.
37. Raponi M, Winkler H, Dracopoli NC. KRAS mutations predict response to EGFR inhibitors. Curr Opin Pharmacol. 2008;8(4):413–8.
38. Kinkade CW, Castillo-Martin M, Puzio-Kuter A, et al. Targeting AKT/mTOR and ERK MAPK signaling inhibits hormone-refractory prostate cancer in a preclinical mouse model. J Clin Invest. 2008;118(9):3051–64.
39. Godin-Heymann N, Ulkus L, Brannigan BW, et al. The T790M "gatekeeper" mutation in EGFR mediates resistance to low concentrations of an irreversible EGFR inhibitor. Mol Cancer Ther. 2008;7(4):874–9.
40. Reed JC. Bcl-2 family proteins. Oncogene. 1998;17(25):3225–36.
41. Reed JC. Apoptosis-targeted therapies for cancer. Cancer Cell. 2003;3(1):17–22.
42. Green DR. At the gates of death. Cancer Cell. 2006;9(5):328–30.
43. Cragg MS, Kuroda J, Puthalakath H, Huang DC, Strasser A. Gefitinib-induced killing of NSCLC cell lines expressing mutant EGFR requires BIM and can be enhanced by BH3 mimetics. PLoS Med. 2007;4(10):1681–9.
44. Insinga A, Monestiroli S, Ronzoni S, et al. Inhibitors of histone deacetylases induce tumor-selective apoptosis through activation of the death receptor pathway. Nat Med. 2005;11(1):71–6.
45. White E, DiPaola RS. The double-edged sword of autophagy modulation in cancer. Clin Cancer Res. 2009;15(17):5308–16.

46. Jin S, White E. Role of autophagy in cancer: management of metabolic stress. Autophagy. 2007;3(1):28–31.
47. Carew JS, Nawrocki ST, Kahue CN, et al. Targeting autophagy augments the anticancer activity of the histone deacetylase inhibitor SAHA to overcome Bcr-Abl-mediated drug resistance. Blood. 2007;110(1):313–22.
48. Bhatt AP, Bhende PM, Sin SH, Roy D, Dittmer DP, Damania B. Dual inhibition of PI3K and mTOR inhibits autocrine and paracrine proliferative loops in PI3K/Akt/mTOR-addicted lymphomas. Blood. 2010;115(22):4455–63.
49. Rahmani M, Anderson A, Habibi JR, et al. The BH3-only protein Bim plays a critical role in leukemia cell death triggered by concomitant inhibition of the PI3K/Akt and MEK/ERK1/2 pathways. Blood. 2009;114(20):4507–16.
50. Shao RG, Cao CX, Shimizu T, O'Connor PM, Kohn KW, Pommier Y. Abrogation of an S-phase checkpoint and potentiation of camptothecin cytotoxicity by 7-hydroxystauro-sporine (UCN-01) in human cancer cell lines, possibly influenced by p53 function. Cancer Res. 1997;57(18):4029–35.
51. Dai Y, Yu C, Singh V, et al. Pharmacological inhibitors of the mitogen-activated protein kinase (MAPK) kinase/MAPK cascade interact synergistically with UCN-01 to induce mito-chondrial dysfunction and apoptosis in human leukemia cells. Cancer Res. 2001;61(13):5106–15.
52. Pei XY, Dai Y, Rahmani M, Li W, Dent P, Grant S. The farnesyltransferase inhibitor L744832 potentiates UCN-01-induced apoptosis in human multiple myeloma cells. Clin Cancer Res. 2005;11(12):4589–600.
53. Dai Y, Chen S, Pei XY, et al. Interruption of the Ras/MEK/ERK signaling cascade enhances Chk1 inhibitor-induced-DNA damage in vitro and in vivo in human multiple myeloma cells. Blood. 2008;112(6):2439–49.
54. Pei XY, Dai Y, Tenorio S, et al. MEK1/2 inhibitors potentiate UCN-01 lethality in human multiple myeloma cells through a Bim-dependent mechanism. Blood. 2007;110(6):2092–101.
55. Rosato RR, Almenara JA, Dai Y, Grant S. Simultaneous activation of the intrinsic and extrin-sic pathways by histone deacetylase (HDAC) inhibitors and tumor necrosis factor-related apoptosis-inducing ligand (TRAIL) synergistically induces mitochondrial damage and apop-tosis in human leukemia cells. Mol Cancer Ther. 2003;2(12):1273–84.
56. Marchion DC, Bicaku E, Daud AI, Richon V, Sullivan DM, Munster PN. Sequence-specific potentiation of topoisomerase II inhibitors by the histone deacetylase inhibitor suberoyla-nilide hydroxamic acid. J Cell Biochem. 2004;92(2):223–37.
57. Workman P, Burrows F, Neckers L, Rosen N. Drugging the cancer chaperone HSP90: com-binatorial therapeutic exploitation of oncogene addiction and tumor stress. Ann N Y Acad Sci. 2007;1113:202–16.
58. Yu C, Rahmani M, Almenara J, et al. Histone deacetylase inhibitors promote STI571-mediated apoptosis in STI571-sensitive and -resistant Bcr/Abl+ human myeloid leukemia cells. Cancer Res. 2003;63(9):2118–26.
59. Fiskus W, Pranpat M, Balasis M, et al. Cotreatment with vorinostat (suberoylanilide hydroxamic acid) enhances activity of dasatinib (BMS-354825) against imatinib mesylate-sensitive or imatinib mesylate-resistant chronic myelogenous leukemia cells. Clin Cancer Res. 2006;12(19):5869–78.
60. Bali P, George P, Cohen P, et al. Superior activity of the combination of histone deacetylase inhibitor LAQ824 and the FLT-3 kinase inhibitor PKC412 against human acute myelogenous leukemia cells with mutant FLT-3. Clin Cancer Res. 2004;10(15):4991–7.
61. Witta SE, Gemmill RM, Hirsch FR, et al. Restoring E-cadherin expression increases sensi-tivity to epidermal growth factor receptor inhibitors in lung cancer cell lines. Cancer Res. 2006;66(2):944–50.
62. Cha TL, Chuang MJ, Wu ST, et al. Dual degradation of aurora A and B kinases by the histone deacetylase inhibitor LBH589 induces G2-M arrest and apoptosis of renal cancer cells. Clin Cancer Res. 2009;15(3):840–50.

63. Dai Y, Chen S, Venditti CA, et al. Vorinostat synergistically potentiates MK-0457 lethality in chronic myelogenous leukemia cells sensitive and resistant to imatinib mesylate. Blood. 2008;112(3):793–804.
64. Chao SH, Price DH. Flavopiridol inactivates P-TEFb and blocks most RNA polymerase II transcription in vivo. J Biol Chem. 2001;276(34):31793–9.
65. Almenara J, Rosato R, Grant S. Synergistic induction of mitochondrial damage and apoptosis in human leukemia cells by flavopiridol and the histone deacetylase inhibitor suberoylanilide hydroxamic acid (SAHA). Leukemia. 2002;16(7):1331–43.
66. Grant S, Kolla S, Sirulnik A, et al. Phase I trial of vorinostat (SAHA) in combinatin with alvocidib (flavopiridol) in patients with refractory, relapsed, or (selected) poor-prognosis AML or refractory anemia with excess blasts-2 (RAEB-2). Blood (Abstr). 2008;112:2986.
67. Dai Y, Rahmani M, Dent P, Grant S. Blockade of histone deacetylase inhibitor-induced RelA/p65 acetylation and NF-{kappa}B activation potentiates apoptosis in leukemia cells through a process mediated by oxidative damage, XIAP downregulation, and c-Jun N-terminal kinase 1 activation. Mol Cell Biol. 2005;25(13):5429–44.
68. Dai Y, Chen S, Kramer LB, Funk VL, Dent P, Grant S. Interactions between bortezomib and romidepsin and belinostat in chronic lymphocytic leukemia cells. Clin Cancer Res. 2008;14(2):549–58.
69. Chen S, Dai Y, Pei XY, Grant S. Bim up-regulation by histone deacetylase inhibitors mediates interactions with the Bcl-2 antagonist ABT-737: evidence for distinct roles for Bcl-2, Bcl-xL and Mcl-1. Mol Cell Biol. 2009;29(23):6149–69.
70. Bali P, Pranpat M, Bradner J, et al. Inhibition of histone deacetylase 6 acetylates and disrupts the chaperone function of heat shock protein 90: a novel basis of antileukemia activity of histone deacetylase inhibitors. J Biol Chem. 2005;280(29):26729–34.
71. Nawrocki ST, Carew JS, Dunner Jr K, et al. Bortezomib inhibits PKR-like endoplasmic reticulum (ER) kinase and induces apoptosis via ER stress in human pancreatic cancer cells. Cancer Res. 2005;65(24):11510–9.
72. Mitsiades CS, Mitsiades NS, McMullan CJ, et al. Transcriptional signature of histone deacetylase inhibition in multiple myeloma: biological and clinical implications. Proc Natl Acad Sci USA. 2004;101(2):540–5.
73. Badros A, Burger AM, Philip S, et al. Phase I study of vorinostat in combination with bortezomib for relapsed and refractory multiple myeloma. Clin Cancer Res. 2009;15(16):5250–7.
74. Dasmahapatra G, Lembersky D, Kramer L, et al. The pan-HDAC inhibitor vorinostat potentiates the activity of the proteasome inhibitor carfilzomib in human DLBCL cells in vitro and in vivo. Blood. 2010;115(22):4478–87.
75. Dai Y, Rahmani M, Grant S. Proteasome inhibitors potentiate leukemic cell apoptosis induced by the cyclin-dependent kinase inhibitor flavopiridol through a SAPK/JNK- and NF-kappaB-dependent process. Oncogene. 2003;22(46):7108–22.
76. Takada Y, Aggarwal BB. Flavopiridol inhibits NF-kappaB activation induced by various carcinogens and inflammatory agents through inhibition of IkappaBalpha kinase and p65 phosphorylation: abrogation of cyclin D1, cyclooxygenase-2, and matrix metalloprotease-9. J Biol Chem. 2004;279(6):4750–9.
77. Grant S, Sullivan D, Roodman D, et al. Phase I trial of bortezomib (NSC 681239) and flavopiridol (NSC 649890) in patients with recurrent or refractory indolent B-cell neoplasms. Blood (Abstr). 2008;112:1573.
78. Perez-Galan P, Roue G, Villamor N, Campo E, Colomer D. The BH3-mimetic GX15–070 synergizes with bortezomib in mantle cell lymphoma by enhancing Noxa-mediated activation of Bak. Blood. 2007;109(10):4441–9.
79. Pei XY, Dai Y, Grant S. The proteasome inhibitor bortezomib promotes mitochondrial injury and apoptosis induced by the small molecule Bcl-2 inhibitor HA14-1 in multiple myeloma cells. Leukemia. 2003;17(10):2036–45.
80. Paoluzzi L, Gonen M, Bhagat G, et al. The BH3-only mimetic ABT-737 synergizes the anti-neoplastic activity of proteasome inhibitors in lymphoid malignancies. Blood. 2008;112(7):2906–16.

81. Trudel S, Li ZH, Rauw J, Tiedemann RE, Wen XY, Stewart AK. Preclinical studies of the pan-Bcl inhibitor obatoclax (GX015–070) in multiple myeloma. Blood. 2007;109(12): 5430–8.

82. Konopleva M, Contractor R, Tsao T, et al. Mechanisms of apoptosis sensitivity and resistance to the BH3 mimetic ABT-737 in acute myeloid leukemia. Cancer Cell. 2006;10(5):375–88.

83. Chen S, Dai Y, Harada H, Dent P, Grant S. Mcl-1 downregulation potentiates ABT-737 lethality by cooperatively inducing Bak activation and Bax translocation. Cancer Res. 2007;67(2):782–91.

84. Lin X, Morgan-Lappe S, Huang X, et al. "Seed" analysis of off-target siRNAs reveals an essential role of Mcl-1 in resistance to the small-molecule Bcl-2/Bcl-X(L) inhibitor ABT-737. Oncogene. 2007;26(27):3972–9.

85. Zhang W, Konopleva M, Ruvolo VR, et al. Sorafenib induces apoptosis of AML cells via Bim-mediated activation of the intrinsic apoptotic pathway. Leukemia. 2008;22(4):808–18.

86. Yu C, Krystal G, Varticovksi L, et al. Pharmacologic mitogen-activated protein/extracellular signal-regulated kinase kinase/mitogen-activated protein kinase inhibitors interact synergistically with STI571 to induce apoptosis in Bcr/Abl-expressing human leukemia cells. Cancer Res. 2002;62(1):188–99.

87. Tai YT, Fulciniti M, Hideshima T, et al. Targeting MEK induces myeloma cell cytotoxicity and inhibits osteoclastogenesis. Blood. 2007;110(5):1656–63.

88. Nguyen TK, Jordan N, Friedberg J, Fisher RI, Dent P, Grant S. Inhibition of MEK/ERK1/2 sensitizes lymphoma cells to sorafenib-induced apoptosis. Leuk Res. 2010;34(3):379–86.

89. Rahmani M, Yu C, Reese E, et al. Inhibition of PI-3 kinase sensitizes human leukemic cells to histone deacetylase inhibitor-mediated apoptosis through p44/42 MAP kinase inactivation and abrogation of p21(CIP1/WAF1) induction rather than AKT inhibition. Oncogene. 2003;22(40):6231–42.

90. Qian J, Zou Y, Rahman JS, Lu B, Massion PP. Synergy between phosphatidylinositol 3-kinase/Akt pathway and Bcl-xL in the control of apoptosis in adenocarcinoma cells of the lung. Mol Cancer Ther. 2009;8(1):101–9.

91. Meloche S, Pouyssegur J. The ERK1/2 mitogen-activated protein kinase pathway as a master regulator of the G1- to S-phase transition. Oncogene. 2007;26(22):3227–39.

92. Bhalla KN. Epigenetic and chromatin modifiers as targeted therapy of hematologic malignancies. J Clin Oncol. 2005;23(17):3971–93.

93. Nebbioso A, Clarke N, Voltz E, et al. Tumor-selective action of HDAC inhibitors involves TRAIL induction in acute myeloid leukemia cells. Nat Med. 2005;11(1):77–84.

94. Stevens FE, Beamish H, Warrener R, Gabrielli B. Histone deacetylase inhibitors induce mitotic slippage. Oncogene. 2008;27(10):1345–54.

95. Glozak MA, Sengupta N, Zhang X, Seto E. Acetylation and deacetylation of non-histone proteins. Gene. 2005;363:15–23.

96. Chen L, Fischle W, Verdin E, Greene WC. Duration of nuclear NF-kappaB action regulated by reversible acetylation. Science. 2001;293(5535):1653–7.

97. Chen LF, Greene WC. Regulation of distinct biological activities of the NF-kappaB transcription factor complex by acetylation. J Mol Med. 2003;81(9):549–57.

98. Zhao Y, Tan J, Zhuang L, Jiang X, Liu ET, Yu Q. Inhibitors of histone deacetylases target the Rb-E2F1 pathway for apoptosis induction through activation of proapoptotic protein Bim. Proc Natl Acad Sci USA. 2005;102(44):16090–5.

99. Fiskus W, Pranpat M, Bali P, et al. Combined effects of novel tyrosine kinase inhibitor AMN107 and histone deacetylase inhibitor LBH589 against Bcr-Abl-expressing human leukemia cells. Blood. 2006;108(2):645–52.

100. Adams J. The development of proteasome inhibitors as anticancer drugs. Cancer Cell. 2004;5(5):417–21.

101. An B, Goldfarb RH, Siman R, Dou QP. Novel dipeptidyl proteasome inhibitors overcome Bcl-2 protective function and selectively accumulate the cyclin-dependent kinase inhibitor p27 and induce apoptosis in transformed, but not normal, human fibroblasts. Cell Death Differ. 1998;5(12):1062–75.

102. Yu C, Rahmani M, Conrad D, Subler M, Dent P, Grant S. The proteasome inhibitor bortezomib interacts synergistically with histone deacetylase inhibitors to induce apoptosis in Bcr/Abl+ cells sensitive and resistant to STI571. Blood. 2003;102(10):3765–74.
103. Miller CP, Ban K, Dujka ME, et al. NPI-0052, a novel proteasome inhibitor, induces caspase-8 and ROS-dependent apoptosis alone and in combination with HDAC inhibitors in leukemia cells. Blood. 2007;110(1):267–77.
104. Oltersdorf T, Elmore SW, Shoemaker AR, et al. An inhibitor of Bcl-2 family proteins induces regression of solid tumours. Nature. 2005;435(7042):677–81.
105. Deng J, Carlson N, Takeyama K, Dal CP, Shipp M, Letai A. BH3 profiling identifies three distinct classes of apoptotic blocks to predict response to ABT-737 and conventional chemo-therapeutic agents. Cancer Cell. 2007;12(2):171–85.
106. Rahmani M, Davis EM, Crabtree TR, et al. The kinase inhibitor sorafenib induces cell death through a process involving induction of endoplasmic reticulum stress. Mol Cell Biol. 2007;27(15):5499–513.
107. Rahmani M, Davis EM, Bauer C, Dent P, Grant S. Apoptosis induced by the kinase inhibitor BAY 43–9006 in human leukemia cells involves down-regulation of Mcl-1 through inhibition of translation. J Biol Chem. 2005;280(42):35217–27.
108. McCubrey JA, Steelman LS, Abrams SL, et al. Roles of the RAF/MEK/ERK and PI3K/PTEN/AKT pathways in malignant transformation and drug resistance. Adv Enzyme Regul. 2006;46:249–79.
109. Poulikakos PI, Zhang C, Bollag G, Shokat KM, Rosen N. RAF inhibitors transactivate RAF dimers and ERK signalling in cells with wild-type BRAF. Nature. 2010;464(7287):427–30.
110. Fisher RI, Miller TP, O'Connor OA. Diffuse aggressive lymphoma. Hematology Am Soc Hematol Educ Program. 2004;221–236.
111. Stommel JM, Kimmelman AC, Ying H, et al. Coactivation of receptor tyrosine kinases affects the response of tumor cells to targeted therapies. Science. 2007;318(5848):287–90.
112. Barabe F, Kennedy JA, Hope KJ, Dick JE. Modeling the initiation and progression of human acute leukemia in mice. Science. 2007;316(5824):600–4.
113. Pardal R, Clarke MF, Morrison SJ. Applying the principles of stem-cell biology to cancer. Nat Rev Cancer. 2003;3(12):895–902.
114. Zhao C, Chen A, Jamieson CH, et al. Hedgehog signalling is essential for maintenance of cancer stem cells in myeloid leukaemia. Nature. 2009;458(7239):776–9.
115. Naka K, Hoshii T, Muraguchi T, et al. TGF-beta-FOXO signalling maintains leukaemia-initiating cells in chronic myeloid leukaemia. Nature. 2010;463(7281):676–80.

Index

D. Gioeli (ed.), *Targeted Therapies: Mechanisms of Resistance*,
Molecular and Translational Medicine, DOI 10.1007/978-1-60761-478-4,
© Springer Science+Business Media, LLC 2011